Erythropoietin

The Johns Hopkins Series in Contemporary Medicine and Public Health

Erythropoietin

Molecular, Cellular, and Clinical Biology

Edited by

Allan J. Erslev, M.D., D.Sc.

Distinguished Professor of Medicine, Department of Medicine
Cardeza Foundation for Hematologic Research
Thomas Jefferson University, Philadelphia, Pennsylvania

John W. Adamson, M.D.

President, New York Blood Center, New York, New York

Joseph W. Eschbach, M.D.

Clinical Professor, Department of Medicine
University of Washington School of Medicine
Seattle, Washington

Christopher G. Winearls, M.B., Ch.B., D.Phil.

Consultant Nephrologist, Renal Unit, Churchill Hospital
Oxford, England

The Johns Hopkins University Press

Baltimore and London

Notice: Readers should scrutinize product information sheets for dosage changes or contraindications, particularly for new or infrequently used drugs.

© 1991 The Johns Hopkins University Press
All rights reserved
Printed in the United States of America

The Johns Hopkins University Press
701 West 40th Street
Baltimore, Maryland 21211
The Johns Hopkins Press Ltd., London

The paper used in this book meets the minimum requirements of the American National Standard for Information Sciences—Permanence of Paper for Printed Library Materials, ANSI Z39.48-1984.

Library of Congress Cataloging-in-Publication Data

Erythropoietin : molecular, cellular, and clinical biology / edited by Allan J. Erslev . . . [et al.]
    p.   cm. — (The Johns Hopkins series in contemporary medicine and public health)
    Includes bibliographical references and index.
    ISBN 0-8018-4221-2 (alk. paper)
    1. Recombinant erythropoietin—Therapeutic use—Testing.   2. Renal anemia—Chemotherapy.
    3. Anemia—Chemotherapy.   4. Erythropoietin.
    I. Erslev, Allan J.   II. Series.
    [DNLM: 1. Erythropoietin—physiology.
    2. Erythropoietin—therapeutic use.   WH 150 E7395]
RC641.7.R44E793   1991
616.1'52061—dc20
DNLM/DLC
for Library of Congress   91-7009

Contents

v

II. Clinical Trials

Contributors

Robert I. Abels, M.D.
Senior Director and Senior Clinical Research Fellow
R. W. Johnson Pharmaceutical Research Institute
Raritan, New Jersey 08869

John W. Adamson, M.D.
President, New York Blood Center
310 East 67th Street
New York, New York 10021

Tadao Akizawa, M.D.
Assistant Professor of Medicine
Fujigaoka Hospital, Showa University
Yokohama, Japan

Joseph A. Boccagno, M.S.
Project Manager
R. W. Johnson Pharmaceutical Research Institute
Raritan, New Jersey 08869

J. Bommer, M.D.
Nephrology Section
Heidelberg University Clinic
Bergheimer Strasse 56a
6900 Heidelberg, Germany

Maurice C. Bondurant, Ph.D.
Associate Professor, Division of Hematology
Department of Medicine
Vanderbilt University School of Medicine
Associate Research Career Scientist
Department of Veterans Affairs, VA Medical Center
Nashville, Tennessee 37203

K. J. Boughton, M.B., Ch.B., M.Med.
Director of Clinical Research
R. W. Johnson Pharmaceutical Research Institute
Don Mills, Ontario M3C 1L9, Canada

Joan M. Brown, R.N.
Clinical Research Coordinator, Division of Nephrology
Lankenau Hospital and Lankenau Medical Research Center
Philadelphia, Pennsylvania 19151

Jeffrey K. Browne, Ph.D.
Director of Product Development
Amgen, Inc.
1840 Dehavilland Drive
Thousand Oaks, California 91320

Jaime Caro, M.D.
Professor, Department of Medicine
Cardeza Foundation for Hematologic Research
Thomas Jefferson University
Philadelphia, Pennsylvania 19107

Gerald A. Coles, M.D.
Consultant Nephrologist
Institute of Renal Disease
Cardiff Royal Infirmary
Cardiff CF2 1SZ, Wales

P. Mary Cotes, M.B., Ph.D.
Haemostasis Research Group
Clinical Research Centre
Watford Road, Harrow
Middlesex HA1 3UJ, England

Alan D. D'Andrea, M.D.
Assistant Professor
Division of Hematology/Oncology
Department of Medicine
Children's Hospital, Dana Farber Cancer Institute
Harvard Medical School
Boston, Massachusetts 02115

Kai-Uwe Eckardt, M.D.
Postdoctoral Fellow
Department of Physiology
University of Zurich
Winterthurstrasse 190
CH-8057 Zurich, Switzerland

Joan C. Egrie, Ph.D.
Head, Laboratory of Stem Cell Biology
Amgen, Inc.
1840 Dehavilland Drive
Thousand Oaks, California 91320

Allan J. Erslev, M.D., D.Sc.
Distinguished Professor of Medicine
Department of Medicine
Cardeza Foundation for Hematologic Research
Thomas Jefferson University
Philadelphia, Pennsylvania 19107

Joseph W. Eschbach, M.D.
Clinical Professor, Department of Medicine
University of Washington School of Medicine
Seattle, Washington 98195

Eugene Goldwasser, Ph.D.
Professor, Department of Biochemistry and Molecular Biology
University of Chicago
920 East 58th Street
Chicago, Illinois 60637

Lawrence T. Goodnough, M.D.
Associate Professor of Medicine and Pathology
Case Western Reserve University School of Medicine
Associate Medical Director of the Blood Bank and Medical Director,
    Component Therapy Center
University Hospitals of Cleveland
2074 Abington Road
Cleveland, Ohio 44106

David H. Henry, M.D.
Clinical Assistant Professor of Medicine
University of Pennsylvania School of Medicine
Hematology/Oncology Division
Graduate Hospital
DSB-Suite 224
19th and South Streets
Philadelphia, Pennsylvania 19146

Yoshihei Hirasawa, M.D.
Executive Vice Director
Shinrakuen Hospital
1-27 Nishiariake-cho
Niigata 950-21, Japan

Rowland T. Hughes, M.R.C.P.
Research Fellow, Department of Haematology
Clinical Research Centre
Northwick Park, London, England

R. David Hutton, F.R.C.Path.
Senior Lecturer, Department of Haematology
Cardiff Royal Infirmary
Cardiff CF2 1SZ, Wales

Simon S. Jones, Ph.D.
Principal Scientist
Genetics Institute, Inc.
87 Cambridgepark Drive
Cambridge, Massachusetts 02140

Mark J. Koury, M.D.
Associate Professor
Division of Hematology, Department of Medicine
Vanderbilt University School of Medicine
Nashville, Tennessee 37232

Stephen T. Koury, Ph.D.
Research Assistant Professor
Division of Hematology, Department of Medicine
Vanderbilt University School of Medicine
Nashville, Tennessee 37232

Sanford B. Krantz, M.D.
Professor and Director, Division of Hematology
Department of Medicine
Vanderbilt University School of Medicine
Department of Veterans Affairs, VA Medical Center
Nashville, Tennessee 37232

Armin Kurtz, M.D.
Assistant Professor
Department of Physiology
University of Zurich
Winterthurstrasse 190
CH-8057 Zurich, Switzerland

Iain C. Macdougall, M.R.C.P.
Clinical Research Fellow
Institute of Renal Disease
Cardiff Royal Infirmary
Cardiff CF2 1SZ, Wales

Teiryo Maeda, M.D.
Principal
Kanto Rosai Nursing School
Kawasaki, Japan

Robert T. Means, Jr., M.D.
Assistant Professor
Division of Hematology, Department of Medicine
Vanderbilt University School of Medicine
Department of Veterans Affairs, VA Medical Center
Nashville, Tennessee 37232

William C. Mentzer, Jr., M.D.
Professor and Director, Division of Hematology
Department of Pediatrics
University of California School of Medicine
Room 6J5, San Francisco General Hospital
1001 Potrero Avenue
San Francisco, California 94110

Nobuhide Mimura, M.D.
President
Sakura National Hospital
Chiba 285, Japan

Norman Muirhead, M.D., M.B., Ch.B., F.R.C.P.(C)
Associate Professor
Division of Nephrology
Department of Medicine
University Hospital
University of Western Ontario
339 Windermere Road
London, Ontario N6A 5A5, Canada

Roderic H. Phibbs, M.D.
Professor and Head, Division of Neonatology
Department of Pediatrics
University of California School of Medicine
Box 0734
San Francisco, California 94143

Sylvia Ramirez, M.S.
Research Fellow, Department of Medicine
Cardeza Foundation for Hematologic Research
Thomas Jefferson University
Philadelphia, Pennsylvania 19107

I. Jon Russell, M.D., Ph.D.
Associate Professor, Division of Clinical Immunology
Department of Medicine
Director, Brady-Green Clinical Research Center
University of Texas Health Science Center
7703 Floyd Curl Drive
San Antonio, Texas 78284

Stephen T. Sawyer, Ph.D.
Research Assistant Professor
Division of Hematology, Department of Medicine
Vanderbilt University School of Medicine
Nashville, Tennessee 37232

Stephen Schuster, M.D.
Assistant Professor
Department of Medicine
Cardeza Foundation for Hematologic Research
Thomas Jefferson University
Philadelphia, Pennsylvania 19107

Paul Scigalla, M.D.
Associate Professor of Medicine
Vice President, Department of Clinical Research
Boehringer Mannheim GmbH
Sandhoferstrasse 116
6800 Mannheim 31, Germany

Kevin M. Shannon, M.D.
Assistant Adjunct Professor
Department of Pediatrics
University of California School of Medicine
San Francisco, California 94143
Attending Physician
Naval Hospital
Oakland, California 94627

Miles H. Sigler, M.D.
Chief, Division of Nephrology
Lankenau Hospital and Lankenau Medical Research Center
Philadelphia, Pennsylvania 19151
Clinical Professor of Medicine
Jefferson Medical College of Thomas Jefferson University
Philadelphia, Pennsylvania 19107

Joseph T. Sobota, M.D.
Executive Vice President and Chief Operating Officer
Chugai-Upjohn, Inc.
6133 North River Road, Suite 800
Rosemont, Illinois 60018
Adjunct Professor, Department of Medicine
Northwestern University Medical School
Chicago, Illinois 60611

Jerry L. Spivak, M.D.
Professor and Director, Division of Hematology
Department of Medicine
Johns Hopkins University School of Medicine
600 North Wolfe Street/Blalock 1033
Baltimore, Maryland 21205

Judith M. Stevens, M.R.C.P.
Research Fellow, Department of Nephrology
Hammersmith Hospital
London, England

H. Stocker, Ph.D.
Director of Biostatistics and Scientific Information
R. W. Johnson Pharmaceutical Research Institute
Cilag AG Research
Basserdorf, Switzerland

E. Sundal, M.D.
Private practice in internal medicine
Toensberg, Norway

Fumimaro Takaku, M.D.
Professor
The Third Department of Internal Medicine
Tokyo University School of Medicine
Tokyo, Japan

Brendan P. Teehan, M.D.
Attending Physician, Division of Nephrology
Lankenau Hospital and Lankenau Medical Research Center
Philadelphia, Pennsylvania 19151
Clinical Professor of Medicine
Jefferson Medical College of Thomas Jefferson University
Philadelphia, Pennsylvania 19107

John D. Williams, M.D.
Senior Lecturer in Nephrology, Institute of Renal Disease
Cardiff Royal Infirmary
Cardiff CF2 1SZ, Wales

Christopher G. Winearls, M.B., Ch.B., D.Phil.
Consultant Nephrologist
Renal Unit
Churchill Hospital
Headington
Oxford OX3 7LJ, England

Frederick Wolfe, M.D.
Clinical Professor, Department of Medicine
University of Kansas School of Medicine
1035 North Emporia, Suite 230
Wichita, Kansas 67214

Gordon G. Wong, D.Phil.
Senior Scientist
Genetics Institute, Inc.
87 Cambridgepark Drive
Cambridge, Massachusetts 02140

Erythropoietin

Chapter 1

Erythropoietin:
From Physiology to Clinical Trials
Via Molecular Biology

Allan J. Erslev

Weakness, shortness of breath, and palpitations have for ages been symptoms experienced by travelers at high altitude and by patients with blood-loss anemia. However, the relationship between these symptoms and impaired transport of oxygen was first clearly expressed in 1863 by Dennis Jourdanet in his monograph somewhat confusingly entitled "De l'Anémie des Altitudes" (Fig 1.1) (1).

Joseph Priestley and Antoine Lavoisier had already shown that oxygen was a vital component of air. In 1845 Heinrich Gustav Magnus (2) demonstrated that oxygen was taken up by blood from air in the lungs, and in 1857 Lothar Meyer showed that it was present in blood both physically absorbed and chemically bound (3). Meyer realized the potential physiologic importance of the chemically bound fraction, but it was not until Hoppe-Seyler in 1862 (4) showed that this fraction was reversibly bound to a red cell pigment, hemoglobin, that the importance of red cells in oxygen transport was generally accepted. Without this latter information, however, Jourdanet, a French physician working in the highlands of Mexico, recognized that some of his patients had the same symptoms as his former anemic patients in Paris, despite the fact that they had a normal or even increased number of red cell corpuscles in their blood. He proposed that both groups of patients were suffering from a lack of oxygen in blood or an anoxemia. This anoxemia could be either hypoxic due to low oxygen pressure or anemic due to a lack of oxygen-carrying red cell corpuscles.

Jourdanet reported these findings to his colleague Paul Bert in Paris. Bert, a student of and later successor to Claude Bernhard at the Sor-

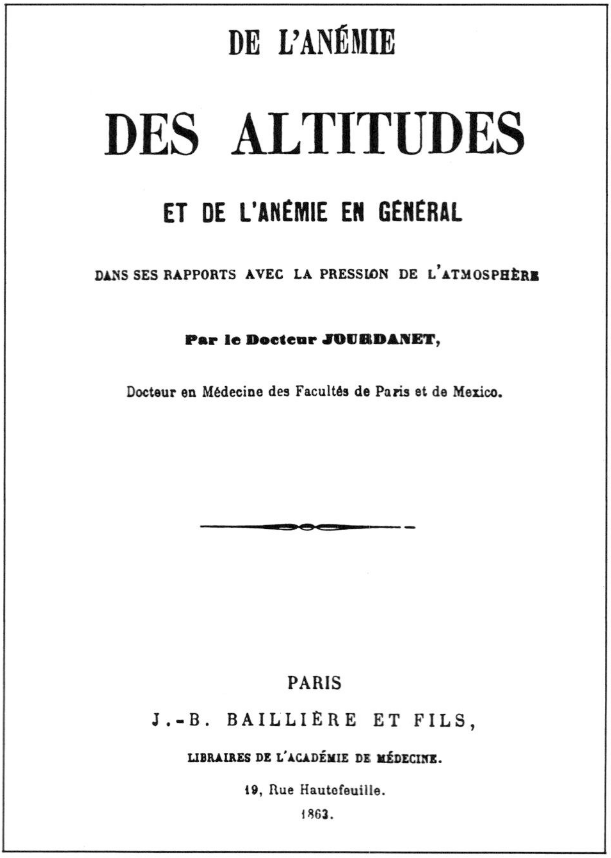

DE L'ANÉMIE

DES ALTITUDES

ET DE L'ANÉMIE EN GÉNÉRAL

DANS SES RAPPORTS AVEC LA PRESSION DE L'ATMOSPHÈRE

Par le Docteur JOURDANET,

Docteur en Médecine des Facultés de Paris et de Mexico.

PARIS

J.-B. BAILLIÈRE ET FILS,

LIBRAIRES DE L'ACADÉMIE DE MÉDECINE.

19, Rue Hautefeuille.

1863.

Figure 1.1. Title page of monograph by Dennis Jourdanet (1863), in which he showed that the "anemic" symptoms of high-altitude dwellers were caused not by a reduction in the hemoglobin concentration but by "hypoxemia."

bonne, was a prominent pulmonary physiologist. He immediately recognized the potential importance of Jourdanet's deductions. They became an important part of his monumental monograph published in 1878, "La Pression Atmospheric" (Fig 1.2) (5), which laid the foundation for modern atmospheric studies and aviation medicine.

Bert was particularly intrigued by Jourdanet's observation that many of his patients had an increased number of red corpuscles in their blood. A few years later Bert found a similar increase in animals living at high altitudes (6). He realized the potential advantage for high-altitude residents of such an increase but felt that this was a fortuitous coincidence and that, if it was induced, it would need generations of high-altitude living to accomplish. This conclusion may in part have been politically motivated because he was strenuously opposed to an attempt by Napoleon III to establish a French empire in the highlands of Mexico. Napoleon obviously did not share this opinion about delayed acclimatization and proceeded with his expansionist adventure, with disastrous, but not oxygen-related, consequences.

The fact that red cell acclimatization was indeed rapid and appropriate was first reported by M. F. Viault in 1890 after a trip by rail from Lima, Peru, to the tin mines of Morochocha at 4400 metres (Fig 1.3)

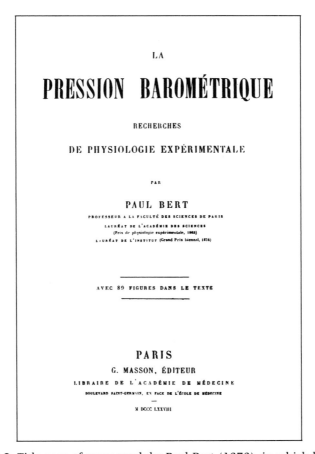

LA

PRESSION BAROMÉTRIQUE

RECHERCHES

DE PHYSIOLOGIE EXPÉRIMENTALE

PAR

PAUL BERT

PROFESSEUR A LA FACULTÉ DES SCIENCES DE PARIS

LAURÉAT DE L'ACADÉMIE DES SCIENCES
(Prix de physiologie expérimentale, 1865)

LAURÉAT DE L'INSTITUT (Grand Prix biennal, 1875)

AVEC 89 FIGURES DANS LE TEXTE

PARIS

G. MASSON, ÉDITEUR

LIBRAIRE DE L'ACADÉMIE DE MÉDECINE

BOULEVARD SAINT-GERMAIN, EN FACE DE L'ÉCOLE DE MÉDECINE

M DCCC LXXVIII

Figure 1.2. Title page of monograph by Paul Bert (1878), in which he described the effect of low barometric pressure on bodily functions and the compensating benefits derived from a high red cell count.

COMPTES RENDUS

HEBDOMADAIRES

DES SÉANCES

DE L'ACADÉMIE DES SCIENCES

PUBLIÉS,

CONFORMÉMENT A UNE DÉCISION DE L'ACADÉMIE

En date du 13 Juillet 1835,

PAR MM. LES SECRÉTAIRES PERPÉTUELS.

TOME CENT-ONZIÈME

JUILLET — DÉCEMBRE 1890.

PARIS

PHYSIOLOGIE EXPÉRIMENTALE. — *Sur l'augmentation considérable du nombre des globules rouges dans le sang chez les habitants des hauts plateaux de l'Amérique du Sud.* Note de M. F. VIAULT, présentée par M. de Lacaze-Duthiers.

	Globules.
A Lima le 4 octobre 1889 (veille de mon départ pour la Cordillère), mon sang contient par millimètre cube	5 000 000
A Morococha le 19 octobre (depuis quinze jours dans la Cordillère)	7 100 000
Dr Mayorga (id.)	7 300 ,00
Mayorca, arriero (depuis trois ans à la mine)	7 840 000
R. Prieto, garçon de cuisine, métis	6 770 000
Dittmann, Allemand, administrateur de la mine	7 920 000
Atchachay, Indien	7 960 000
Margarita, Indienne	7 080 000
Charpentier, fils de Français, majordome	6 000 000
Rossi, Italien, à la Oroya	6 320 000
Mon sang le 27 octobre	8 00, 000
Dr J. Mayorga, id.	7 440 000
Jeune chienne vigoureuse	9 000 000
Coq d'un an vigoureux	6 000 000
Lama mâle	16 000 000

Figure 1.3. The article by M. Viault (1890) included a table depicting the increase in red cell counts experienced by the author and his companions after arrival at Morococha (at 4400 metres), as well as the red cell counts of indigenous natives and animals.

(7). He found an increase in red cell count from 5 million/mm^3 at sea level to 7 million after 2 weeks in Morochocha and 8 million after 3 weeks.

In 1893 a similar but less pronounced increase was reported by F. Miescher, the discoverer of deoxyribonucleic acid (DNA), to occur in patients who entered the sanatorium in Arosa in the Alps in which he himself was seeking a cure for tuberculosis (Fig 1.4) (8). Miescher discussed the possible reason for this fortunate augmentation of oxygen transport and, as a believer in the invigorating and healing effect of hy-

poxia, he suggested that hypoxia directly stimulates the marrow to produce more red cells. At that time it was also believed, but less clearly
expressed, that the increase in red cell production observed after blood-
loss anemia was mediated by a similar direct hypoxic stimulation.

This hypothesis was difficult to prove or disprove and in 1906 it was
replaced by an alternate hypothesis based on an indirect stimulation of
red cell production (Fig 1.5) (9). Paul Carnot, professor of clinical medicine at the Sorbonne, with his assistant, C. Deflandre, infused normal
rabbits with a few millilitres of serum obtained from moderately anemic
donor rabbits and observed an amazing change in the recipients. In
one rabbit with a preinjection red cell count of 5.5 million/mm³, the
count rose on the next day to 8 million/mm³ and on the third day to 12
million/mm³.

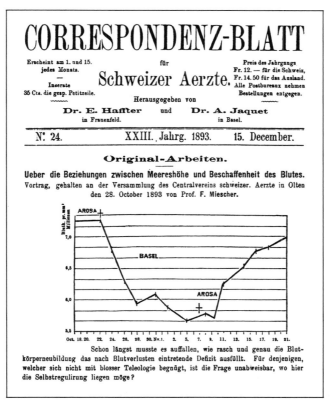

Figure 1.4. The article by F. Miescher (1893) included a figure relating red
cell counts to altitude and a question about the nature of the regulation of
red cell production.

COMPTES RENDUS

HEBDOMADAIRES

DES SÉANCES

DE L'ACADÉMIE DES SCIENCES

PUBLIÉS,

CONFORMÉMENT A UNE DÉCISION DE L'ACADÉMIE

En date du 13 Juillet 1835,

PAR MM. LES SECRÉTAIRES PERPÉTUELS.

—•—

TOME CENT QUARANTE-TROISIÈME.

JUILLET — DÉCEMBRE 1906.

PHYSIOLOGIE. — *Sur l'activité hémopoïétique du sérum au cours de la régénération du sang.* Note de M. Paul Carnot et de Mlle Cl. Deflandre, présentée par M. Bouchard.

Figure 1.5. The article by Paul Carnot and C. Deflandre (1906) claiming to have demonstrated a hemopoietin in anemic plasma.

This spectacular result started a 40-year quest by investigators all over the globe to reproduce and expand on the Carnot-Deflandre study and to identify this "hemopoietin" (10). Some results were tantalizing (11) but irreproducible, and eventually most investigators accepted the conclusion reached by Gordon and Dubin in 1934 (12) that a circulating hemopoietin did not exist.

The concept of a humoral mediator, however, was revived by Kurt Reissmann in 1950 using a parabiotic technique interestingly enough designed by Paul Bert 80 years before (Fig 1.6) (13). Reissmann showed that, if one partner of a parabiotic rat pair is rendered hypoxic, both partners will respond with an accelerated rate of red cell production. A perceptive review of red cell production by Grant and Root (14) led Erslev to repeat the Carnot and Deflandre study using very large amounts of serum obtained from severely anemic rabbits (Fig 1.7) (15). A significant reticulocytosis ensued. After the total infusion of 650 ml of anemic plasma over a 3-week period, the hematocrit rose from about 40 percent to more than 55 percent. The infusion of similar amounts of plasma obtained from normal rabbits had no erythropoietic effect. In a companion study published shortly afterward (16), a similar response was observed in *Macaca mulatta* monkeys given infusions of large amounts of anemic plasma. These results showed directly the existence of a stimulating plasma factor that previously, as a hypothetical entity, had been given the name *erythropoietin* (17).

BLOOD

The Journal of Hematology

VOL. V, NO. 4   APRIL, 1950

STUDIES ON THE MECHANISM OF ERYTHROPOIETIC STIMULATION IN
PARABIOTIC RATS DURING HYPOXIA

By Kurt R. Reissmann, M.D.

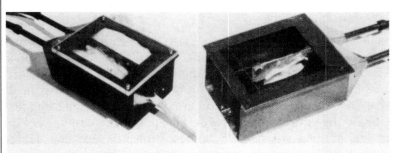

Fig. 1.—Breathing chamber for exposing parabiotic rats to different oxygen levels.

Figure 1.6. The article by Kurt Reissmann (1950) included a picture of the parabiotic rat pair used to show the presence of a red cell-stimulating plasma factor.

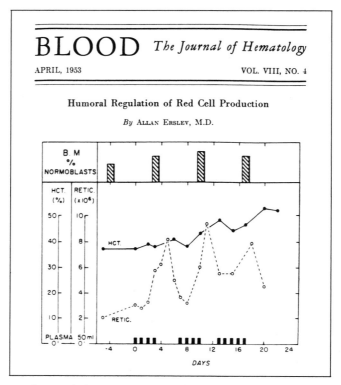

Figure 1.7. The article by Allan Erslev (1953) included a graph demonstrating the erythropoietin effect of the injection of large amounts of "anemic" plasma in rabbits.

The following year Stohlman et al. (18) and Schmid and Gilbertsen (19), in almost identical observations, showed that hypoxia does not have a direct stimulating effect on the bone marrow. They measured erythropoietic activity in the sternum and compared it to that in the iliac crest in two patients with ductus arteriosis and reversed blood flow. They found the same degree of erythropoietic activity despite very different arterial oxygen tensions. With these studies the question of direct vs. indirect stimulation was put to rest. Research during the following years was directed toward elucidating the origin, action, and biochemistry of the erythropoietic hormone.

In 1957 Leon Jacobson and his young co-workers, Goldwasser, Fried, and Plzak, showed that nephrectomized rats fail to produce erythro-

NATURE   March 23, 1957

Role of the Kidney in Erythropoiesis

L. O. JACOBSON
E. GOLDWASSER
W. FRIED
L. PLZAK

Argonne Cancer Research Hospital and
Departments of Medicine and Biochemistry,
University of Chicago,
Chicago, Illinois.   Jan. 7.

Table 1. EFFECT OF NEPHRECTOMY ON ERYTHROPOIETIN PRODUCTION
IN RATS

Condition of donor	Stimulus	Assay of plasma (percentage of Iron-59 incorporated into RBC)
Normal	Cobalt	9·8
Nephrectomized	Cobalt	2·4
Ureters ligated	Cobalt	5·5
Control	(Saline)	2·6
Normal (hæmatocrit 25)	Bleeding	15·4
Nephrectomized (hæmatocrit 33)	Bleeding	6·0
Adrenalectomized (hæmatocrit 35)	Bleeding	11·3
Control	(Saline)	6·9

Figure 1.8. The article by Leon Jacobson and associates (1957) included a table suggesting a renal origin of erythropoietin.

poietin in response to a hypoxic stimulus whereas ureter-ligated rats respond almost normally (Fig 1.8) (20). The data convinced most investigators that erythropoietin was synthesized by the kidney, and subsequent studies showed low erythropoietin levels in anemic patients with chronic kidney disease (21). These studies were facilitated by an improved bioassay that replaced laborious reticulocyte counting with the measurement of red cell incorporation of radioactive iron (22). A subsequent improvement was the use as recipients of mice with polycythemia-induced suppression of endogenous erythropoietin production (23,24). The use of such assays and the distribution (sponsored by the National Institutes of Health) of crude urinary erythropoietin obtained from patients with aplastic anemia or even hookworm anemia led to rapid progress in our understanding of the biology of this new

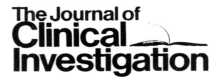

BLOOD
The Journal of
The American Society of Hematology

VOL. 71, NO 2 (pp 273-538)   FEBRUARY 1988

Localization of Erythropoietin Synthesizing Cells in Murine Kidneys By In Situ Hybridization

By Stephen T. Koury, Maurice C. Bondurant, and Mark J. Koury

The Journal of Clinical Investigation

February 1988   Volume 81, Number 2, Pages 277-634

Peritubular Cells Are the Site of Erythropoietin Synthesis in the Murine Hypoxic Kidney

Catherine Lacombe,* Jean-L. Da Silva,‡ Patrick Bruneval,‡ Jean-G. Fournier,§ Françoise Wendling,* Nicole Casadevall,* Jean-P. Camilleri,‡ Jean Bariety,‡ Bruno Varet,* and Pierre Tambourin*
Institut National de la Santé et de la Recherche Médicale (INSERM) U152, CNRS UA 628, Hôpital Cochin, 75014 Paris, France; ‡INSERM U28, Hôpital Broussais, 75014 Paris, France; and §INSERM U43, Hôpital St. Vincent de Paul, 75014 Paris, France

Figure 1.9. Stephen Koury and associates (1988) and Catherine Lacombe and associates (1988) demonstrated a peritubular origin of renal erythropoietin.

hormone. A number of national and international conferences devoted to erythropoietin took place, an international reference standard was established in England and distributed to workers throughout the world (25), and in 1970 an influential monograph by Krantz and Jacobson (26) could list 1400 references to erythropoietin-related research.

At that point the tempers of investigators were ignited by an attractive but divisive new hypothesis. This hypothesis proposed that erythropoietin was not synthesized by the kidney but was produced elsewhere, presumably by the liver, and was first activated in the blood stream by a renal enzyme generated in the kidneys by hypoxia (27). This enzyme was termed *erythrogenin,* and the hypothesis rapidly gained ground because of its cascade nature, similar to that which activates angiotensin and many other biologic compounds. Nevertheless, the data supporting the hypothesis were difficult to reproduce, and it was eventually abandoned when isolated kidneys perfused with saline were found to synthesize erythropoietin (28) and when erythropoietin was found to be present in renal extracts (29). Subsequent studies using the tools of molecular biology convincingly showed that the gene for erythropoietin is expressed in the kidneys (30–32) and that its product is fully active without the need for additional modification.

Why the kidney should be the main source of erythropoietin is still not clear but, as an organ controlling the volume and pressure of circulating blood, it may be well suited also to control the red cell mass (33). The kidney apparently contains an oxygen-sensing device capable of activating the gene for erythropoietin. Recent studies provided tantalizing clues about this oxygen sensor and its erythropoietin-producing target. The oxygen sensor seems to be a heme protein responding to the oxygen tension by signal-producing allosteric modifications (34). The targets have been identified by in situ hybridization studies to be interstitial cells lying in close proximity to the proximal tubular cells in the cortex (35,36) (Fig 1.9).

Measurement of erythropoietin titers of blood in patients with conditions characterized by changes in oxygen transport in general support the concept that a renal oxygen sensor controls erythropoietin synthesis and red cell production. Decreased oxygen transport (as in anemia or secondary polycythemia) leads to an exponential increase in titers, whereas increased oxygen transport (as after hypertransfusion or in polycythemia vera) leads to decreased titers (37,38). These observations resulted in the construction of a hypothetical feedback circuit linking the bone marrow to the kidney and mediated in one direction by red cell-bound oxygen and in the opposite direction by erythropoietin.

The liver, however, also plays a role in the synthesis of erythropoietin, as shown most convincingly by the low levels of sustained erythropoietin synthesis and red cell production observed in anephric individuals. It is estimated that 10 to 15 percent of circulating erythropoietin in adults is derived from the liver, either from hepatocytes or from Kupffer cells (39). During fetal life, hepatic synthesis of erythropoietin is predominant, with a switch to renal production first occurring around the time of birth (40).

Early studies showed that the action of erythropoietin is directed at primitive, still-undifferentiated cells (23,41,42). Subsequent studies outlined the hierarchy of red cell development from multipotential stem cells via erythroid-committed progenitor cells and erythroid precursor cells to mature red cells and showed that erythropoietin acts primarily

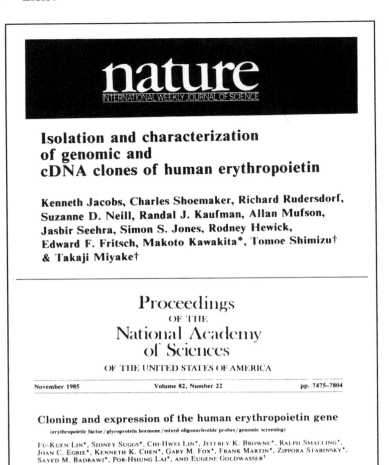

Figure 1.10. Kenneth Jacobs and associates (1985) and Fu-Kuen Lin and associates (1985) described the cloning and expression of the erythropoietin gene.

on the progenitor cells. It seems that erythropoietin has a growth-promoting effect on all progenitor cells as well as on early precursor cells but that its regulatory action is directed exclusively at the late progenitor cells, the colony-forming units-erythroid (CFU-E) (43). Receptors on these cells have been identified (44), and studies are in progress to elucidate the specific biologic action of the erythropoietin-receptor complex (45).

In the late 1970s, erythropoietin was purified and isolated (46), leading to the development of an easy and accurate radioimmune assay (47). Biochemical identification, primarily by Goldwasser and his group (46), established it as a glycoprotein consisting of 165 amino acids and containing 40 percent carbohydrate. The carbohydrate moiety determines in vivo viability but apparently has no effect on biologic activity. The amino acid domain responsible for this activity is still not known, but identification of part of the amino acid sequence led in 1985 to the construction of short oligonucleotide probes and the isolation of the gene (48,49). The gene was then cloned and expressed in Chinese hamster ovary cells (Fig 1.10), resulting in mass production of the hormone and in turn permitting clinical trials.

The Lancet · Saturday 22 November 1986

| EFFECT OF HUMAN ERYTHROPOIETIN DERIVED FROM RECOMBINANT DNA ON THE ANAEMIA OF PATIENTS MAINTAINED BY CHRONIC HAEMODIALYSIS | CHRISTOPHER G. WINEARLS[1]   DESMOND O. OLIVER[2]
MARTIN J. PIPPARD[1]   CECIL REID[3]
MICHAEL R. DOWNING[4]   P. MARY COTES[3] |

The New England
Journal of Medicine

Copyright, 1987, by the Massachusetts Medical Society

| Volume 316 | JANUARY 8, 1987 | Number 2 |

CORRECTION OF THE ANEMIA OF END-STAGE RENAL DISEASE WITH RECOMBINANT HUMAN ERYTHROPOIETIN

Results of a Combined Phase I and II Clinical Trial*

JOSEPH W. ESCHBACH, M.D., JOAN C. EGRIE, PH.D., MICHAEL R. DOWNING, PH.D., JEFFREY K. BROWNE, PH.D., AND JOHN W. ADAMSON, M.D.

Figure 1.11. Christopher Winearls and associates (1986) and Joseph Eschbach and associates (1987) showed the therapeutic benefits of treating dialysis patients with recombinant human erythropoietin.

Previously, a number of exploratory studies in nephrectomized animals had suggested that erythropoietin could be a valuable therapeutic tool in uremic patients. However, the results published in late 1986 by Winearls et al. (50) and in early 1987 by Eschbach et al. (51) (Fig 1.11) were dramatic beyond anyone's dreams. They showed convincingly that the anemia of chronic renal failure is primarily due to erythropoietin deficiency and that the correction of this anemia rectifies many symptoms formerly attributed to azotemia per se.

The following chapters are written by basic scientists and clinical investigators whose work has changed erythropoietin from a dimly envisioned growth factor to a mass-produced renal hormone and brought it from the laboratory to the bedside. These chapters vividly describe its present use in the "cure" of the anemia associated with chronic renal disease and its future potential for reducing transfusion dependency and enhancing the quality of life in patients with many other kinds of anemia.

REFERENCES

1. Jourdanet D. De l'anemie des altitudes et de l'anemie en general dans ses rapports avec la pression de l'atmosphere. Paris: Baillière, 1863.

2. Magnus G. Über das Absorptionvermögen des Blutes für Sauerstoff. Ann Physik und Chemie 1845;66:177.

3. Meyer L. Die Gase des Blutes. Göttingen: Dieterich, 1857.

4. Hoppe-Seyler, F. Über die Chemischen und Optischen Eigenschaften des Blutfarbstoffe. Virchows Arch 1864;23:446–9.

5. Bert P. La pression barometrique. Paris: Masson et Cie, 1878.

6. Bert P. Sur la richesse en hemoglobine du sang des animaux vivant sur les hauts lieux. C R Acad Sci (Paris) 1882;94:805–7.

7. Viault F. Sur l'augmentation considerable du nombre des globules rouges dans le sang chez les habitants des haut plateaux de l'Amerique du Sud. C R Acad Sci (Paris) 1890;111:917–8.

8. Miescher F. Ueber die Beziehungen zwischen Meereshohe und Beschaffenheit des Blutes. Korresp-Bl Schweiz Arz 1893;23:809–30.

9. Carnot P, Deflandre C. Sur l'activité hemopoietique de serum au cours de la regeneration du sang. C R Acad Sci (Paris) 1906;143:384–6.

10. Thorling EB. The history on the early theories of humoral regulation of the erythropoiesis. Danish Med Bull 1969;16:159–164.

11. Krumdich N. Erythropoietin substance in the serum of anemic animals. Proc Soc Exp Biol & Med 1943;81:14–17.

12. Gordon AS, Dubin M. On the alleged presence of "hemopoietine" in the blood serum of rabbits either rendered anemic or subjected to low pressures. Am J Physiol 1934;107:704–8.

13. Reissmann KR. Studies on the mechanism of erythropoietic stimulation in parabiotic rats during hypoxia. Blood 1950;5:372–80.

14. Grant WC, Root WS. The relation of O_2 in bone marrow blood to post-hemorrhagic erythropoiesis. Am J Physiol 1947;150:618–27.

15. Erslev AJ. Humoral regulation of red cell production. Blood 1953; 8:349–571.

16. Erslev AJ, Lavietes PH, van Wagenen G. Erythropoietic stimulation induced by "anemic serum." Proc Soc Exp Biol Med 1953;83:548–50.

17. Bonsdorff E, Jalavisto E. A humoral mechanism in anoxic erythrocytosis. Acta Physiol Scand 1948;16:150–70.

18. Stohlman F Jr, Rath CE, Rose JC. Evidence for a humoral regulation of erythropoiesis. Blood 1954;9:721–33.

19. Schmid R, Gilbertsen AS. Fundamental observations on the production of compensatory polycythemia in a case of patent ductus arteriosus with reversed blood flow. Blood 1955;10:247–51.

20. Jacobson LO, Goldwasser E, Fried W, Plzak L. Role of the kidney in erythropoiesis. Nature 1957;179:633–4.

21. Gallagher NJ, McCarthy JM, Lange RD. Observations on erythropoietic stimulating factor (ESF) in the plasma of uremic and non-uremic anemia patients. Ann Intern Med 1960;52:1201–12.

22. Plzak LF, Fried W, Jacobson LO, Bethard WF. Demonstration of stimulation of erythropoiesis by plasma from anemic rats using Fe^{59}. J Lab Clin Med 1955;46:671–8.

23. Jacobson LO, Goldwasser E, Gurney CW. Transfusion-induced polycythaemia as a model for studying factors influencing erythropoiesis. In: Wolstenholme GEW, O'Conner M, eds. Haemopoiesis. Ciba Foundation Symposium. London: Churchill, 1960:423–52.

24. Cotes PM, Bangham DR. Bioassay of erythropoietin in mice made polycythaemic by exposure to air at a reduced pressure. Nature 1961;191: 1065–7.

25. Cotes PM, Bangham DR. The international reference preparation of erythropoietin. Bull WHO 1966;35:751.

26. Krantz SB, Jacobson LO. Erythropoietin and the regulation of erythropoiesis. Chicago: University of Chicago Press, 1970;11–2.

27. Contrera JF, Gordon AS, Weintraub AH. Extraction of an erythropoietin-producing factor from a particular fraction of rat kidney. Blood 1966; 28:330–43.

28. Erslev AJ. In vitro production of erythropoietin by kidneys perfused with a serum-free solution. Blood 1974;44:77–85.

29. Fried W, Barone-Varelas J, Berman M. Detection of high erythropoietin titers in renal extracts of hypoxic rats. J Lab Clin Med 1981;97:82–6.

30. Bondurant M, Koury M. Anemia induces accumulation of erythropoietin in RNA in the kidneys and liver. Mol Cell Biol 1986;6:2731–3.

31. Beru N, McDonald J, Lacombe C, Goldwasser E. Expression of the erythropoietin gene. Mod Cell Biol 1986;6:2571–5.

32. Schuster SJ, Wilson JH, Erslev AJ, Caro J. Physiologic regulation and tissue localization of renal erythropoietin messenger RNA. Blood 1987;70: 316–8.

33. Erslev AJ, Caro J, Besarab A. Why the kidney? Nephron 1985;41:213–6.

34. Goldberg MA, Dunning SP, Bunn HT. Regulations of the erythropoietin

gene: evidence that the oxygen sensor is a hemeprotein. Science 1988;242:
1412–5.

35. Lacombe C, DaSilva JL, Bruneval P, et al. Peritubular cells are the site
of erythropoietin synthesis in the murine hypoxic kidney. J Clin Invest 1988;
81:620–3.

36. Koury ST, Bondurant MC, Koury MJ. Localization of erythropoietin
synthesizing cells in murine kidneys by in situ hybridization. Blood 1988;
71:524–7.

37. Adamson JW. The erythropoietin/hematocrit relationship in normal and
polycythemic man: implications for marrow regulation. Blood 1968;32:597–
609.

38. Erslev AJ, Caro J, Miller O, Silver R. Plasma erythropoietin in health
and disease. Ann Clin Lab Sci 1980;10:250–7.

39. Fried W. The liver as a source of extrarenal erythropoietin. Blood
1972;40:671–7.

40. Zanjani ED, Poster J, Burlington H, Mann LI, Wasserman LR. Liver as
the primary site of erythropoietin formation in the fetus. J Lab Clin Med
1977;89:640–4.

41. Erslev AJ. The effect of anemic anoxia on the cellular development of
nucleated red cells. Blood 1959;14:386–98.

42. Alpen EL, Cranmore D. Observations on the regulation of erythropoiesis and on cellular dynamics by Fe^{59} autoradiography. In: Stohlman F, ed. The
kinetics of cellular proliferation. New York: Grune and Stratton, 1959;290–
300.

43. Spivak JL. The mechanism of actions of erythropoietin. Int J Cell Cloning 1986;4:139–66.

44. Sawyer ST, Krantz SB, Goldwasser E. Binding and receptor-mediated
endocytosis of erythropoietin in Friend virus-infected erythroid cells. J Biol
Chem 1987;262:5554–62.

45. D'Andrea AD, Lodish HF, Wong GG. Expression cloning of the murine
erythropoietin receptor. Cell 1989;57:277–85.

46. Miyake T, Kung CKH, Goldwasser E. Purification of human erythropoietin. J Biol Chem 1977;252:5558–64.

47. Garcia JF, Sherwood J, Goldwasser E. Radioimmunoassay for erythropoietin. Blood Cells 1979;5:405–19.

48. Jacobs K, Shoemaker C, Rudersdorf R, et al. Isolation and characterization of genomic and cDNA clones of human erythropoietin. Nature 1985;
313:806–10.

49. Lin FK, Suggs S, Lin C-H, et al. Cloning and expression of the human
erythropoietin gene. Proc Natl Acad Sci USA 1985;82:7580–4.

50. Winearls CG, Oliver DO, Pippard M, et al. Effect of human erythropoietin derived from recombinant DNA on the anemia of patients maintained
by chronic hemodialysis. Lancet 1986;2:1175–81.

51. Eschbach JW, Egrie JC, Downing MR, et al. Correction of the anemia
of end-stage renal disease with recombinant human erythropoietin. N Engl J
Med 1987;316:73–8.

I. Molecular and Cellular Biology

Chapter 2

The Molecular Biology
of Erythropoietin

Joan C. Egrie and Jeffrey K. Browne

The isolation of human erythropoietin gene clones has enabled the development of erythropoietin for use as a therapeutic, facilitated structural analysis of the hormone, and made possible the study of the regulation of its expression. Physiologic control of the red blood cell mass has been known for over 100 years and was first postulated to be under humoral control in 1906 (1). It was not until the mid-20th century, however, that the existence of erythropoietin, a hormone specifically regulating the rate of erythropoiesis, was confirmed (2–4). The biochemical properties of erythropoietin were studied by indirect methods (5–7) until 1978, when the successful isolation of pure human erythropoietin from the urine of aplastic anemia patients (8) made direct analysis possible. Purification of the hormone from natural sources (e.g., serum from normal or anemic individuals) has not been possible due to the low circulating concentrations of erythropoietin (0.1–100 ng of erythropoietin vs. 70 mg of total protein per ml of serum). The sole starting material from which isolation of the endogenous hormone has been successful is the urine from aplastic anemia patients. This urine is greatly enriched in erythropoietin content, but its scarcity has precluded the development of erythropoietin from a natural source for use as a therapeutic.

In the 1980s the nucleic acid sequences encoding human, cynomolgus monkey, and mouse erythropoietin were isolated, characterized, and compared. The isolation of each was accomplished by somewhat different methods. The cloning strategies and comparisons of the structure and genetic organization of the three isolated erythropoietin gene sequences are reviewed below.

The Isolation of the Erythropoietin Gene Clones

Isolation of an erythropoietin gene clone, which was first reported in 1984 (9), was difficult because of the limited amount of data on the primary structure of human erythropoietin and the lack of a known source of erythropoietin messenger ribonucleic acid (mRNA). No cell lines that produced significant amounts of erythropoietin and therefore could be used as a source of mRNA had been described. In addition, although the kidney and fetal liver had been identified as the probable sites of erythropoietin synthesis (10), it was not known if induction of erythropoietin production by hypoxia in these organs was due to an increase in the transcription rate of the erythropoietin gene (and thereby an increase in the steady state mRNA level), release of stored erythropoietin, or activation of an inactive erythropoietin precursor (11–13).

As a consequence, a variety of different cloning strategies were simultaneously pursued. The approach that led to the successful cloning of the first erythropoietin gene sequence relied on obtaining protein sequence information from the limited quantities of purified human urinary erythropoietin which were available. Amino acid sequence data were obtained both from the amino terminus of erythropoietin and from internal tryptic fragments. Mixed oligonucleotides, containing all possible sequences that could code for selected amino acid sequences, were synthesized and used as hybridization probes to screen a λ bacteriophage human genomic gene library. In addition, these probes were also used to screen a cynomolgus monkey complementary deoxyribonucleic acid (cDNA) library constructed from kidney mRNA isolated from a monkey made anemic by phenylhydrazine treatment (14,15).

A flow diagram of the schema used to isolate human erythropoietin genomic gene clones and cynomolgus monkey erythropoietin cDNA clones is shown in Figure 2.1. From the available amino acid sequence data, two peptides, which were derived from internal tryptic fragments and had relatively low codon degeneracy, were selected, and mixed oligonucleotide pools corresponding to these sequences were synthesized. Each set of oligonucleotide probes contained a pool of 128 sequences. One probe mixture contained 20-nucleotide-long oligonucleotides containing all possible coding sequences for an internal heptapeptide, and the second mixture contained 17-nucleotide-long oligonucleotides directed against the coding sequence for a hexapeptide (16). Screening of the human gene library for a single copy gene was difficult because of the complexity of the human genome and the short length and high

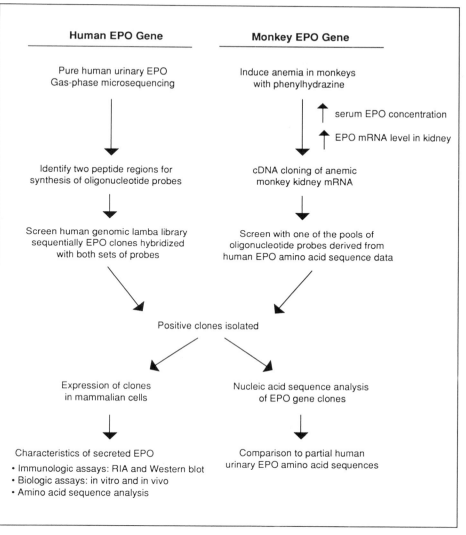

Figure 2.1. Cloning strategy for human genomic and monkey cDNA erythropoietin (EPO) clones. *Source: Reference 18. Copyright © 1985 by Alan R. Liss, Inc. Reprinted by permission of Wiley-Liss, a division of John Wiley and Sons, Inc.*

degeneracy of the oligonucleotide probe mixtures. For this reason, sequential hybridization of the human gene library with the two sets of non-overlapping probes was used to facilitate identification of the erythropoietin gene. As only the erythropoietin gene clones should be able to hybridize with both probe mixtures, this technique eliminated many of the false positives that were obtained when each probe mixture was used alone (16,17).

The clones identified by sequential hybridization with the oligonucleotide probes were verified to encode human erythropoietin by two approaches: first, by comparing the amino acid sequence predicted by the clones to the partial amino acid sequence of purified human urinary erythropoietin and, second, by expressing the gene clones in mammalian cells and demonstrating that they directed the synthesis of a glycoprotein with the structural, immunologic, and biologic properties of human erythropoietin (16–20).

A cynomolgus monkey erythropoietin cDNA clone was isolated from an anemic monkey kidney cDNA library using the mixed oligonucleotide probes derived from the amino acid sequence of human erythropoietin (14,15) (Fig 2.1). This heterologous approach required that the monkey and human erythropoietin amino acid sequence be essentially identical over the region for which the nucleic acid probes were constructed. In addition, this approach required that erythropoietin mRNA be enriched in the kidneys of anemic monkeys. Animals made anemic by treatment with phenylhydrazine were shown to have increased serum erythropoietin levels as measured by radioimmunoassay and Western blot analysis (18). Furthermore, Northern blot analysis indicated that the increase in circulatory erythropoietin levels was, in fact, due to an increase in the steady state level of erythropoietin mRNA (14,15,18). In contrast, erythropoietin mRNA was not detected in kidney RNA isolated from normal animals.

Northern blot analysis also demonstrated that the 20-nucleotide-long but not the 17-nucleotide-long probe mixture was able to cross-hybridize with monkey erythropoietin mRNA (15,18). It was later determined that, although there is 92 percent amino acid sequence homology between human and monkey erythropoietin, the second set of probes failed to cross-hybridize because of a single amino acid sequence difference between human and monkey in the region corresponding to the probe (tryptophan 88 in human erythropoietin vs. phenylalanine in monkey erythropoietin) (15). The 20-nucleotide-long probe mixture was therefore used to screen the anemic monkey kidney cDNA library. The monkey cDNA clones were confirmed by gene sequencing and by demonstrating that the clones directed the synthesis of erythropoietin when transfected into mammalian cells (15).

With the isolation of the initial erythropoietin genomic gene clones, it then became possible to isolate additional examples of human gene clones and erythropoietin gene clones from other species (21,22). Human erythropoietin cDNA clones have been isolated using genomic gene clone probes from human fetal liver (17) or from recombinant mammalian cells expressing a transfected human erythropoietin gene (16). Murine erythropoietin gene clones were isolated using human (23) or monkey (24) gene clones as probes.

The Structure of the Erythropoietin Gene

The human erythropoietin gene comprises five exons and four introns. One of the intervening sequences occurs within the sequence encoding the signal peptide. Thus, the first exon, which is very guanine-cytosine-rich, codes for a relatively long 5' untranslated region and four amino acids of the signal peptide. Schematic diagrams of the human erythropoietin gene and of the predicted mRNA transcript are shown in Figure 2.2. The nucleotide sequence of the human genomic gene and the amino acid sequence of the primary translation product are shown in Figure 2.3. The intron/exon junction sites were deduced by comparison with the sequence of human and monkey cDNA clones and with the amino acid sequence of purified recombinant human erythropoietin and urinary-derived erythropoietin (25). The sequence around the splice junction conforms to the consensus splice rules (26).

The basic organization of the erythropoietin genomic genes is similar between species, with the intervening sequences being located in the same relative positions for the human and mouse genes (16,17,23). The most conserved region between the two genes has 90 percent sequence homology and is located directly upstream from the transcriptional start site (23). The first exon for human, monkey, and mouse erythropoietin also shows similarities, being guanine-cytosine-rich and having a longer than usual 5' untranslated region. There is a significant degree of homology (65 percent) throughout the first intron of the human and mouse erythropoietin genes, and the intron lengths are nearly identical (559 vs. 554 base pairs) (23). It is conceivable that sequences within the first intervening sequence may serve a regulatory function, but this has not as yet been tested. In contrast, the size and sequence of the second, third, and fourth introns is highly divergent between human and mouse. A comparison of the sequences of the erythropoietin gene

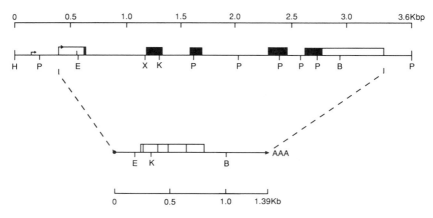

Figure 2.2. Map of the human erythropoietin gene. Exons are indicated by boxes; the solid areas indicate the approximate position of the coding portion of the gene. The two horizontal arrows indicate the two most prominent transcription initiation sites (28). The first exon is shown beginning at the major transcription initiation site. The restriction endonuclease sites are abbreviated: B is *Bgl* II, H is *Hin*d III; E is *Bst* E II, K is *Kpn* I, P is *Pst* I, X is *Xba* I. Map distances are indicated in kilobasepairs (Kbp). A map of the major mRNA transcript is also shown.

and erythropoietin protein for the three species is presented in Table 2.1.

There is only a single copy of the human, monkey, and mouse erythropoietin gene (15,16,23). There is no evidence, by low stringency Southern blot hybridization, of an erythropoietin-related gene family or of any pseudogenes (16). The human erythropoietin gene has been mapped to chromosome 7pter-q22, and the mouse gene has been mapped to chromosome 5 (27). Within the coding region, the sequence homology between human and mouse erythropoietin and between mouse and monkey erythropoietin is 80 percent, whereas between human and monkey erythropoietin it is 94 percent (15,23,24).

The predicted size of the major human erythropoietin mRNA transcript, based on the major transcription initiation site (28–30) and the known polyadenylation site (16,17) is approximately 1390 nucleotides. The major inducible transcription start site, as mapped by Semenza et al. (28–30), is at nucleotide 388 in Figure 2.3. This corresponds to the transcription start site described for the mouse erythropoietin mRNA transcript (23) and the 5′ end of the cynomolgus monkey erythropoi-

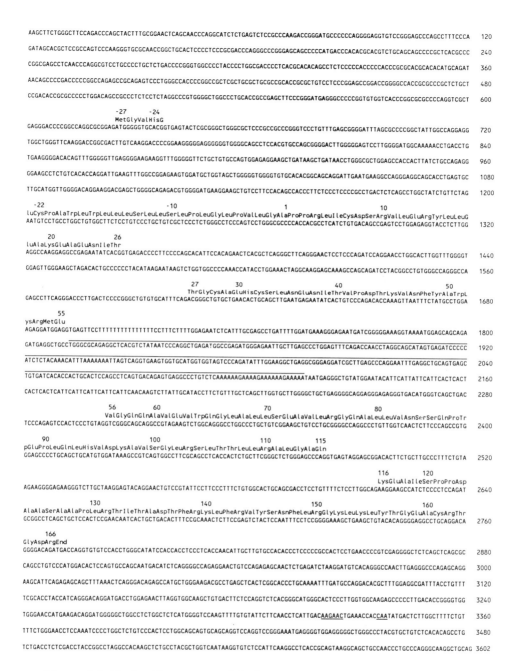

Figure 2.3. Nucleotide sequence of the human erythropoietin gene. The sequence of the 193-amino acid primary translation product is shown. The NH$_2$ terminus of the mature protein begins at amino acid 1. An Alu repeat found in the third intron is overlined. The putative polyadenylation signal and the polyadenylation site are underlined. *Source: Reference 16*

Table 2.1. A Comparison of Human, Monkey, and Mouse Erythropoietin Gene and Protein Sequences

	Human	Monkey	Mouse
Nucleic acid			
Introns/exons	4/5	?	4/5
	Intron 1 in		Intron 1 in
	signal peptide		signal peptide
Chromosome	7	?	5
mRNA size	~1390 bp	~1462 bp	?
Sequence homology			
cDNA vs. human	—	~94%	~80% (predicted)
cDNA vs. monkey	~94%	—	~80% (predicted)
Consensus polyadenylation			
sequence	None	None	None
Protein			
Primary translation product	193 aa	192 aa	192 aa
Signal peptide	27 aa	24 aa	26 aa
Mature protein			
Predicted	166 aa	168 aa	166 aa
Isolated	165 aa*	?	?
Cysteines			
Number	4	5	4
Position relative			
to human erythropoietin	7,29,33,161	7,29,33,139,161	7,29,139,161
Disulfide bonds	7-161, 29-33	?	?
Carbohydrate			
N-linked			
Number	3	3	3
Position relative			
to human erythropoietin	24,38,83	24,38,83	24,38,83
O-linked			
Number	1	?	?
Position	126	?	?
Amino acid homology			
vs. human	—	92%	79%
vs. monkey	92%	—	79%

*COOH-terminal arginine removed post-translationally from both urinary-derived human erythropoietin and recombinant erythropoietin expressed in Chinese hamster ovary but not BHK cells.

etin cDNA clone (14). Using ribonuclease protection assays of RNA isolated from various tissues of transgenic mice carrying the human
erythropoietin genomic gene, as well as analysis of Hep3B liver cells
and human fetal liver RNA, investigators have mapped several additional transcription initiation start sites (28). These additional start sites
map to nucleotides 105, 118, 123, 135, 141, and 151 in Figure 2.3,
with the site at nucleotide 151 being the most prominent. The sites at
nucleotides 151 and 388 both increase in the liver when the erythropoietin gene transcript is induced by hypoxia. It is not known whether
the 5' set of transcription initiation sites is used in the kidney; these
upstream start sites have been described only in liver cell lines or in
cells from the liver of transgenic mice which failed to produce erythropoietin in the kidney in response to hypoxia. Transcription initiation
sites further upstream have not been found in the transgenic mice that
carry up to 6 kilobasepairs of DNA 5' to the start of the gene. To date,
studies mapping the exact transcriptional start site within the human
erythropoietin gene using human tissue source mRNA have not been
performed.

The polyadenylation site has been mapped to nucleotide 3341-2 (Fig
2.3) based on the 3' end of the human erythropoietin cDNA clones
(16,17). The 3' end of the monkey cDNA clone is at the analogous position (14). The sequence upstream of the polyadenylation site does not
contain a consensus A_2TA_3 polyadenylation signal in human, monkey,
or mouse genes. However, an A_2GA_2C is found approximately 11 base
pairs upstream of the polyadenylation site in both the human and cynomolgus monkey sequences. In Chinese hamster ovary cells transfected with the human erythropoietin genomic gene, the 3' end of the
major transcript maps to this same position. In addition, a minor transcript, using a polyadenylation site approximately 2 kilobasepairs further downstream, is also observed (unpublished observations). Because
of the lack of a consensus polyadenylation signal, read-through transcripts are not unexpected. Longer transcripts, utilizing a downstream
polyadenylation site, have not been observed in human cells, although
they may be present below the limits of detection.

Translation of the human erythropoietin gene begins at the second
ATG codon in the mRNA. The upstream ATG is in a different reading
frame from that of the erythropoietin gene and would code for only a
short peptide. The upstream ATG is preserved in both the monkey and
mouse genes, and in each case it would code for a 13- or 14-amino acid
peptide, which is out of frame with the erythropoietin gene (15,24).
Each of the ATG codons fits only marginally with the translation ini-

tiation consensus sequence found adjacent to the initiating codon (31). The effect, if any, on translation attenuation by the upstream ATG is not known.

The primary translation product of the human gene is predicted by the nucleotide sequence to be 193 amino acids. The first 27 amino acids are predominantly hydrophobic, consistent with a signal sequence directing the nascent polypeptide chain to the endoplasmic reticulum. The size of the mature protein has been determined to be 165 amino acids, one residue shorter than the predicted length (25,32,33). Amino acid sequence analysis of both recombinant erythropoietin expressed by Chinese hamster ovary cells (32,33) and human urinary erythropoietin (25) indicate that the COOH-terminal arginine residue is missing from the isolated mature protein. Direct sequence analysis of human erythropoietin mRNA has shown that the transcript does code for an arginine at position 193, which is consistent with the observation that recombinant erythropoietin expressed by BHK cells is a 166-amino acid protein containing the terminal arginine (22). At present, it is not known if this post-translational modification occurs as a result of intracellular or extracellular processing. Because the recombinant erythropoietin expressed by both transfected BHK and Chinese hamster ovary cells is biologically active, neither the presence nor the absence of the COOH-terminal arginine is required for biologic activity (22). Whether the COOH-terminal arginine is present in mature monkey or mouse erythropoietin is not known.

The monkey erythropoietin gene encodes a protein of 192 amino acids, one shorter than that encoded by the human erythropoietin gene. The cDNA sequence of cynomolgus monkey erythropoietin indicates that exon 5 is shorter at its 5' end by one codon; thus, the amino acid corresponding to lysine 116 of human erythropoietin is not present in the monkey sequence (14). The deletion of this amino acid may be due to an alteration in splicing of the mRNA. As determined by direct amino acid sequencing of the recombinant monkey erythropoietin expressed in Chinese hamster ovary cells, the amino terminus of monkey erythropoietin contains an additional three amino acids, Val-Pro-Gly, compared with human erythropoietin. This indicates that the site of cleavage by the signal peptide processing enzyme is different and that there are 24 amino acids in the monkey signal peptide instead of the 27 amino acids cleaved from human erythropoietin. The alteration in the cleavage site may be due to changes around the amino terminus of the monkey protein. Of the first 50 amino acid residues of the monkey primary translation product, there are only two changes. These are a valine (monkey -8) vs. leucine (human -11) and a proline (monkey $+2$) vs. leuine (human -2). Preliminary evidence suggests that it is the substitution of proline for leucine which is responsible for the altered cleavage (unpublished observations). Thus, the mature monkey protein is predicted to contain 168 amino acids.

The mouse erythropoietin sequence encodes a 192-amino acid primary translation product. The mouse leader sequence is predicted to be 26 amino acids, one shorter than that of human erythropoietin, because of a 3-nucleotide deletion in the gene occurring at a position corresponding to human amino acid -17 (23,24). To date, there have been no amino acid sequence studies on natural or recombinant mouse erythropoietin, and the predicted length of the mature protein is 166 amino acids. Figure 3.1 in the following chapter by Dr. Goldwasser shows a comparison of the amino acid sequences of human, monkey, and mouse erythropoietin.

As suggested above, the amino acid sequence is moderately conserved between species (24). The overall homology at the amino acid sequence level is 92 percent between human and cynomolgus monkey, 79 percent between human and mouse, and 79 percent between monkey and mouse (14,23,24). Thus, the primary translation products of human and monkey erythropoietin differ at 16 positions, and those of human and mouse differ at 41 positions. Within the region predicted for the mature protein, there are 15 amino acid differences between human and monkey erythropoietin and 33 between human and mouse erythropoietin. This approximate 20 percent sequence difference does not lead to species specificity because human and monkey erythropoietin are both biologically active on mouse marrow. The regions of greatest sequence divergence are located near the carbohydrate sites. The secondary structure for one of the variable regions (around amino acid 32) is predicted to be conserved. The second variable region is in a segment predicted to be an external nonstructural loop (amino acids 76 to 90) (24) and is around a conserved N-linked carbohydrate addition site at position 83. A third variable region is located between amino acids 118 and 135, which surround the O-linked glycosylation site. Only three amino acid residues vary among human, monkey, and mouse erythropoietin; these correspond to positions 32, 88, and 95 of the human protein.

Estimates of evolution rates from the sequences of human, monkey, and mouse erythropoietin indicate 1.3×10^{-9} amino acid substitutions per site per year. This is faster than the rate of evolution of rapidly evolving proteins, such as the fibrinopeptides (9×10^{-9} substitutions/site/

year), much more rapid than slowly evolving proteins such as the histones (0.006×10^{-9} substitutions/site/year), and approximately equal to the rate of evolution of α and β globin (24). The incidence of silent or conservative substitutions is three- to sevenfold greater than that for replacement substitutions (24).

The mature human and mouse erythropoietin proteins have four cysteine residues, whereas monkey erythropoietin has five. The four cysteine amino acids in the human protein, which occur at positions 7, 29, 33, and 161, are conserved in the monkey hormone; the fifth cysteine in the monkey protein is at a position corresponding to amino acid 139 of the human protein (14). In mouse erythropoietin, the three cysteines corresponding to amino acids 7, 29, and 161 of the human protein are conserved, and the fourth cysteine is located at position 139 (23,24), corresponding to the position of one of the cysteines in the monkey protein. Analysis of the human protein has shown that disulfide bridges are formed between the cysteines at residues 7 and 161 and between the cysteines at residues 29 and 33 (34) (Fig 2.4). The position of the disulfide bridges in monkey and mouse erythropoietin are not known.

Carbohydrate Structure

In contrast to the cysteine residues, the number and position of Asn X Ser/Thr consensus sites for N-linked carbohydrate addition is invariant between the human, monkey, and mouse genes. The results of enzymatic deglycosylation experiments of human urinary and recombinant erythropoietin indicate that complex carbohydrate is present on each of the three potential N-glycosylation sites (19) (Fig 2.5) and that there is also a single site of O-linked glycosylation (20) (Fig 2.6). In the human, the N-linked carbohydrate sites are located at positions 24, 38, and 83 and the O-linked glycosylation site is mapped to serine 126 (25). It is not known whether monkey or mouse erythropoietin contains O-linked carbohydrate, but the amino acid sequence of monkey erythropoietin is identical to that of human erythropoietin around serine 126. In contrast, the amino acid sequence for mouse erythropoietin in this region is different.

It has been known for some time that erythropoietin is a highly glycosylated molecule, in which the carbohydrate moieties constitute approximately 39 percent of the total mass of the hormone (8,34). The carbohydrate fine structure, however, has only recently been investigated. The N-linked oligosaccharide structures of urinary derived-human erythropoietin (35,36) and recombinant human erythropoietin

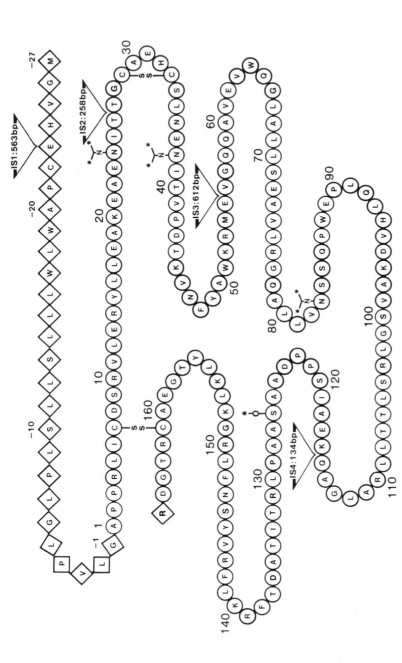

Figure 2.4. Amino acid sequence of human erythropoietin. The sequence of the 193-amino acid primary translation product is presented in one-letter code. The 27-amino acid signal peptide and the COOH-terminal arginine, which are removed postranslationally, are indicated by diamonds. The amino acids present in the 165-amino acid mature protein are circled. The disulfide linkages and the position of the four intervening sequences are presented. The N-linked (*N*) and the O-linked (O-*) glycosylation sites are designated. *Source: Reference 20*

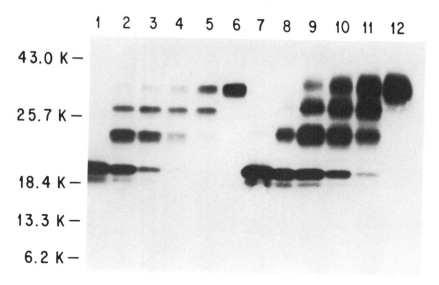

Figure 2.5. Western blot analysis of a time course of digestion of both human urinary and recombinant human erythropoietin with *N*-glycanase. Purified human urinary erythropoietin (lanes 1–6) and purified recombinant human erythropoietin (lanes 7–12) were digested with *N*-glycanase. Samples were removed at the following times after enzyme addition: 0 hour (lanes 6 and 12), 0.5 hour (lanes 5 and 11), 1 hour (lanes 4 and 10), 2 hours (lanes 3 and 9), 4 hours (lanes 2 and 8), and 8 hours (lanes 1 and 7). The enzyme digestion was stopped by boiling the samples in Laemmli sample buffer.
Source: Reference 19

expressed in a variety of host cells (35–38) have been determined. The carbohydrate structures described for human urinary erythropoietin are shown in Figure 2.7. Approximately 65 percent of the oligosaccharides on human urinary erythropoietin are tetra-antennary, with a small proportion containing one (6.9 percent) or two (0.6 percent) additional lactosamine repeats. The balance of the oligosaccharides are triantennary (23.6 percent) or biantennary (9 percent) structures. Approximately 82 percent of the oligosaccharides are fucosylated on the reducing *N*-acetylglucosamine residue.

Although the role of the carbohydrate structure in the function of erythropoietin is not fully understood, the conservation of glycosylation sites suggests that they have an important functional role. The glycosylation of erythropoietin is important for its biosynthesis, secretion, and biologic activity (39–48). Inhibition of carbohydrate synthesis by

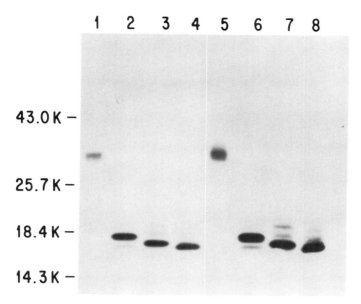

Figure 2.6. Western blot analysis of enzymatically deglycosylated human urinary erythropoietin (lanes 1–4) and recombinant human erythropoietin (lanes 5–8). Samples were either untreated (lanes 1 and 5) or digested sequentially with endoglycosidase F (lanes 2 and 6), followed by neuraminidase (lanes 3 and 7) and then *O*-glycanase (lanes 4 and 8). *Source: Reference 20*

treatment of cultured cells with tunicomycin inhibits erythropoietin secretion. In addition, the removal of any of the glycosylation sites by site-directed mutagenesis results in either a decrease in the efficiency of erythropoietin expression or a decrease in its biologic activity (40). Erythropoietin that is enzymatically deglycosylated is inactive *in vivo* but retains its receptor binding activity and *in vitro* biologic activity (39,40). The terminal sialic acids and the degree of branching of the oligosaccharides both have an important role in determining the level of *in vivo* bioactivity (41). Desialyted erythropoietin is inactive *in vivo* (40,42–44), apparently because of its rapid clearance from the circulation by hepatic galactose receptors (45–47). Recombinant human erythropoietin enriched in tetra-antennary oligosaccharides has greater *in vivo* activity and lower *in vitro* biologic activity than recombinant erythropoietin enriched in biantennary structures (41). Polylactosamine repeats, in contrast (which are found on approximately 7.5 percent of the tetra-antennary oligosaccharides), may decrease the *in vivo*

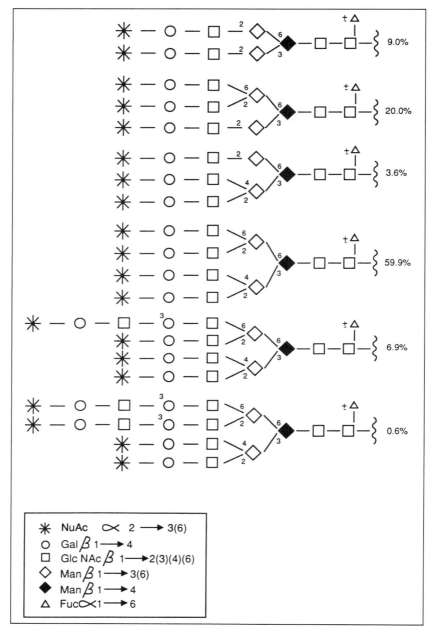

Figure 2.7. Structure of asparagine-linked carbohydrates and the frequency at which they occur in human urinary erythropoietin (35). *Data from Reference 35*

activity of erythropoietin because of a more rapid clearance from the serum (47).

Conclusion

Limited structural information and the lack of erythropoietin-producing cell lines made the cloning of the erythropoietin gene particularly difficult and made necessary the optimization of methods to permit the isolation of a single copy gene from a genomic library using multiple DNA probes. Once the technology was developed and appropriate DNA probe sequences were identified, the cloning of the human erythropoietin genomic gene, as well as the genes for monkey and mouse erythropoietin, was accomplished. Isolation of these erythropoietin-encoding gene clones has advanced our knowledge of the molecular biology and structural biochemistry of the hormone and permitted the development of recombinant erythropoietin for use in the treatment of anemia.

ACKNOWLEDGMENTS

We thank Pamm Deluca and Hillary Markowitz for their help in the preparation of this manuscript and Julie Heuston for the artwork.

REFERENCES

1. Carnot P, Deflandre C. Sur l'activité hematopoietique des differents organes au cours de la regeneration du sang. C R Acad Sci 1906;143:432–5.
2. Reissman KR. Studies on the mechanism of erythropoietic stimulation in parabiotic rats during hypoxia. Blood 1950;5:372–80.
3. Erslev AJ. Humoral regulation of red cell production. Blood 1953; 8:349–57.
4. Stohlman F, Rath CE, Rose JC. Evidence for humoral regulation of erythropoiesis: studies on a patient with polycythemia secondary to regional hypoxia. Blood 1954;9:721–4.
5. O'Sullivan MB, Chiba Y, Gletich GJ, Linman JW. Some molecular characteristics of human urinary erythropoietin determined by gel filtration and density gradient ultracentrifugation. J Lab Clin Med 1970;75:771–9.
6. Shelton RN, Ichiki AT, Lange RD. Physiocochemical properties of erythropoietin: isoelectric focusing and molecular weight studies. Biochem Med 1975;12:45–54.
7. Rosse WF, Berry RJ, Waldmann TA. Some molecular characteristics of erythropoietin from difference sources determined by inactivation by ionizing radiation. J Clin Invest 1963;42:124–9.

8. Miyake T, Kung CKH, Goldwasser E. Purification of human erythropoietin. Biol Chem 1977;252:5558–64.

9. Lin FK, Lai PH, Smalling R, et al. Cloning and expression of monkey and human erythropoietin gene. Exp Hematol 1984;12:357.

10. Jacobson LO, Goldwasser E, Fried W, Plzak LF. Role of the kidney in erythropoiesis. Nature 1957;179:633–4.

11. Peschle C, Condorelli M. Biogenesis of erythropoietin: evidence for proerythropoietin in a subcellular fraction of the kidney. Science 1975;190:910–2.

12. Gordon AS, Cooper GW, Zanjani ED. The kidney and erythropoiesis. Semin Hematol 1967;4:337–58.

13. Fyhrquist F, Rosenlof K, Gronhagen-Riska C, Hortling L, Tikkanen I. Is renin substrate an erythropoietin precursor? Nature 1984;308:649–52.

14. Lin FK, Lin CH, Lai PH, et al. Cloning of the monkey erythropoietin gene. J Cell Biochem 1984;8:45.

15. Lin FK, Lin CH, Lai PH, et al. Monkey erythropoietin gene: cloning, expression and comparison with the human erythropoietin gene. Gene 1986;44:201–9.

16. Lin FK, Suggs S, Lin CH, et al. Cloning and expression of the human erythropoietin gene. Proc Natl Acad Sci USA 1985;82:7580–4.

17. Jacobs K, Shoemaker C, Rudersdorf R, et al. Isolation and characterization of genomic and cDNA clones of human erythropoietin. Nature 1985;313:806–10.

18. Egrie JC, Browne J, Lai P, Lin FK. Characterization of recombinant monkey and human erythropoietin. In: Stanatoyannopoulos G, Nienhuis AW, eds. Experimental Approaches for the Study of Hemoglobin Switching. New York: Alan R. Liss, 1985:339–50.

19. Egrie JC, Strickland TW, Lane J, et al. Characterization and biological effects of recombinant human erythropoietin. Immunobiology 1986;72:213–24.

20. Browne JK, Cohen AM, Egrie JC, et al. Erythropoietin: gene cloning, protein structure, and biological properties. Cold Spring Harbor Symp Quant Biol 1986;51:693–702.

21. Powell JS, Berkner KL, Lebo RV, Adamson JW. Human erythropoietin gene: high level expression in stably transfected mammalian cells and chromosome localization. Proc Natl Acad Sci USA 1986;83:6465–9.

22. Goto M, Akai K, Murakami A, et al. Production of recombinant human erythropoietin in mammalian cells: host-cell dependency of the biological activity of the cloned glycoprotein. Biotechnology 1988;6:67–71.

23. Shoemaker CB, Mitsock LD. Murine erythropoietin gene: cloning, expression, and human gene homology. Mol Cell Biol 1986;6:849–58.

24. McDonald JD, Lin FK, Goldwasser E. Cloning, sequencing, and evolutionary analysis of the mouse erythropoietin gene. Mol Cell Biol 1986;6:842–8.

25. Lai PH, Everett R, Wang FF, Arakawa T, Goldwasser E. Structural characterization of human erythropoietin. J Biol Chem 1986;261:3116–21.

26. Mount SM. A catalog of splice junction sequences. Nucleic Acids Res 1982;10:459–72.

27. Watkins PC, Eddy R, Hoffman N, et al. Regional assignment of the erythropoietin gene to human chromosome region 7pter-q22. Cytogenet Cell Genet 1986;42:214–8.

28. Semenza GL, Dureza RC, Traystman MD, Gearhart JD, Antonarakis SE. Human erythropoietin gene expression in transgenic mice: multiple transcription initiation sites and cis acting regulatory elements. Mol Cell Biol 1990; 10:930–8.

29. Semenza GL, Dureza RC, Traystman MD, Gearhart JD, Antonarakis SE. Different DNA sequences control liver versus kidney expression of the human erythropoietin gene in transgenic mice [Abstract]. Am J Hum Genet 1989; 45:A116.

30. Semenza GL, Traystman MD, Gearhart JD, Antonarakis SE. Polycythemia in transgenic mice expressing the human erythropoietin gene. Proc Natl Acad Sci USA 1989;86:2301–5.

31. Kozak M. Compilation and analysis of sequences upstream from the translational start site in eukaryotic mRNAs. Nucleic Acids Res 1984;12: 857–72.

32. Vapnek D, Egrie JC, Browne JK, et al. Comparative studies of natural and recombinant human erythropoietin. In: Therapeutic peptides and proteins: assessing the new technologies. Cold Spring Harbor, New York: Cold Spring Harbor Laboratory, 1988:241–56. (Banbury Report 29).

33. Recny MA, Scoble HA, Kim Y. Structural characterization of natural human urinary and recombinant DNA-derived erythropoietin. Identification of des-arginine 166 erythropoietin. J Biol Chem 1987;262:17156–63.

34. Davis JM, Arakawa T, Strickland TW, Yphantis DA. Characterization of recombinant human erythropoietin produced in Chinese hamster ovary cells. Biochemistry 1987;26:2633–8.

35. Takeuchi M, Takasaki S, Miyazaki H, et al. Comparative study of the asparagine-linked sugar chains of human erythropoietins purified from urine and the culture medium of recombinant Chinese hamster ovary cells. J Biol Chem 1988;263:3657–63.

36. Tsuda E, Goto M, Mirakami A, et al. Comparative structural study of N-linked oligosaccharides of urinary and recombinant erythropoietins. Biochemistry 1988;27:5646–54.

37. Sasaki H, Bothner B, Dell A, Fukuda M. Carbohydrate structure of erythropoietin expressed in Chinese hamster ovary cells by a human erythropoietin cDNA. J Biol Chem 1987;262:12059–76.

38. Sasaki H, Ochi N, Dell A, Fukuda M. Site-specific glycosylation of human recombinant erythropoietin: analysis of glycopeptides at each glycosylation site by fast atom bombardment mass spectrometry. Biochemistry 1988; 27:8618–26.

39. Dordal MS, Wang FF, Goldwasser E. The role of carbohydrate in erythropoietin action. Endocrinology 1985;116:2293–9.

40. Tsuda E. Kawanishi G, Ueda M, Masuda S, Sasaki R. The role of carbohydrate in recombinant human erythropoietin. Eur J Biochem 1990;188: 405–12.

41. Takeuchi M, Inoue N, Strickland TW, et al. Relationship between sugar chain structure and biological activity of recombinant human erythropoietin produced in Chinese hamster ovary cells. Proc Natl Acad Sci USA 1989; 86:7819–22.

42. Goldwasser E, Kung CK, Eliason J. On the mechanism of erythropoietin-induced differentiation. 13. The role of sialic acid in erythropoietin action. J Biol Chem 1974;;249:4202–6.

43. Lowry PH, Keighley G, Borsook H. Inactivation of erythropoietin by neuraminidase and mild substitution reactions. Nature 1960;185:102–3.

44. Lukowsky WH, Painter RH. Studies on the role of sialic acid in the physical and biological properties of erythropoietin. Can J Biochem 1972;50:909–17.

45. Spivak JL, Hogans BB. The in vivo metabolism of recombinant human erythropoietin in the rat. Blood 1989;73:90–9.

46. Fukuda M, Sasaki H, Fukuda MN. Erythropoietin metabolism and the influence of carbohydrate structure. Contrib Nephrol 1989;76:78–89.

47. Fukuda MN, Sasaki H, Lopez L, Fukuda M. Survival of recombinant erythropoietin in the circulation: the role of carbohydrates. Blood 1989;73:84–9.

48. Dube S, Fisher JW, Powell JS. Glycosylation at specific sites of erythropoietin is essential for biosynthesis, secretion, and biological function. J Biol Chem 1988;263:17516–21.

Chapter 3

The Structure-Function Relationship of Erythropoietin

Eugene Goldwasser

After several decades of research on erythropoietin, the question of what structural features of this glycoprotein are responsible for its remarkable biologic activity is beginning to yield to the experimental approach. The reasons for the acceleration in our understanding lie in the ready availability of pure, recombinant erythropoietin and its gene (1– 5) and the ability to manipulate its structure by recombinant DNA methods. In this chapter the emphasis, except where indicated to the contrary, will be on human erythropoietin.

Interpretation of the molecular properties of human erythropoietin should include distinguishing between the two forms that have been studied in some detail, recombinant (rHuEpo) and urinary. The most evident difference between the two lies in their specific activities. The accepted, average potency of urinary erythropoietin is 80,000 to 130,000 units/mg of protein (6), whereas rHuEpo has about twice that specific activity (7). The basis for this difference is not yet clear because both forms have the same primary protein structure and very similar, if not identical, carbohydrate structure.

The Primary Structure

The amino acid sequences of erythropoietin from three species—human, old-world monkey, and mouse—are known. For the last two, the sequences were derived from the DNA sequence (3–5); for human erythropoietin, it was determined by direct sequencing (8) and from the gene sequence (1,2). The amino acid sequences are shown in Figure 3.1. Counting the carboxy-terminal arginine, there are 193 amino

```
        -20              -10            -1
Hu  MGVHECPAWLWLLLSLLSLPLGLPVLG
Mk  MGVHECPAWLWLLLSLVSLPLGLPVPG
Ms  MGVPERPT—LLLLLSLLLIPLGLPVLC


    +1          10              20      *        30        * 40
Hu  APPRLICDSRVLERYLLEAKEAENITTGCAEHCSLNENIT
Mk  APPRLICDSRVLERYLLEAKEAENVTTGCSESCSLNENIT
Ms  APPRLICDSRVLERYILEAKEAENITMGCAEGPRLSENIT


    41          50              60        70            80
Hu  VFDTKVNFYAWKRMEVGQQAVEVWQGLALLSEAVLRGQAL
Mk  VFDTKVNFYAWKRMEVGQQAVEVWQGLALLSEAVLRGQAV
Ms  VFDTKVNFYAWKRMEVEEQAIEVWQGLSLLSEAILQAQAL


    81  *      90             100          110          120
Hu  LVNSSQPWEPLQLHVDKAVSGLRSLTTLLRALGAQKEAIS
Mk  LANSSQPFEPLQLHMDKAVSGLRSITTLLRALGAQ—EAIS
Ms  LANSSQPPETLQLHIDKAISGLRSLTSLLRVLGAQKELMS


    121     *  130            140          150          160
Hu  PPDAASAAPLRTITADTFRKLFRVYSNFLRGKLKLYTGEA
Mk  PPDAASAAPLRTITADTFCKLFRVYSNFLRGKLKLYTGEA
Ms  LPDTTPPAPLRTLTVDTFCKLFRVYANFLRGKLKLYTGEV


    161
Hu  CRTGDR
Mk  CRRGDR
Ms  CRRGDR
```

Figure 3.1. The amino acid sequences of human (Hu), monkey (Mk), and mouse (Ms) erythropoietins. * = glycosylation site, — = missing residue.

acids, including a 27-residue leader sequence, in human erythropoietin and 192 amino acids in monkey and mouse erythropoietin; the leader sequence in monkey erythropoietin is also 27 residues long and that in mouse erythropoietin is 26. There is evidence that for both recombinant and urinary erythropoietin the carboxy-terminal arginine predicted from the DNA sequence is absent, having been split off by an enzyme (9).

In monkey erythropoietin, residue 116, which is a lysine in human erythropoietin, is missing. In mouse erythropoietin, however, residue −2 (tryptophan) is missing.*

A very high degree of conservation (4) is seen in comparisons of the three erythropoietin sequences: between monkey and human, 177 res-

*The numbering used in this chapter starts at the first residue of the mature (processed) human protein, with the leader sequence assigned negative numbers.

idues are identical; between mouse and human, 152 residues are identical, and between monkey and mouse, 151 are identical. Of the 15 residues that differ between human and monkey erythropoietins, 8 of the replacements are conservative. Similarly, in the comparison of human and mouse erythropoietins, 19 of the 41 replacements are conservative, whereas 14 of the 40 monkey-mouse replacements are conservative. This sample of species is far too small to permit many conclusions about the evolutionary history of erythropoietin and to infer important structural features from conserved sequences, but it does suggest that little of the erythropoietin primary structure is dispensable.

Human and mouse erythropoietins have four cysteine residues, and monkey erythropoietin has five. Human erythropoietin has no free sulfhydryls (10), and so there must be two disulfide bonds. The disulfide structure of human erythropoietin has been determined; cysteine 7 is linked to cysteine 161, and the cysteines at positions 29 and 33 are linked (10,11). Neither monkey nor mouse erythropoietin has been purified and studied; therefore, disulfide linkages are not known. By analogy one could infer that, for both monkey and mouse erythropoietins, cysteines 7 and 161 are linked and that, if there is a second disulfide in mouse erythropoietin, it would have to be between cysteines 29 and 139. In monkey erythropoietin it is not known whether cysteine 29 is bonded to 33, as in human erythropoietin, or to cysteine 139, as might be the case for mouse erythropoietin. These questions will be answered when the nonhuman erythropoietins are expressed in sufficient quantity to permit conventional protein chemistry. A similar structure has been proposed by Bazan (31).

The Secondary Structure

The three primary structures available at present have been analyzed by the Chou-Fasman method of predicting secondary structure (12). Even though such predictions are of limited use, in the absence of more reliable data regarding the folding of the erythropoietin molecule some features are worth comment. The Chou-Fasman method shows a considerable degree of conservation of helical structures for the three sequences (Fig 3.2). With this method of analysis, the exon-intron boundaries, which generally demark the domain structures of proteins, show interruption of helical structures by the splice junctions. These are at amino acid positions −23, 26–27, 55–56, and 115–116. An alter-

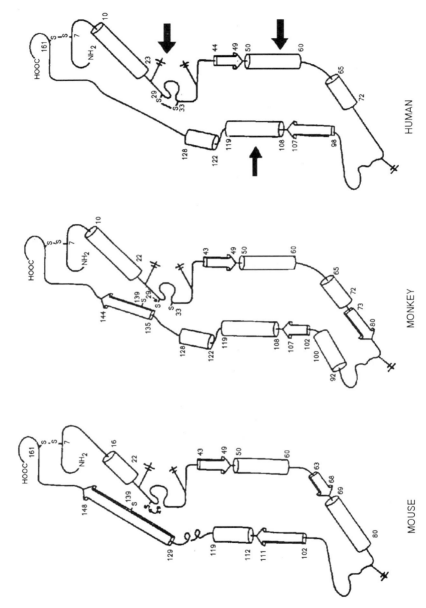

Figure 3.2. Predicted secondary structures of mouse, monkey, and human erythropoietins. The arrows indicate intron-extron boundaries. *Source: Reference 4*

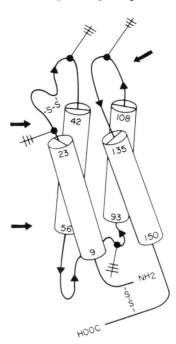

Figure 3.3. Predicted four-helix bundle structure of human erythropoietin. The arrows indicate intron-extron boundaries. *Source: Data from Reference 13*

native algorithim predicts that human erythropoietin has a four-helical bundle structure with paired amphiphilic helices (K. Berndt, E. T. Kaiser, and F. Kezdy, unpublished communication). This model (Fig 3.3) has the exon-intron boundaries in the nonhelical regions.

The region 29 to 33 is of some interest, involving (as mentioned above) a disulfide bond forming a loop with three residues between the cysteines. These three residues are not conserved in the three sequences, but the loop conformation, at least for human and mouse erythropoietins, is conserved because of the replacement of cysteine 33 by a proline. There is also the possibility that in monkey erythropoietin the disulfide bridge is between residues 29 and 33, yielding a loop, as in human erythropoietin. The probable conservation of this feature of secondary structure suggests that it might be important in biologic function.

These considerations of secondary structure are clearly based on incomplete evidence. We will have to wait for the crystallization of erythropoietin and the solution of its structure before understanding its true three-dimensional array.

Physical Properties

Molecular size determinations of impure erythropoietin preparations have been reported to range from 23 kd to 62 kd. The protein portion of erythropoietin has a formula weight of 18,399 (8) with the carboxy-terminal arginine or 18,243 without it. The molecular size of the intact glycoprotein determined by sedimentation equilibrium is 30,400 (13). Using 18.24 kd for the protein molecular mass of the des-arginine form, one can calculate that erythropoietin consists of 60% protein and 40% carbohydrate.

Studies of circular dichroism spectra and fluorescence quenching suggest that there is an α helix content of about 50% and that the three tryptophan residues are all in the same environment or that the ultraviolet absorption may be predominantly due to one of the residues (13). In this same study the data were interpreted to suggest that residues 48 to 70 and 88 to 102 were in α helical array. The first of these helices would contain tryptophan 64 in a hydrophobic segment of the molecule; the second would contain tryptophan 88 in a similar region, leaving tryptophan 51 available to interact with the solvent. These suggested helical regions agree roughly with the structure predicted in Figure 3.3, but only the first of them agrees with the Chou-Fasman prediction (Fig 3.2).

The Stokes' radius determined from hydrodynamic methods (32Å) is considerably larger than that calculated from the molecular mass (20.2Å), indicating that there is a fairly large hydration shell around the protein due to the carbohydrate or that the molecule is elongated rather than spherical (15).

Carbohydrate Structure

The amino acid sequence shows three sites of possible N-glycosylation, and the evidence derived from experiments with *N*-glycanase (16) shows that all three sites—asparagines 24, 38, and 83—are glycosylated. Other data (8) indicate that serine 126 is a site of O-glycosylation. It is interesting in this regard that mouse erythropoietin has a proline at position 126 rather than a serine; whether there is an O-linked oligosaccharide is not yet known. The oligosaccharide structures of rHuEpo have been determined (15,16), and one of the predominant sugar chains is illustrated in Figure 3.4. Essentially the same carbohydrate structures were described for urinary erythropoietin, which has

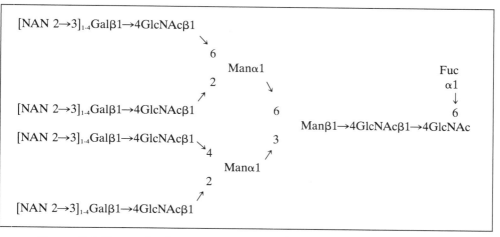

Figure 3.4. The predominant tetraantennary oligosaccharide chain in erythropoietin. Fuc = fucose, Gal = galactose, GlcNAc = *N*-acetylglucosamine, Man = mannose, NAN - *N*-acetylneuraminic acid (sialic acid).

a slight difference in sialic acid content (15), and for rHuEpo expressed in human β-lymphoblastoid cells (17).

Studies of urinary erythropoietin showed that removal of the carbohydrate resulted in the loss of about one-half of the biologic activity measured in vitro (18). Deglycosylation, however, also resulted in the formation of a biologically inactive aggregate representing about 80 percent of the original urinary erythropoietin treated. The remaining monomeric urinary erythropoietin having 50 percent of the biologic activity has, therefore, two- to threefold increased potency. A similar finding when the terminal sialic acids were removed was reported some years ago (19). When asialo erythropoietin or aglyco erythropoietin was assayed in vivo, there was essentially no activity detected. A plausible explanation for the results with asialo erythropoietin was based on the existence of a liver receptor for asialo glycoprotein that cleared the modified erythropoietin from the circulation in vivo (19). No explanation for the results with aglyco erythropoietin has been offered.

More recently, a different rHuEpo preparation derived from Chinese hamster ovary cells was shown to consist of two forms, one with predominantly biantennary oligosaccharides and one with tetra-antennary sugar chains (20). When compared with conventional rHuEpo, the biantennary form had only about 14 percent of the activity measured in vivo and threefold higher activity when assayed in vitro. The tetra-antennary form had essentially the same activity by both assay methods as did the "standard" erythropoietin. There seems to be a correlation with content of tetra-antennary oligosaccharide and in vivo activity, but the mechanisms underlying these effects are not at all understood.

Erythropoietin expressed by insect cells using a baculovirus vector has less carbohydrate than that expressed by mammalian cells (M_r 26,000). It has full activity when assayed in vitro but no activity in vivo. When treated with N-glycanase, it loses about 80 percent of its in vitro activity (21). This finding may be due to aggregation of the deglycosylated erythropoietin, if one may draw an analogy with rHuEpo expressed by Chinese hamster ovary cells or with urinary erythropoietin.

Structure-Function Studies

Inactivation studies with reagents of well-defined specificity have led to fragmentary information on structural requirements for the activity of urinary erythropoietin. Acylation of sulfhydryls after reduction caused loss of activity of urinary erythropoietin (10), as did iodination and substitution on amino groups (22). Similar experiments with rHuEpo indicated that both carboxyl and amino groups are required for activity of an unspecified preparation of rHuEpo and for an impure preparation of urinary erythropoietin (23).

No definitive study of the chemistry of the active site (or sites) of erythropoietin has yet been published, although older data derived by the use of highly impure erythropoietin or urinary erythropoietin indicated that tryptophan (25), tyrosine, and or amino groups (22) may be required for biologic activity.

Analysis of the amino acid sequence of erythropoietin by the method of Hopp and Woods (25) shows a mean hydrophilicity value of 1.83 for the region 18–23 (E A K E A E), which represents a probable antigenic site. Studies using rabbit antisera raised against synthetic peptides conjugated to limpet hemocyanin indicate that an antibody made to the amino-terminal 26 residues does not impair biologic function (26). Of five other antibodies made similarly against synthetic peptides, only those raised against residues 99–118 and 111–129 had any inhibitory effect on erythropoietin action. These regions of the erythropoietin protein lack tryptophan and tyrosine, although there is one lysine at residue 116. In a very recent paper, study with monoclonal antierythropoietins showed that residues 1–20 do not seem to be associated with binding to specific erythropoietin receptors. Similarly, none of the eight (nine if reduced) fragments derived from endoprotease-Lys-c digestion competed for receptor binding. Other monoclonal antibodies, presumably recognizing "nonsequential, conformation-dependent epitopes," do inhibit binding of erythropoietin to its receptor (27). An interpretation of these seemingly inconsistent observations is still not possible, except that much more data are needed for the assignment of biologic activity to specific chemical features of the erythropoietin molecule.

Some information has been derived from site-directed mutagenesis experiments using the ratio of activity by an in vitro assay to activity by radioimmunoassay to indicate biologic function (28). The substitution of leucine at residue 2 for proline had no effect on activity, nor did phenylalanine at 49 for tyrosine or glutamic acid at 52 for lysine. The replacement of cysteine 33 with proline (as in the mouse) caused a decrease in the ratio of biologic activity to immunoreactivity. This result could indicate that the small disulfide loop formed is not exactly replaced by putting in a turn in the peptide chain with a proline. Alternatively, the presence of the free thiol in the modified erythropoietin may permit inactive aggregate formation by interchain disulfide bond formation. It might also suggest that pure mouse erythropoietin could have a lower potency than human erythropoietin.

When one of the three asparagines that are linked to carbohydrate (asparagine 24) was replaced by glutamine, there was significantly decreased biologically active erythropoietin secreted by BHK cells transfected with the modified human erythropoietin gene (29). In contrast, replacement of asparagines 38 or 83 by glutamine and replacement of serine 126 by glycine resulted in essentially no secretion of active erythropoietin. In the case of the modified residue 24, there was no decrease in immunoreactive material secreted by the cells. For the other three mutations, however, very little, if any, immunoreactive material was secreted. For each of the mutants, transcription of the erythropoietin gene was not affected.

The use of scanning mutants to determine which regions of the structure are responsible for biologic activity has recently been reported (30). A construct of the human erythropoietin complementary DNA driven by the strong adenovirus promoter was expressed in COS cells, and deletion mutants were studied. Block deletions of residues 9–21, 48–64, 83–98, 142–150, 151–157, and 151–165 resulted in complete loss of both biologic and immunologic activity. When residues 111–119 were deleted, full activity by both assays was retained.

Conclusion

It is clear that the last few years of research have resulted in an increase of several orders of magnitude in our knowledge of erythropoietin chemistry over that known from the first 80 years of study. It is also quite clear that much remains to be done before the relationship between glycoprotein structure and the remarkable ability to induce red cell differentiation can be understood in satisfying molecular detail.

ACKNOWLEDGMENTS

The work reported from this laboratory was done under grants HL21676 and HL30121 from the National Institutes of Health. The author acknowledges with gratitude the essential secretarial help of Mrs. Betty Kniaz.

REFERENCES

1. Lin FK, Suggs S, Lin CH, et al. Cloning and expression of the human erythropoietin gene. Proc Natl Acad Sci USA 1985;82:7580–4.

2. Jacobs K, Shoemaker C, Rudersdorf R, et al. Isolation and characterization of genomic and cDNA clones of human erythropoietin. Nature 1985; 313:806–10.

3. Lin FK, Lin CH, Lai PH, et al. Monkey erythropoietin gene: cloning expression and comparison with the human erythropoietin gene. Gene 1986; 44:201–9.

4. McDonald J, Lin FK, Goldwasser E. Cloning, sequencing and evolutionary analysis of the mouse erythropoietin gene. Mol Cell Biol 1986;6:842–8.

5. Shoemaker CB, Mistock LD. Murine erythropoietin gene: cloning, expression, and human gene homology. Mol Cell Biol 1986;6:849–58.

6. Miyake T, Kung CKH, Goldwasser E. Purification of human erythropoietin. J Biol Chem 1977;252:5558–64.

7. Browne JK, Cohen AM, Egrie JC, et al. Erythropoietin: gene cloning, protein structure and biological properties. Cold Spring Harbor Symp Quant Biol 51;1986:693–702.

8. Lai PH, Everett R, Wang FF, Arakawa T, Goldwasser E. Structural characterization of human erythropoietin. J Biol Chem 1986;26:3116–21.

9. Recny MA, Scoble HA, Kim Y. Structural characterization of natural human urinary and recombinant DNA-derived erythropoietin. J Biol Chem 1987;262:17156–63.

10. Wang FF, Kung CKH, Goldwasser E. Some chemical properties of human erythropoietin. Endocrinology 1985;116:2286–92.

11. Sytkowski AJ. Denaturation and renaturation of human erythropoietin. Biochem Biophys Res Commun 1980;96:143–9.

12. Chou PY, Fasman GD. Empirical prediction of protein conformation. Annu Rev Biochem 1978;47:251–76.

13. Davis JM, Arakawa T, Strickland TW, Yphantis DA. Characterization of recombinant human erythropoietin produced in Chinese hamster ovary cells. Biochemistry 1987;26:2633–8.

14. Egrie J, Strickland TW, Lane J, et al. Characterization and biological effects of recombinant human erythropoietin. Immunobiology 1986;172:213–24.

15. Takeuchi M, Takasaki S, Miyazaki H, et al. Comparative study of the asparagine-linked sugar chains of human erythropoietin purified from urine and the culture medium of recombinant Chinese hamster ovary cells. J Biol Chem 1988;263:3657–63.

16. Sasaki H, Bothner B, Dell A, Fukuda M. Carbohydrate structure of erythropoietin expressed in Chinese hamster ovary cells by a human erythropoietin cDNA. J Biol Chem 1987;262:12059–76.

17. Yanagi H, Yoshima T, Ogawa I, Okamoto M. Recombinant human erythropoietin produced by Namalwa cells. DNA 1989;8:419–27.

18. Dordal MS, Wang FF, Goldwasser E. The role of carbohydrates in erythropoietin action. Endocrinology 1985;116:2293–9.

19. Goldwasser E, Kung CKH, Eliason JF. On the mechanism of erythropoietin induced differentiation: XII. The role of sialic acid in erythropoietin action. J Biol Chem 1974;249:4202–6.

20. Takeuchi M, Inoue N, Strickland T, et al. Relationship between sugar chain structure and biological activity of recombinant human erythropoietin produced in Chinese hamster ovary cells. Proc Natl Acad Sci USA 1989;86:7819–22.

21. Wojchowski DM, Orkin SH, Sytkowski AJ. Active human erythropoietin expressed in insect cells using a baculovirus vector: a role for N-linked oligosaccharide. Biochim Biophys Acta 1987;910:224–32.

22. Goldwasser E. Erythropoietin and red cell differentiation. In: Cunningham D, Goldwasser E, Watson J, Fox CF, eds. Control of cellular division and development. New York: AR Liss, 1981:487–94.

23. Wojchowski DM, Caslake L. Biotinylated recombinant human erythropoietins: bioactivity and utility as receptor ligands. Blood 1989;74:952–8.

24. Lowy P, Keighly G. Inactivation of erythropoietin by Koshland's tryptophan reagent and by membrane filtration. Biochim Biophys Acta 1968;160:413–9.

25. Hopp TP, Woods KR. Prediction of protein antigenic determinants from amino acid sequences. Proc Natl Acad Sci USA 1981;78:3824–8.

26. Sytkowski AJ, Donahue KA. Immunochemical studies of human erythropoietin using site-specific anti-peptide antibodies. J Biol Chem 1987; 262:1161–5.

27. D'Andrea AD, Szklut PJ, Lodish HF, Alderman EM. Inhibition of receptor binding and neutralization of bioactivity by anti-erythropoietin monoclonal antibodies. Blood 1990;75:874–80.

28. Lin FK. The molecular biology of erythropoietin. In: Rich IN, ed. Molecular and cellular aspects of erythropoietin and erythropoiesis. New York: Springer, 1987:23–36.

29. Dube S, Fisher JW, Powell JS. Glycosylation at specific sites of erythropoietin is essential for biosynthesis, secretion and biological function. J Biol Chem 1988;263:17516–21.

30. Boissel JP, Bunn HF. Erythropoietin structure-function relationships. In: Daniak N, Cronkite EP, McCaffrey R, Shadduck RK, eds. The biology of hematopoiesis. New York: Wiley-Liss, 1990;227–32.

31. Bazan JF. Haemopoetic receptors and helical cytokines. Immunol Today 1990;11:350–54.

Chapter 4

The Regulation of
Erythropoietin Gene Expression

Jaime Caro, Stephen Schuster, and
Sylvia Ramirez

Erythropoietin is the glycoprotein growth factor that regulates the rate of red cell production by stimulating the proliferation and differentiation of erythroid precursor cells. It forms part of a regulatory feedback system that adapts the circulating red cell mass to the physiologic need for oxygen by the tissues (1). As shown in Figure 4.1, erythropoietin acts as the humoral link between oxygen sensing in the kidney and red cell production by the bone marrow. The role of the kidney in the production of erythropoietin was suggested early in 1957 by Jacobson and co-workers in studies with nephrectomized animals (2). It was not until the cloning of the erythropoietin gene (3,4), however, that the direct participation of the kidney in erythropoietin synthesis was clearly established. Although extrarenal sites of erythropoietin production also exist in the adult animal, they probably do not account for more than

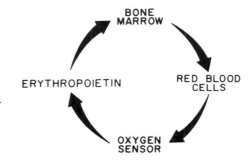

Figure 4.1. Schematic representation of the feedback system that regulates the production of erythropoietin.

15 percent of the total production of erythropoietin (5). During fetal life, however, the contribution of extrarenal erythropoietin production seems to be, at least in some species, more important (see Chapter 5). The main source of extrarenal production of erythropoietin is the liver (6). Although other sources of extrarenal erythropoietin may exist, their physiologic significance has yet to be proved.

The cloning of the erythropoietin gene represents a great advance in the field because it has permitted determination of the precise amino acid sequences of the erythropoietin molecule and allowed studies that eventually will clarify the mechanisms that regulate erythropoietin synthesis and secretion.

The Expression of the Erythropoietin Gene

Erythropoietin production is greatly stimulated by anemic or hypoxic hypoxia and also by pharmacologic doses of cobalt chloride. In patients with different types of anemias, erythropoietin levels increase exponentially, and levels about 1000 times higher than normal are found in cases of severe anemia (7). In experimental animals, exposure to hypobaric hypoxia produces an intense stimulation of erythropoietin, and this animal model is reliable and effective for the study of erythropoietin gene expression (8). As shown in Figure 4.2, erythropoietin levels in rats exposed to 0.4 atm begin to increase in the kidney at about 1 hour after stimulation, and erythropoietin continues to accumulate during the 4 hours of the experiment. Plasma erythropoietin levels, with a minor delay, follow the changes in the kidney. These changes in erythropoietin content in the kidney correlate with the changes in erythropoietin-specific messenger RNA (mRNA) measured in RNA extracted from similarly hypoxic-treated animals. Figure 4.3 shows that erythropoietin mRNA, which is undetectable in normal kidneys, becomes detectable at about 1 hour of stimulation and peaks at 4 hours of continuous hypoxia. Discontinuation of the hypoxic stimulus causes a rapid decay in erythropoietin mRNA, which again becomes undetectable about 3 hours into the poststimulation period. It thus seems that erythropoietin production is regulated at the level of its specific mRNA and that these levels follow very closely the degree of tissue hypoxia. The erythropoietin mRNA seems to have a very short half-life, a property that allows for very tight control of erythropoietin production when the hypoxic stimulus is discontinued. Injection of pharmacologic doses of cobalt, which greatly stimulates erythropoietin production, also produces accumulations of erythropoietin mRNA in the kidneys,

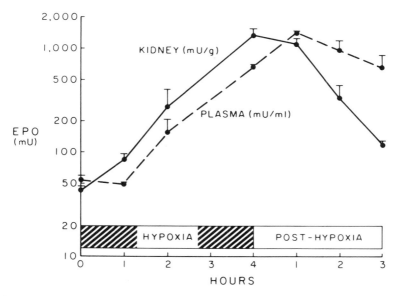

Figure 4.2. Levels of erythropoietin (EPO) in the plasma and kidneys of rats exposed to hypoxia (0.4 atm) for various periods.

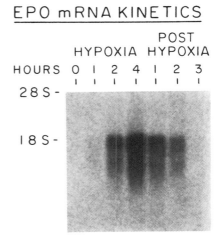

Figure 4.3. Levels of erythropoietin (EPO) mRNA in the kidneys of rats exposed to acute hypoxia for various periods.

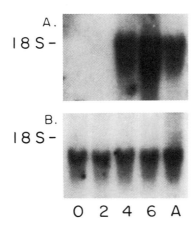

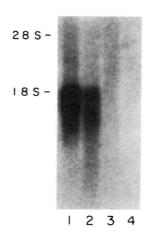

Figure 4.4. Levels of erythropoietin mRNA in the kidneys of rats after the injection of cobalt (6 mg/100 g). Samples of RNA were taken 0, 2, 4, and 6 hours after injection. A, Erythropoietin mRNA; B, glyceraldehyde-3-phosphate dehydrogenase mRNA.

Figure 4.5. Northern blot analysis of erythropoietin mRNA obtained from hypoxic whole rat kidney (1), hypoxic nonglomerular fraction (2), hypoxic glomerular fraction (3), and normal whole kidney (4).

as shown in Figure 4.4. In the case of cobalt stimulation there is a delay of about 4 hours between the injection of cobalt and the appearance of detectable levels of erythropoietin mRNA. This delay in the effect of cobalt may be related to the mechanisms of oxygen sensing, which probably involves the presence of a heme-containing protein (9). The demonstration of erythropoietin mRNA in kidneys of stimulated animals has settled an old controversy that questioned the direct role of the kidney in erythropoietin production by postulating an indirect mechanism of activation of a plasma erythropoietin precursor.

Northern blot analysis of RNA extracted from different tissues of similarly hypoxic, cobalt-treated animals also showed erythropoietin mRNA expression in the liver, whereas all other organs studied were negative. It thus seems that erythropoietin gene expression is highly tissue specific and, in the adult animal, is restricted mainly to the kidney and to a lesser extent to the liver. The specific cells in the kidney or liver responsible for erythropoietin production are still a matter of some controversy. Separation of hypoxic kidneys into their glomerular and nonglomerular fractions showed that erythropoietin mRNA was present only in the nonglomerular fraction, suggesting an extraglomerular origin of renal erythropoietin (8) (see Fig 4.5). The precise localization of erythropoietin-producing cells was further studied by in situ hybridization techniques, and both Koury et al. (10) and Lacombe et al. (11) identified cortical interstitial cells, probably endothelial, as the erythropoietin-producing cells in the kidney. However, a recent report by Maxwell et al. (12), also using in situ hybridization, suggested the proximal tubule as the site of origin of erythropoietin. This report is supported by studies by DaSilva et al., who showed that tumor parenchymal cells are the source of erythropoietin in human renal cancers associated with erythrocytosis (13).

Studies on the hepatic origin of erythropoietin have been more difficult because of the scarcity of the erythropoietin messenger in that organ. Lacombe (14) reported, using a metrizamide gradient separation technique, that erythropoietin-producing cells were contained in the small cell, nonhepatocyte fraction of hypoxic mouse livers. Kurtz et al. (15), using in situ hybridization, reported positive erythropoietin signal in periportal interstitial cells of stimulated livers from neonatal (11-day-old) rats. On the other hand, regulated expression of erythropoietin was described in the human hepatoma cell lines Hep3B and HepG2 derived from hepatocytes (16). These cell lines respond to hypoxia and cobalt in vitro with increased erythropoietin production and accumulation of erythropoietin mRNA. They are currently utilized extensively for studies regarding the regulation of erythropoietin gene expression. Figure 4.6 shows the time course of erythropoietin mRNA accumulation of Hep3B cells exposed to 1 percent O_2 in vitro. As observed, these results are very similar to those shown in Figure 4.3 regarding the response to hypoxia of rat kidneys in vivo.

Transcriptional Control of Erythropoietin Gene Expression

The role of transcriptional control in the erythropoietin response to hypoxia or cobalt stimulation was studied by "run-on" experiments conducted in isolated nuclei derived from normal and stimulated rat kidneys (17). These experiments measured the rate of RNA synthesis by the incorporation of uridine triphosphate labeled with phosphorus 32 into primary RNA transcripts initiated in vivo and elongated in vitro during a short incubation period. Labeled transcripts obtained from normal and hypoxic rat kidney nuclei were hybridized against erythropoietin DNA immobilized in nitrocellulose, and the dot blot hybrid-

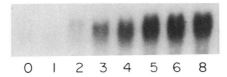

Figure 4.6. Levels of erythropoietin mRNA from Hep3B cells exposed to hypoxia (1 percent O_2) for various lengths of time.

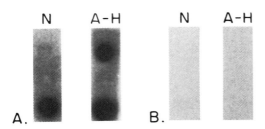

Figure 4.7. The effect of hypoxia on the transcription rate of the erythropoietin gene (run on). Nuclei were isolated from normal (N) or hypoxic (A-H) rat kidneys and allowed to incorporate uridine [^{32}P]triphosphate in the absence (A) or presence (B) of α-amanitin. The labeled transcripts were hybridized against erythropoietin complementary deoxyribonucleic acid (cDNA) (upper lane), control plasmid (middle lane), and glyceraldehyde-3-phosphate dehydrogenase cDNA (lower lane).

HOURS

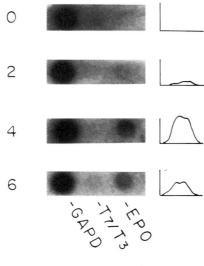

Figure 4.8. The transcription rate of the erythropoietin gene in rat kidneys at various points after the injection of cobalt chloride (run on). The labeled transcripts were hybridized against glyceraldehyde-3-phosphate dehydrogenase (GAPD), control T_7/T_3 plasmid, and erythropoietin (EPO) cDNA. The right panel shows densitometric scanning of erythropoietin gene blots.

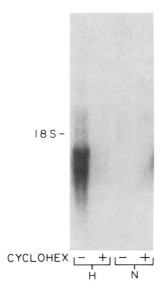

18S−

CYCLOHEX ┌─ +┐┌─ +┐
          └─┬─┘└─┬─┘
            H   N

Figure 4.9. Northern blot analysis of erythropoietin mRNA obtained from normal (N) or hypoxic (H) rat kidneys in the presence (+) or absence (−) of cycloheximide.

izations are shown in Figure 4.7. Nuclei isolated from normal kidneys show a barely detectable hybridization signal, whereas nuclei obtained from hypoxic animals show a clearly demonstrable signal. Both normal and hypoxic nuclei give positive hybridization with the control housekeeping glyceraldehyde phosphate dehydrogenase gene. The transcriptional signal is completely abolished by low doses of α-amanitin, a phenomenon characteristic of polymerase II-dependent genes.

Similar transcriptional activation of the erythropoietin gene is observed in animals given injections of cobalt, as shown in Figure 4.8. This figure also shows that the delay in mRNA accumulation corresponds to the delay in transcription activation.

The requirement for protein synthesis in activation of the erythropoietin gene was studied with the use of the protein synthesis inhibitor cycloheximide. As shown in Figure 4.9, injection of cycloheximide almost completely abolishes expression of the erythropoietin gene in response to hypoxia. Run-on analysis showed that this effect of cycloheximide on mRNA accumulation was secondary to specific inhibition of transcription of the erythropoietin gene.

It thus seems that erythropoietin gene responses are regulated primarily at the level of transcription and that this response requires the presence of active protein synthesis. Whether these proteins are necessary for the mechanism of transcription itself or are involved in the mechanisms of oxygen sensing is still unknown.

Post-transcriptional regulation mechanisms affecting the stability of the erythropoietin messenger may also possibly exist as part of the response to hypoxia. Erythropoietin mRNA has a very short half-life and, as has been shown for other growth factors, changes in messenger stability could represent a very effective way to increase the levels of mRNA rapidly upon stimulation. The half-life of the erythropoietin mRNA is greatly prolonged after the addition of RNA synthesis inhibitors like actinomycin D. It is not yet clear, however, whether changes of mRNA stability do indeed occur in the physiologic response to anemia or hypoxia.

Mechanisms of Oxygen Sensing

Although it has long been known that tissue hypoxia is the main stimulus for erythropoietin production, very little was known regarding the mechanisms of oxygen sensing and transduction. Observations by Goldberg et al. (9) in the erythropoietin-producing Hep3B cells provided exciting information on the possible nature of the oxygen sensor. Their data suggested that the oxygen sensor is a heme-containing protein that is exquisitely sensitive to the variations in oxygen tension at which the erythropoietin-producing cells are continuously exposed. When the oxygen tension is low, the heme protein is in the deoxy-conformation and will, by still-unknown mechanisms, stimulate erythropoietin gene expression. Conversely, when the oxygen tension is sufficiently high, the heme protein is in the inactive oxy-conformation and will not stimulate erythropoietin production (see schema in Fig 4.10). As mentioned, the mechanisms by which the conformational changes in this heme protein result in changes in activity of the erythropoietin gene are still only speculative. When erythropoietin-producing cells are exposed to high concentrations of cobalt, this metal could substitute for iron in the porphyrin ring and lock the heme moiety in the deoxy or active conformation, thereby stimulating erythropoietin production. Other metals that can substitute for iron in the porphyrin ring, such as nickel or manganese, also stimulate erythropoietin production. Exposure of the cells to carbon monoxide, which mimicks oxygen in the heme moiety, abolishes the response to hypoxia. This effect of carbon monoxide was not observed in cobalt-treated cells because cobalt does not bind carbon monoxide. All of the experimental data are very sup-

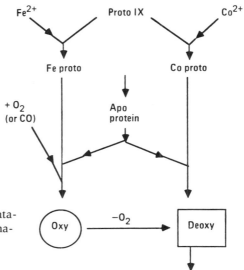

Figure 4.10. Schematic representation of the oxygen-sensing mechanism. *Source: Reference 18*

portive of the heme protein theory, and we hope that more data on the actual structure and properties of this oxygen sensor will become available in the near future.

Regulatory Elements in Erythropoietin Gene Expression

Studies of the regulation of gene transcription in eukaryotic systems identified two major classes of transcriptional control elements in genomic DNA, promoters and enhancers. Promoter sequences are located proximal or 5' to the transcription start site. They are typically about 100 to 200 base pairs in length and usually have a common organization, including an adenine-thymidine-rich region ("TATA" box) located 25 to 30 base pairs upstream from the start site. In addition they contain other upstream sequence elements known as upstream promoter elements, which regulate the rate of transcription. Enhancer sequences, like upstream promoter elements, modulate the rate of transcription but can function over greater distances and in an orientation-independent manner. It is now clear that frequency of initiation of mRNA synthesis depends also on the presence of specific proteins that interact with these regulatory genomic sequences and ultimately determine the rate of transcription.

The functional organization of the erythropoietin gene is still largely unknown, as are the regulatory transcriptional factors that may regulate the response to hypoxia. Comparison of mouse and human erythropoietin gene sequences reveals a high degree of homology not only in the coding sequences but also in the 5' flanking, 3' untranslated, and intron I sequences (19,20). The evolutionary conservation of these sequences suggests that these regions probably contain important genomic regulatory elements. The most highly conserved region of the erythropoietin gene is found in the putative promoter sequences immediately upstream of the transcription start site. The conserved sequences are very GC rich and do not contain clearly identifiable equivalents to the canonical TATA box or the CAAT sequences at -80. Although there is a sequence that is moderately equivalent to the TATA box, at position -30, it is believed that the erythropoietin promoter may resemble more the structure of the so-called housekeeping genes (19).

The precise regulatory sequences responsible for the tissue specificity and responsiveness to hypoxia of the erythropoietin gene have not yet been clearly identified. However, transient transfection experiments and the use of transgenic mice models provided initial evidence for regions required for the regulated expression of the erythropoietin gene. Semenza et al. (21) reported that transgenic mice carrying a 4-kilobasepair (kb) fragment of the human erythropoietin gene with 0.4 kb of 5' flanking and 0.7 kb of 3' flanking sequences express the erythropoietin gene and have increased erythropoietin production that results in secondary erythrocytosis. In these animals the erythropoietin gene was expressed in organs that normally produce erythropoietin, like the kidney and liver, but also in other tissues that do not normally express the erythropoietin gene. Moreover, induction by hypoxia was encountered only in the liver and not in the kidney, where maximal erythropoietin production normally takes place. These results suggested that the 4-kb microinjected DNA fragment contained some regulatory elements that allowed inducible expression in the liver but lacked others that conferred responsiveness in the kidney. They also suggested that it lacked elements that restricted expression to only these two organs because the erythropoietin gene also was expressed in several other tissues. A more recent report (22) using a larger 6-kb 5' flanking region of the human erythropoietin gene in transgenic mice showed that these animals express the erythropoietin gene only in the liver and that this expression is regulated by anemia or by the injection of cobalt. Surprisingly, even with this large genomic fragment, no expression was observed in the kidney. Therefore, it seems that DNA sequences that control inducible kidney expression may map further upstream of 6 kb in the 5' flanking or further downstream of 0.7 kb in the 3' flanking regions. These data also suggest that different regulatory transacting factors may mediate the hypoxic responsiveness in kidney and liver.

Imagawa et al., using a reporter gene under the control of erythropoietin genomic sequences, have found regulated response to hypoxia when transfected into Hep3B cells (23). The regulatory sequences were included within 400 bp of 5' flanking, exon and intron I and untranslated region of exon V of the human erythropoietin gene. Results from our laboratory using an erythropoietin mini-gene construct have shown hypoxia responsiveness confined to a genomic fragment containing 400 bp of 5' upstream and 600 bp of 3' downstream flanking regions. This construct has shown hypoxia responsiveness when transfected into Hep3B cells but no response when transfected into the non-erythropoietin-producing Hela cell line. Deletion analysis of the 5' and 3' flanking regions in this mini-gene construct has determined the presence of an enhancer type element in the 3' flanking region of the human erythropoietin gene which appears responsible for hypoxia responsiveness (24). This element is active in Hep3B cells; however, because of lack of appropriate renal cells, it cannot yet be assessed whether the same element is active in kidney cells.

REFERENCES

1. Schuster SJ, Caro J, Erslev AJ. Erythropoietin: current concepts and future prospects. Hematol Pathol 1987;1:193–201.

2. Jacobson LD, Goldwasser E, Fried W, Plzak L. Role of the kidney in erythropoietin. Nature 1957;179:633–4.

3. Jacobs K, Shoemaker C, Rudersdorf R, et al. Isolation and characterization of genomic and cDNA clones of human erythropoietin. Nature 1985; 313:806–10.

4. Lin FK, Suggs S, Lin CH, et al. Cloning and expression of the human erythropoietin gene. Proc Natl Acad Sci USA 1985;82:7580–4.

5. Erslev AJ, Caro J, Kansu E, Silver R. Renal and extrarenal erythropoietin production in anaemic rats. Br J Haematol 1980;45:65–72.

6. Zanjani ED, Poster J, Burlington H, Mann LI, Wasserman LR. Liver as the primary site of erythropoietin formation in the fetus. J Lab Clin Med 1977;89:640–4.

7. Erslev AJ, Wilson J, Caro J. Erythropoietin titers in anemic, nonuremic patients. J Lab Clin Med 1987;109:429–33.

8. Schuster SJ, Wilson JH, Erslev AJ, Caro J. Physiologic regulation and

tissue localization of renal erythropoietin messenger RNA. Blood 1987;70: 316–8.

9. Goldberg MA, Dunning SP, Bunn HF. Regulation of the erythropoietin gene: evidence that the oxygen sensor is a heme protein. Science 1988;242: 1412–5.

10. Koury ST, Bondurant MC, Koury MJ. Localization of erythropoietin synthesizing cells in murine kidneys by in situ hybridization. Blood 1988; 71:524–7.

11. Lacombe C, DaSilva, J-L, Bruneval P, et al. Peritubular cells are the site of erythropoietin synthesis in the murine hypoxic kidney. J Clin Invest 1988; 81:620–3.

12. Maxwell AP, Lappin TR, Bridges JM, McGeown MC. Erythropoietin production in kidney tubular cells. Br J Haematol 1990;74:535–9.

13. DaSilva J-L, Lacombe C, Bruneval P, et al. Tumor cells are the site of erythropoietin synthesis in human renal cancers associated with polycythemia. Blood 1990;75:577–82.

14. Lacombe C. Response and adaptation to hypoxia: organ to organelle. Oxford, England: Oxford University Press (in press).

15. Kurtz A, Eckard K-U, Newmann R, Kaissling B, Lehir M, Bauer C. Site of erythropoietin formation. Contrib Nephrol 1989;76:14–20.

16. Goldberg MA, Glass GA, Cunningham JM, Bunn HF. The regulated expression of erythropoietin by two human hepatoma cell lines. Proc Natl Acad Sci USA 1987;84:7972–6.

17. Schuster SJ, Badiavas EV, Costa-Giomi P, Weinmann R, Erslev AJ, Caro J. Stimulation of erythropoietin gene transcription during hypoxia and cobalt exposure. Blood 1989;73:13–6.

18. Goldberg M, Imagawa S, Dunning S, Bunn F. Oxygen sensing and erythropoietin gene regulation. Contrib Nephrol 1989;76:39–51.

19. Shoemaker CB, Mitsock LD. Murine erythropoietin gene: cloning, expression and human gene homology. Mol Cell Biol 1986;6:849–58.

20. McDonald J, Lin FK, Goldwasser E. Cloning, sequencing and evolutionary analysis of the mouse erythropoietin gene. Mol Cell Biol 1986;6: 842–8.

21. Semenza GL, Traystman MD, Gearhart JD, Antonarakis SE. Polycythemia in transgenic mice expressing the human erythropoietin gene. Proc Natl Acad Sci USA 1989;86:2301–5.

22. Semenza G, Dureza R, Traystman M, Gearhart J, Antonarakis S. Human erythropoietin gene expression in transgenic mice: multiple transcription initiation sites and cis-acting regulatory elements. Mol Cell Biol 1990;10:930–8.

23. Imagawa S, Goldberg M, Doweiko J, Bunn F. Regulatory elements of the erythropoietin gene. Blood 1991;77:278–85.

24. Beck I, Ramirez S, Weinmann R, Caro J. Functional analysis of erythropoietin gene reveals hypoxia responsive element at the 3′ flanking region. Clin Research 1991 abstract. (In press.)

Chapter 5

The Biogenesis of Erythropoietin in Vivo

Stephen T. Koury, Mark J. Koury, and Maurice C. Bondurant

Many studies have indicated that the kidneys (1,2) are the major or-gans responsible for the production of erythropoietin in adult mam-mals. The liver was also demonstrated to be involved in the production of erythropoietin in fetal sheep (3) and adult rats (4–6). Various meth-ods have been used in an attempt to determine which type of cells in the kidney produce erythropoietin. Several groups used antibodies to localize erythropoietin to glomeruli in sheep (7), humans (8), and dogs (9). Another method used was the identification of erythropoietin im-munologically in fractionated kidneys. Caro and Erslev (10) used a siev-ing procedure to separate kidneys from anemic rats into tubular and glomerular fractions and measured the erythropoietin in each fraction. They found that the tubular fraction contained four to five times as much erythropoietin as the glomerular fraction, indicating that the cells that produced erythropoietin could be separated from glomeruli. How-ever, another group of investigators fractionated kidneys from anemic rats and found erythropoietin associated with the glomerular fraction (although the amount of erythropoietin in the nonglomerular fraction was not given) (11). A third approach was to grow cells from kidney explants and assay for erythropoietin in the culture medium. Using such a technique, Kurtz et al. (12) proposed that mesangial cells were the source of erythropoietin in the kidney.

The conflicting results outlined above reveal the limitations of the experimental methods used in those studies. Because erythropoietin circulates in the plasma and is excreted in urine, immunolocalization of erythropoietin within the glomerulus could have been an artifact due

65

to filtration rather than being the result of synthesis within the glomerulus. In fact, immunolocalization of erythropoietin anywhere in the kidney must be viewed with caution unless the erythropoietin is specifically localized within the Golgi or endoplasmic reticulum by immunoelectron microscopy. To date no one has been able to perform such a study. The fractionation experiments are limited because they can enrich only for either tubules or glomeruli and do not account for the cellular elements in the interstitial space. The use of explanted cells in culture is limited by the purity of the cell population. Even though the majority of cells in a culture may be of a particular cell type, a small number of contaminant cells might account for the erythropoietin in the culture media. Cloning of the murine erythropoietin gene (13,14) has made it possible to use the mouse as an experimental model system to study the biogenesis of erythropoietin in vivo and to determine the sites of erythropoietin production.

The Production of Erythropoietin by the Kidney and Liver

Initial experiments in our laboratory were performed to determine which tissues contain erythropoietin messenger ribonucleic acid (mRNA) (15). The rationale for this approach was that organs containing the mRNA for erythropoietin were likely to be those in which erythropoietin is synthesized. The model system for this study and most of the subsequent ones described in this manuscript was the phlebotomized mouse. With this model, hematocrit values can be precisely controlled and similar hematocrits can be obtained from one experiment to the next. RNA was isolated from various organs of anemic (hematocrit, 20 percent) or normal (hematocrit, 50 percent) mice, separated on agarose gels, transferred to nitrocellulose sheets, and hybridized with a nick-translated ^{32}P-labeled probe specific for erythropoietin mRNA. Figure 5.1 summarizes the results. Erythropoietin mRNA was easily detected using 30 μg of total RNA isolated from anemic kidneys and had a size of about 2 kilobases (lanes 3 and 8). With the use of 2.5 μg of polyadenylated RNA (lane 1), the kidney erythropoietin mRNA was even more obvious. Normal kidneys did not have detectable amounts of erythropoietin mRNA unless 25 μg of polyadenylated RNA was analyzed (lane 2). It was estimated that there was at least a 200-fold increase in erythropoietin mRNA in response to anemia as compared to normal mice. Erythropoietin mRNA was detectable within 1.5 hours of the last bleed used to induce anemia and revealed a maximal plateau

Figure 5.1. Analysis of organs expressing erythropoietin mRNA. Autoradiograms of nitrocellulose blots of formaldehyde-agarose gels containing RNAs from various organs that were hybridized with a probe specific for erythropoietin mRNA. Lane 1, 2.5 μg of polyadenylated RNA from anemic kidney; lane 2, 25 μg of polyadenylated RNA from nonanemic kidney; lanes 3 and 8, 30 μg of total RNA from anemic kidney; lane 4, 25 μg of polyadenylated RNA from nonanemic liver; lane 5, 25 μg of polyadenylated RNA from anemic liver; lane 6, 25 μg of polyadenylated RNA from anemic spleen; lane 7, no RNA. *Source: Data from Reference 15*

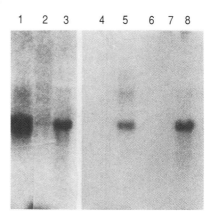

level within 4 to 8 hours that was stable over the next 24 hours (15). In contrast to the kidney, no erythropoietin mRNA was detectable in the liver when 30 μg of total RNA was analyzed (15). Erythropoietin mRNA was detectable in anemic liver only when 25 μg of polyadenylated RNA was used (lane 5). No other tissue analyzed, including spleen (lane 6), brain, skeletal muscle, and lung (not shown), contained erythropoietin mRNA. These initial results demonstrated that only kidney and liver contained erythropoietin mRNA. Similar results were obtained by Beru et al. (17).

The Production of Erythropoietin during Development

A further study was performed to quantitate erythropoietin production in the kidney and liver during murine development. It had been suggested that the liver is the major organ responsible for erythropoietin production during fetal and early postnatal life and that the kidney becomes the major source of the hormone after the early postnatal period (3). With the murine model, erythropoietin mRNA levels were determined from day 14 of fetal gestation through a 60-day-old adult (18) (Table 5.1). Normal (nonanemic) fetal livers contained a trace amount of erythropoietin mRNA at day 14 of gestation, but no erythropoietin mRNA could be detected on days 15 to 19 of gestation. However, erythropoietin mRNA was detectable in kidneys of anemic fetal mice at day

Table 5.1. Relative Amounts of Erythropoietin mRNA in Kidneys and Livers of Mice

Age, d	Erythropoietin mRNA/ µg total RNA*		Relative Erythropoietin mRNA†	
	Kidney	Liver	Kidney	Liver
Anemic postnatal‡				
2	0.245	0.006	11	3
9	2.05	0.125	232	88
16	2.41	0.129	319	100
30	5.26	0.100	863	89
60	1.00	0.015	212	16
Normal postnatal				
2	Und§	Und		
9	0.004	Und	0.5	
16	0.007	Und	0.9	
30	0.037	Und	6.1	
60	0.002	Und	0.4	
Fetal¶				
14		0.004		0.1
16		Und		
19	Und	Und		
(19 d anemic)	0.011	Und	0.2	

Source: Data from Reference 18
*Erythropoietin mRNA values are expressed relative to anemic adult (60 d) kidney, which is assigned a value of 1.00.
†Relative erythropoietin mRNA is the product of erythropoietin mRNA/µg total RNA and total µg of RNA per 2 kidneys or 1 liver. The average quantities of total RNA in µg per 2 kidneys or 1 liver in postnatal mice were, respectively: 2 d, 42 and 424; 9 d, 113 and 704; 16 d, 133 and 758; 30 d, 164 and 885; 60 d, 212 and 1071. Average for 2 kidneys in day 19 gestation fetal mice was 22 µg and fetal liver at day 14 of gestation was 30 µg.
‡Anemic postnatal mice have hematocrits of 16–22%.
§Und, undetectable by methods used (<0.002 of adult anemic kidney).
¶Ages for fetuses are days of gestation; fetal kidneys cannot be identified before day 17; anemic fetuses have hematocrits of 25–28%.

19 of gestation but not in livers of the same animals. Thus, it seems that in mice the liver produces a small amount of erythropoietin during the early stages of gestation but none during the later stages of gestation. However, the mother seems to contribute erythropoietin to the fetal circulation in rodents. This is supported by the observation that erythropoietin can be transferred to the fetus from the mother (18) and by the demonstration of erythropoietin receptors in the placentas of mice and rats (19). From day 19 of fetal gestation through adulthood, murine kidneys produce a significantly greater amount of erythropoietin than does the liver. An altered responsiveness to anemia was found in neo-

natal mice aged 9 through 30 days. Kidneys and livers from these mice produced severalfold more erythropoietin mRNA per μg of total RNA than did those of 60-day-old mice bled to similar hematocrits (Table 1). Caro et al. (16) also found hyperproduction of renal erythropoietin in rats during the first month of life. This increased responsiveness may be due to the anemia of juvenile mice during this period of life. They do not reach hematocrit values of close to 50 percent until 30 to 60 days of age. Another reason for the increased responsiveness may be that the kidneys undergo a rapid increase in size during the same period. It is possible that a growing kidney may produce an increased amount of erythropoietin much as does a regenerating liver (6).

These results quantitating the production of erythropoietin during fetal and postnatal development are in conflict with those obtained in sheep (3). It may be that the larger sheep fetus requires its own source of erythropoietin to support erythropoiesis, whereas the smaller fetuses of mice and rats get enough erythropoietin from their mothers during late gestation to drive normal erythropoiesis. However, our results suggest that it may be worthwhile to reinvestigate the role of the kidney in erythropoietin production in response to anemia during late fetal life in larger animals.

The Localization of Erythropoietin-producing Cells in the Kidney by in Situ Hybridization

The studies described above clearly demonstrated that the kidney is the primary source of erythropoietin production and that the liver also produces erythropoietin but to a much lesser extent. However, these studies did not answer the question of which cells in these organs produced erythropoietin. Schuster et al. (20) fractionated hypoxic rat kidneys into tubular and glomerular fractions and probed for erythropoietin mRNA. They found that erythropoietin mRNA was associated with the tubular fraction, but they could not determine whether the erythropoietin-producing cells were tubule cells or some cell in the peritubular interstitium. To localize erythropoietin-producing cells more specifically, Koury et al. performed in situ hybridization on formaldehyde-fixed, paraffin-embedded sections of anemic and nonanemic murine kidneys using a ^{35}S-labeled complementary RNA probe specific for erythropoietin mRNA (21). The location of erythropoietin-producing cells was determined using a double staining technique. Emulsion-coated slides containing the sections were developed and stained with hematoxylin and eosin, and erythropoietin-producing cells were photomicrographed. The slides were then destained and restained using the periodic acid-Schiff technique, and the same areas were photomicrographed again. Staining with the periodic acid-Schiff technique removed silver grains from the emulsion and allowed visualization of the tubular basement membrane. With this technique it was possible to determine that erythropoietin-producing cells were found outside the basement membrane of tubules and thus were interstitial (21). It is possible, however, clearly to identify the erythropoietin-producing cells as interstitial without performing periodic acid-Schiff staining (Figure 5.2). Tubular epithelial cells were never observed to contain erythropoietin mRNA. The erythropoietin-producing cells were found in the cortex and outer medulla. Lacombe et al. (22) came to the same conclusion about the erythropoietin-producing cells in the kidney using in situ hybridization without the double staining technique. The specific type of cell producing erythropoietin could not be determined by morphologic criteria (21), but it has been proposed that it is the peritubular capillary endothelial cell (22). Eckardt et al. (23) used in situ hybridization to identify erythropoietin-producing cells in human polycystic kidneys. They found that isolated cells within the stroma of the cyst wall were the sites of erythropoietin production, suggesting that interstitial cells are the site of erythropoietin production within the human kidney as well. The production of erythropoietin by malignant tumors in human kidneys has also been reported (24).

Recently, investigators using in situ hybridization and immunolocalization reported that tubular epithelial cells produced erythropoietin in mice (25). However, the use of ^{32}P-labeled probes with their high-energy β emissions and their consequent loss of resolving capability in autoradiograms, as well as the above-described problems associated with erythropoietin detection by immunologic means, make these results difficult to interpret. Because of these methodologic problems, the autoradiographic signals were scattered over some interstitial, tubular, and glomerular cells. On the other hand, the immunologic signals in the same kidneys were found uniformly in all tubular cells and to a lesser extent in most glomeruli. Thus, the conclusions of Maxwell et al. (25) about erythropoietin-producing cells being of tubular origin are, in our opinion, incorrect. Another report that macrophages produce erythropoietin in vitro (26) was not well controlled and has not been confirmed in vivo. Thus, the significance of this observation remains unknown.

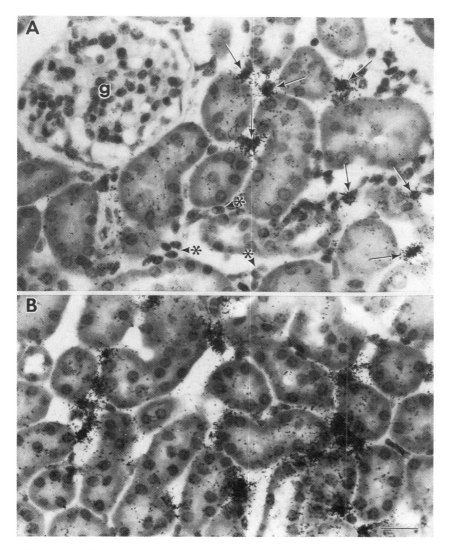

Figure 5.2. Identification of EPO-producing cells in the kidney by *in situ* hybridization. A. EPO-producing cells overlaid with silver grains are found only in the interstitium (arrows). Tubule cells and glomerular cells (g) are negative. Note that there are numerous interstitial cells which do not produce EPO, some examples of which are indicated (*). B. Another area of higher EPO-producing cell density. Again, all EPO-producing cells are in the interstitium between tubules. Bar = 20 μm. Section thickness is 3 μm.

The Correlation of the Number of Erythropoietin-producing Cells with the Hematocrit, Serum Erythropoietin Level, and Amount of Erythropoietin mRNA

When periodic acid-Schiff-stained sections were compared with their matched hematoxylin and eosin-stained sections containing silver grains, it became obvious that not all interstitial cells were producing erythropoietin (21). In fact, it appeared that a minority of the total interstitial cell population was producing erythropoietin. A study was undertaken to determine the percentage of interstitial cells involved in the production of erythropoietin and whether that percentage would change in response to different severities of anemia (27). The relationship between the number of interstitial cells producing erythropoietin and the severity of anemia was studied using two experimental approaches. In the first approach, groups of mice were bled to three levels of acute anemia: slight (hematocrits of 36 to 37 percent), moderate (hematocrits of 24 to 25 percent), and severe (hematocrits of 13 to 15 percent). Normal mice had hematocrits of 49 to 50 percent. Eight hours after bleeding, the animals were killed and their kidneys were removed for analysis. In the second approach, a large group of mice was bled to achieve a severe anemia (hematocrit of 15 to 20 percent) and then several animals were killed at intervals as their hematocrits returned to normal values. The times of sacrifice after the induction of anemia were 24, 36, 46, 60, 70, 96, and 168 hours. In both approaches, the kidneys were processed for in situ hybridization and the serum was analyzed for the concentration of circulating erythropoietin. Mice with similar hematocrits were killed, and RNA was collected from their kidneys for analysis of erythropoietin mRNA levels using Northern blots. The number of erythropoietin-producing cells per cm^2 of cortex on 5-μm tissue sections was calculated in the in situ autoradiograms and plotted against the hematocrit of the mouse from which the kidneys were taken. As can be seen in Figures 5.3 and 5.4, the number of erythropoietin-producing cells varies exponentially in an inverse manner with hematocrit, regardless of whether the hematocrit was the result of an acute bleed (Fig 5.3) or of the recovery from a severe acute bleed (Fig 5.4). In addition, serum erythropoietin levels and the relative amount of erythropoietin mRNA correlated directly with the number of erythropoietin-producing cells under both sets of conditions (27). Extremely rare erythropoietin-producing interstitial cells could be found in non-anemic kidney, suggesting that interstitial cells are responsible for pro-

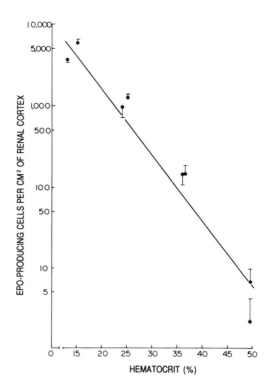

Figure 5.3. The exponential increase in the number of erythropoietin (EPO)-producing cells with decreasing hematocrit. Data are the mean values ± SEM of quadruplicate determinations per mouse. *Source: Reference 27*

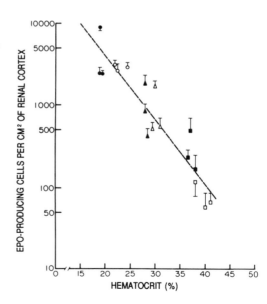

Figure 5.4. The exponential decrease in the number of erythropoietin (EPO)-producing cells with increasing hematocrit during the recovery from anemia. Data are means ± SEM of quadruplicate determinations per mouse. Three mice were used at each of the following times after the acute bleed: closed circle, 24 hours; open circle, 48 hours; closed triangle, 60 hours; open triangle, 72 hours; closed square, 96 hours; open square, 168 hours. *Source: Reference 27*

ducing the erythropoietin that drives normal erythropoiesis. These results strongly suggest that erythropoietin-producing cells are either "on" or "off." As anemia becomes more severe, more cells are recruited to produce erythropoietin. When anemia abates because of erythrocyte production, however, increasing numbers of cells turn off their production of erythropoietin. When erythropoietin-producing cells are "turned on," they all seem to contain the same, fixed amount of erythropoietin mRNA. This conclusion is supported by the following findings: (a) individual erythropoietin-producing cells have a similar silver grain distribution in autoradiograms regardless of the severity of anemia or whether they are found in nonanemic mice and (b) the ratio of total erythropoietin mRNA levels to the number of erythropoietin-producing cells is constant at all levels of anemia and throughout the recovery of anemia (27). As described above, the relationship between the number of erythropoietin-producing cells and hematocrit does not depend on whether that hematocrit was achieved by an acute bleed or during recovery from an even lower hematocrit. This shows that, under the conditions tested, no compensatory mechanism other than hematocrit played a role in erythropoietin production.

The Distribution of Erythropoietin-producing Cells in the Kidney

The distribution of erythropoietin-producing cells within the kidney cortex was determined in response to slight, moderate, or severe anemia (27). In response to a slight or moderate anemia, erythropoietin-producing cells were not randomly distributed in the cortex but rather were mostly in small clusters. The clusters were larger in moderately anemic mice, but in both cases the clusters were found predominantly in the inner aspect of the cortex near the cortico-medullary boundary. Erythropoietin-producing cells were more uniformly distributed throughout the inner cortex and outer medulla in severely anemic mice. It was estimated that 20 to 30 percent of the total interstitial cell population of the inner cortex produced erythropoietin and that less than 10 percent of the interstitial cells in the subcapsular cortex produced erythropoietin. These observations demonstrate that erythropoietin-producing cells represent only a subset of the total interstitial cell population even at the most severe level of anemia obtained in the study. Thus, erythropoietin-producing cells may represent a specialized cell type within the cortical interstitium rather than a generalized cell type such as a peritubular capillary endothelial cell (22). The results further demonstrate that the hypoxic stimulus responsible for "turning on" erythropoietin-producing cells is not uniformly distributed throughout the cortex. The small groups of erythropoietin-producing cells found in slightly or moderately anemic mice suggest that the hypoxic stimulus reaches threshold values for turning on erythropoietin-producing cells in focal areas or that cells in different areas have different threshold values. As the anemia becomes more severe, these areas increase in size and number until the entire inner cortex becomes involved.

The finding in the above-mentioned study concerning the "on" or "off" nature of erythropoietin production by individual cells and the data supporting the hypoxic stimulus reaching a threshold level for turning on erythropoietin-producing cells are consistent with the findings of Goldberg et al. concerning the hypoxia-regulated expression of the erythropoietin gene in a human cell line (28). Goldberg et al. found negligible erythropoietin production in vitro until a threshold level of 1 to 2 percent oxygen was reached, whereupon an abrupt increase in erythropoietin production was found. All of the cells in the in vitro situation were exposed to the same level of hypoxia; within the kidney in vivo, however, the hypoxic stimulus varies throughout the cortex.

What is the nature of these foci of erythropoietin-producing cells? Serial section analysis confirmed that the foci of erythropoietin-producing cells are indeed isolated from one another in three dimensions (29). In addition, Koury et al. found that the majority of erythropoietin-producing cells are adjacent to proximal convoluted tubules as opposed to other segments of the nephron (29). These findings are in agreement with those of Eckardt et al., who found that erythropoietin production is directly related to proximal tubule function (30). Koury et al. are presently performing reconstructions from the serial sections to determine whether the foci of erythropoietin-producing cells occur around the proximal convoluted tubules of individual nephrons or whether the foci interact with proximal convoluted tubules of multiple nephrons.

Two models can be proposed to explain the focal recruitment of erythropoietin-producing cells within the kidney (31). The actual mechanism could involve either of these models or some combination of the two. In the first model, the focal areas of hypoxia might arise as a result of constriction of a small artery just proximal to the capillary bed in the hypoxic area. This constriction could be active in an attempt to shunt arterial blood in response to the anemia or could simply be due to the anatomical presence of a narrow vessel supplying that capillary bed. In the second model, O_2 consumption by renal tubule cells at a more proximal site supplied by a microvascular bed would utilize the majority of O_2 available for delivery in that bed, resulting in hypoxia at sites more distal in the supply distribution of that same bed.

Erythropoietin-producing Cells in the Liver

The site of erythropoietin production within the liver is still unknown, but both Kuppffer cells and hepatocytes (32) have been proposed to be involved. The liver is responsible for only 10 to 15 percent of total erythropoietin production (18,33) (Table 5.1) in the adult. Considering how much larger is the liver than the two kidneys combined, the erythropoietin mRNA accumulation per producing cell in the liver may be much lower than that per interstitial cell in the kidney. Alternatively, if the hepatic erythropoietin-producing cell has an accumulation per cell similar to that of the renal interstitial cell, then these cells must be very rare in the liver. Our recent in situ hybridization results demonstrate that the majority of erythropoietin-producing cells in the liver are hepatocytes, but that a small subset of nonepithelial cells produce erythropoietin as well (34).

REFERENCES

1. Jacobson DO, Goldwasser E, Fried W, Plzak L. Role of the kidney in erythropoiesis. Nature 1957;179:633–4.
2. Mirand EA, Prentice TC. Presence of plasma erythropoietin in hypoxic rats with and without kidneys and or spleen. Proc Soc Exp Biol Med 1957; 96:49–51.
3. Zanjani ED, Poster J, Burlington H. Liver as the primary site of erythropoietin formation in the fetus. J Lab Clin Med 1977;89:640–4.
4. Anagnostou A, Schade S, Barone J, Fried W. Effects of partial hepatectomy on extrarenal erythropoietin production in rats. Blood 1977;50:457–62.
5. Caro J, Zon L, Silver R, Miller O, Erslev AJ. Erythropoietin in liver tissue extracts and in liver perfusates from hypoxic rats. Am J Physiol 1983;244: E431–4.
6. Naughton BA, Kaplan SM, Roy M, Burdowski AJ, Gordon AS, Piliero SJ. Hepatic regeneration and erythropoietin production in the rat. Science 1977;196:301–2.
7. Fisher JW, Taylor E, Porteous DD. Localization of erythropoietin in glomeruli of sheep kidney by fluorescent antibody technique. Nature 1965; 205:611–2.
8. Mori S, Saito T, Morishita Y, et al. Glomerular epithelium as the main locus of erythropoietin in human kidney. J Exp Med 1985;55:69–70.

9. Busuttil RW, Roh BL, Fisher JW. Localization of erythropoietin in the glomerulus of the hypoxic dog's kidney using a fluorescent antibody technique. Acta Haematol (Basel) 1972;47:238–42.

10. Caro J, Erslev AJ. Biologic and immunologic erythropoietin in extracts from hypoxic whole rat kidneys and in their glomerular and tubular fractions. J Lab Clin Med 1984;103:922–31.

11. Jelkman W, Kurtz A, Bauer C. Extraction of erythropoietin from isolated renal glomeruli of hypoxic rats. Exp Hematol 1983;11:581–8.

12. Kurtz A, Jelkmann W, Bauer C. Mesangial cells derived from rat glomeruli produce an erythropoiesis stimulating factor in cell culture. FEBS Lett 1982;137:129–32.

13. McDonald JD, Lin FK, Goldwasser E. Cloning, sequencing, and evolutionary analysis of the mouse erythropoietin gene. Mol Cell Biol 1986;6:842–9.

14. Shoemaker CB, Mistock LD. Murine erythropoietin gene: cloning, expression and human gene homology. Mol Cell Biol 1986;6:849–58.

15. Bondurant MC, Koury MJ. Anemia induces accumulation of erythropoietin mRNA in the kidney and liver. Mol Cell Biol 1986;6:2731–3.

16. Caro J, Erslev AJ, Silver R, Miller O, Birgegard G. Erythropoietin production in response to anemia of hypoxia in the newborn rat. Blood 1982; 60:984–8.

17. Beru NJ, McDonald J, Lacombe C, Goldwasser E. Expression of the erythropoietin gene. Mol Cell Biol 1986;6:2571–5.

18. Koury MJ, Bondurant MC, Graber SE, Sawyer ST. Erythropoietin messenger RNA levels in developing mice and transfer of ^{125}I-erythropoietin by the placenta. J Clin Invest 1988;82:154–9.

19. Sawyer ST, Krantz SB, Sawada K. Receptors for erythropoietin in mouse and human erythroid cells and placenta. Blood 1989;74:103–9.

20. Schuster SJ, Wilson JH, Erslev AJ, Caro J. Physiologic regulation and tissue localization of renal erythropoietin messenger RNA. Blood 1987;70: 316–8.

21. Koury ST, Bondurant MC, Koury MJ. Localization of erythropoietin synthesizing cells in murine kidneys by in situ hybridization. Blood 1988; 71:524–7.

22. Lacombe C, DaSilva J-L, Bruneval P, et al. Peritubular cells are the site of erythropoietin synthesis in the murine hypoxic kidney. J Clin Invest 1988; 81:620–3.

23. Eckardt KU, Mollman M, Neumann R, et al. Erythropoietin in polycystic kidneys. J Clin Invest 1989;84:1160–6.

24. DaSilva J-L, Lacombe C, Bruneval P, et al. Tumor cells are the site of erythropoietin synthesis in human renal cell cancers associated with polycythemia. Blood 1990;75:577–82.

25. Maxwell AP, Lappin TRJ, Johnston CF, et al. Erythropoietin production in kidney tubular cells. Br J Haematol 1990;74:535–9.

26. Vogt C, Penz S, Rich IN. A role for macrophage in normal hemopoiesis: III. In vitro and in vivo erythropoietin gene expression in macrophages detected by in situ hybridization. Exp Hematol 1989;17:391–7.

27. Koury ST, Koury MJ, Bondurant MC, Caro J, Graber SE. Quantitation of erythropoietin-producing cells in the kidneys of mice by in situ hybridization: correlation with hematocrit, renal erythropoietin messenger RNA and serum erythropoietin concentration. Blood 1989;74:645–51.

28. Goldberg MA, Glass GA, Cunningham JM, Bunn HF. The regulated expression of erythropoietin by two human hepatoma cell lines. Proc Natl Acad Sci USA 1988;84:7972–6.

29. Koury ST, Thamer SL, Koury MJ, Bondurant MC. Erythropoietin-producing interstitial cells are primarily found adjacent to proximal tubules in murine kidneys. Blood 1989;74:18a.

30. Eckardt K-U, Kurtz A, Bauer C. Regulation of erythropoietin formation is related to proximal tubular function. Am J Physiol 1989;256:F942–7.

31. Koury MJ, Koury ST, Bondurant MC, Graber SE. Correlation of the molecular and anatomical aspects of renal erythropoietin production. Contrib Nephrol 1989;76:24–32.

32. Fried W, Barone-Varelas J, Morley C. Factors that regulate extrarenal erythropoietin production. Blood Cells 1984;10:287–304.

33. Erslev AJ, Caro J, Kausu E, Silver R. Renal and extrarenal erythropoietin production in anemic rats. Br J Haematol 1980;45:65–72.

34. Koury ST, Bondurant MC, Koury MJ, Semenza GL. Localization of cells producing erythropoietin in murine liver by in situ hybridization. Blood 1991 (in press).

Chapter 6

Renal Function and Oxygen Sensing

Armin Kurtz and Kai-Uwe Eckardt

The production of erythropoietin in vivo is influenced by a number of physiologic parameters generated either by the supply of oxygen or by the consumption of oxygen (1). The supply of oxygen is determined primarily by the oxygen-transport capacity of the blood, by the arterial oxygen tension (P_{O_2}), and by the oxygen affinity. The oxygen-transport capacity of the blood is normally measured by the hemoglobin concentration. A decrease in hemoglobin levels (anemia) is known to be associated with exponential increases in the production of erythropoietin, whereas an increase in hemoglobin is associated with a decreased production of erythropoietin.

With normal oxygen-carrying capacity of the blood, the supply of oxygen to the tissues is determined by the arterial oxygen saturation of the hemoglobin, which in turn depends primarily upon the alveolar oxygenation. Consequently, the production of erythropoietin is inversely and exponentially related to the alveolar and arterial oxygen tension (2). Although even isolated perfused kidneys respond to arterial hypoxia with an increase in erythropoietin production (3,4), in vivo stimulation of erythropoietin formation by hypoxia can be virtually neutralized by polycythemia (5). This suggests that neither the oxygen-carrying capacity nor the arterial oxygen tension alone is the major determinant of erythropoietin formation. Rather, the major determinant is the oxygen content of the blood, which is the product of both parameters.

The oxygen supply to the tissues is further influenced by the oxygen affinity of the hemoglobin. An increase in oxygen affinity (i.e., a left shift of the oxygen binding curve) impedes oxygen unloading in the

79

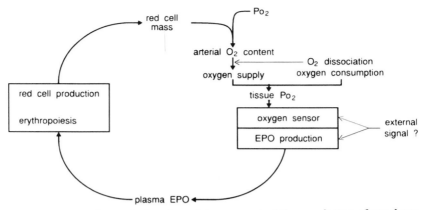

Figure 6.1. A schematic drawing of the concept of the regulation of renal production of erythropoietin (EPO) by the oxygen demand/supply ratio in the kidney.

tissues and thus reduces the oxygen supply. Because of the shape of the oxygen binding curve, this reduction in the oxygen supply is only partially counterbalanced by an increased arterial oxygen saturation and causes increased production of erythropoietin (6). A decrease in oxygen affinity has the opposite effect and increases the oxygen supply.

From these observations it has been inferred that the supply of oxygen to the tissues is the main physiologic factor controlling the production of erythropoietin. With a more or less constant rate of oxygen consumption by the tissues, changes in the oxygen supply lead to concordant changes in the local tissue oxygen tensions, and it seems reasonable to assume that the interstitial tissue oxygen tension is the primary signal for the oxygen-sensing mechanism.

Obviously, the tissue Po_2 must be registered and transduced into signals regulating the production of erythropoietin. These processes have been summarized under the "oxygen sensor" function controlling the formation of erythropoietin (Fig 6.1). Our knowledge of the sensing mechanisms, however, is rather incomplete. It is the aim of this chapter to bring together pieces of the mosaic of information about this oxygen sensor and its structural and functional basis.

A fundamental question relates to the localization of the oxygen sensor. Because our knowledge of the regulation of the hepatic production of erythropoietin is much less than our knowledge of the regulation of renal production and because, at least in adults, the kidney is by far the more important production site, we shall focus on the production of erythropoietin by the kidney and on the immediate question of whether the oxygen sensor governing the renal formation of erythropoietin is located intra- or extrarenally.

The existence of a controlling extrarenal sensor is supported by the observation that a selective reduction in the renal oxygen supply, brought about by a severe reduction in the renal blood flow, leads to only a slight increase in the renal formation of erythropoietin (7,8), despite a dramatic drop in oxygen tension (9). In contrast, a reduction in the systemic oxygen supply due to decreased hemoglobin levels may increase the formation of erythropoietin by a factor of thousands (10).

When looking for a possible extrarenal oxygen sensor, it seems reasonable to search in the nervous system. However, the classic chemoreceptors seem not to be involved in controlling the production of erythropoietin because ablation of the carotid bodies does not significantly influence erythropoietin formation (11). It also seems as if the efferent autonomic nervous system (in particular, the sympathetic nerves that represent the vast majority of nerve fibers in the kidney) does not play an essential role in the oxygen-dependent control of erythropoietin production. Thus, neither blockers of catecholamine receptors nor renal denervation consistently attenuates or even blocks the production of erythropoietin (1,3,4). Moreover, studies after kidney transplantation showed that the transplanted kidney without neural input is able to increase its rate of erythropoietin production in response to anemia (12,13). It seems unlikely therefore that a possible extrarenally located oxygen sensor controls renal erythropoietin production via the nervous system. However, we cannot definitively rule out the existence of an extrarenal sensor that humorally interacts with the kidney.

On the other hand, a number of findings indicate that the essentials of oxygen sensing lie within the kidney itself. The release of erythropoietin can be induced in vitro in kidneys isolated from normoxic animals and perfused under hypoxic conditions (3). As there is no evidence for erythropoietin precursors or for erythropoietin stores in the kidneys, it can be inferred from these experiments that it is possible to induce the renal formation of erythropoietin in vitro by hypoxia. This conclusion is corroborated by a recent demonstration that hypoxic perfusion of kidneys taken from normoxic animals leads to the accumulation of erythropoietin mRNA in the isolated perfused kidney to an extent found under in vivo conditions (4).

Furthermore, a lack of erythropoietin formation despite reductions

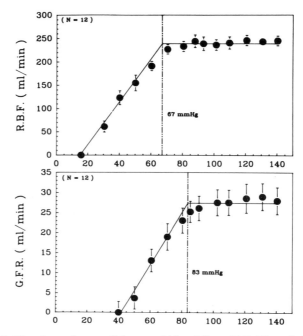

Figure 6.2. The dependency of the renal blood flow (R.B.F.) and glomerular filtration rate (G.F.R.) on the arterial pressure in awake dogs. *Source: Adapted from Reference 14*

in renal blood flow does not necessarily exclude an intrarenal location of the oxygen sensor because a severe reduction in the renal blood flow interferes with a number of renal functions, the integrity of which may be a prerequisite for effective oxygen sensing. For example, both the demand for and the supply of oxygen in the kidney seem to be related to the renal blood flow (Fig 6.2). Consequently, a reduction in the renal blood flow not only reduces the oxygen supply to the kidneys but also reduces the glomerular filtration and in consequence tubular work, a fact that may be of importance for oxygen sensing (7).

If we accept that the oxygen sensor is located in the kidney, we are confronted with the question of how an organ that is known to be lux- uriously supplied with oxygen can sense the overall balance between the oxygen demand and the oxygen supply. To answer this question, we first have to consider the functional anatomy and physiology of the kidney.

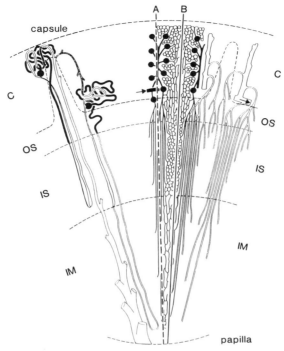

Figure 6.3. A schematic drawing of the functional anatomy of the kidney. On the left are the tubular structures; on the right are the vascular structures. The arterial parts of the vasculature are indicated by solid and the venous parts by open structures. The dashed arcs in the cortex represent cortical medullary rays. Lines A and B indicate the section lines for the oxygen tension profiles shown in Figure 6.5. C, cortex; OS, outer stripe of outer medulla; IS, inner stripe of outer medulla; IM, inner medulla. *Source: Adapted from References 15 and 16*

The Functional Anatomy of the Kidney

The Tubules

Renal tissue can be divided into three parts that are functionally linked: the nephrons, containing all types and parts of the tubules; the renal vasculature, with arteries, capillaries, and veins; and the renal interstitium (Fig 6.3). The segmentation of the nephron provides the basis for the division of the kidney into four zones: the cortex, the outer medulla with an outer and an inner stripe, and the inner medulla (i.e., papilla). Each nephron originates from a glomerulus, from which the plasma ultrafiltrate is drained into Bowman's capsule. The wall of Bowman's capsule continues into the proximal tubule, which is convoluted at its beginning and straight at its end. The proximal tubule proceeds into the descending part of the thin limb of Henle, and the transition marks the border between the outer and inner stripe of the outer medulla.

The extensions of the thin loops of Henle are variable. Those of short-loop nephrons extend only into the deeper parts of the inner stripe of the outer medulla. Those of long-loop nephrons reach the inner medulla (i.e., papilla). The thin ascending loop of Henle then continues into the thick ascending limb of Henle. The border between the inner and outer medulla is defined by the transition site of the two parts of the long loops of Henle. The thick limb continues into the distal tubule, which is convoluted over its whole length. At the contact site between the thick limb and the distal tubule, the tubule touches its parent glomerulus at a specialized area named the macula densa. The distal tubule system feeds via the connecting tubules into the collecting duct system, which extends through all zones of the kidney and which finally releases the tubular fluid into the renal pelvic cavity.

The renal cortex, which makes up about 80 percent of the total renal mass, can be subdivided into two parts: the medullary rays and the cortical labyrinths. The medullary rays contain all cortical straight nephron segments, including the straight parts of the proximal tubules, the loops of Henle, and the collecting ducts. The cortical labyrinth, on the other hand, contains the glomeruli, the convoluted parts of the proximal tubules, and the distal tubules.

The functions of the kidney are well distributed among the different parts of the nephron. About 75 percent of the primary glomerular ultrafiltrate, which makes up about 50 nl/minute/glomerulus, is reabsorbed by the proximal tubule. Moreover, the proximal tubule almost completely reabsorbs filtered substrates such as glucose, amino acids, and fatty acids. The main task of the thin limb of Henle's loop is to reabsorb water by a countercurrent system. The main task of the thick limb is to reabsorb sodium chloride (about 10 percent of the filtered load). Apart from reabsorbing the rest of the filtered sodium chloride, the distal tubules and the collecting ducts secrete protons and potassium into the urine and reabsorb water. As a result, more than 99 percent of the filtered sodium and water are reabsorbed during the tubular passage.

Mainly because of the active reabsorptive functions of the nephrons, the kidney has a high rate of energy consumption. Although the kidney accounts for only approximately 0.5 percent of the body weight, it accounts for approximately 10 percent of the total oxygen consumption by the body under basal conditions. More than 80 percent of the oxygen consumed by the kidney is normally required by sodium reabsorption (17), which is quantitatively by far the most important transport function of the renal tubules. The rest of the oxygen consumed by the kidney is required for synthetic functions, including gluconeogenesis, which takes place in the proximal tubules (18–21). Interestingly, the metabolic costs of sodium reabsorption in the various nephron segments are inversely related to their capacity to transport sodium. Thus, although the amount of sodium reabsorbed by the different nephron segments varies markedly, the absolute energy requirement for sodium transport of the different tubular segments is rather constant. The sodium reabsorption rates for the proximal tubules, thick limb of Henle, distal tubule, and collecting duct are 75, 10, 10, and 5 percent of the filtered load, respectively. The minimum energy requirements for the reabsorption of one equivalent of sodium, however, have a corresponding ratio of 0.07:0.4:0.55:1 (18). The low specific energy requirement for sodium reabsorption of the proximal tubule results from its favorable electrochemical gradient for sodium and from its favorable permeability properties. It has been calculated that about two thirds of the sodium reabsorption by the proximal tubule is passive (22,23), and it is thought that only sodium bicarbonate is actively reabsorbed (24).

The energy required for sodium reabsorption results predominantly from oxidative phosphorylation. The substrates used for oxidative adenosine triphosphate (ATP) generation vary among the different nephron segments. The proximal tubule utilizes succinate, glutamate, glutamine, α-ketoglutarate, and malate, but not glucose, as substrates. The thick limb of Henle, on the other hand, utilizes glucose and lactate together with glutamine, glutamate, α-ketoglutarate, and palmitate as fuel (25). Also, anaerobic metabolism of glucose occurs in the kidney (in particular, in the inner stripe of the outer medulla and in the inner medulla). The capability of utilizing glucose to generate energy is also reflected by the activities of the key enzymes for glycolysis. The failure of the proximal tubule to utilize glucose as a fuel may represent a precaution taken by nature. Apart from hepatocytes, the proximal tubules are the only sites of gluconeogenesis in the body. It has been calculated that they contribute about 25 percent to the blood glucose level (26). Up to 25 percent of the total renal oxygen consumption can be used for gluconeogenesis by the proximal tubules under certain conditions. In consequence, the failure to utilize glucose prevents the proximal tubule from consuming a fuel synthesized and also reabsorbed for the use of the whole organism. On the other hand, it renders the proximal tubules very sensitive to oxygen deficiency because they have no means of generating energy anaerobically (17).

The Vasculature

The energy requirement of the nephron is met by the renal vasculature, which delivers substrates and oxygen to the different nephron segments (15). In brief, the renal artery divides into branches, which then enter the renal tissue at the border between the cortex and the outer medulla (Fig 6.3). They follow an arclike course and are called arcuate arteries. They give rise to the interlobular arteries, which ascend radially within the cortical labyrinth. The cortex is dense with arteries. The renal interlobular and arcuate veins accompany their corresponding arteries. The contact between the arteries and their veins is very narrow, and it is believed that these contact areas provide the basis for effective preglomerular oxygen and carbon dioxide shunting (27). As a consequence, the oxygen tension is lower in the renal cortical parenchyma than in the renal vein (28), whereas the opposite holds for the carbon dioxide tension (29).

The afferent arterioles arise from the interlobular arteries and supply the glomeruli with blood for plasma ultrafiltration. A human kidney contains about 1 million glomeruli; a rat kidney, about 30,000. The efferent arterioles drain the glomeruli and supply all tubules with blood in a characteristic fashion. Basically, a distinction between efferent arterioles of superficial, midcortical, and juxtamedullary glomeruli is important (Fig 6.4).

The superficial efferent arterioles spread out to the kidney surface before dividing. The branches of these efferent arterioles form capillary plexuses around the structures in the superficial cortical labyrinth (i.e., convoluted proximal tubules and distal tubules). These plexuses then feed into the interlobular veins. The branches of efferent arterioles from the midcortical glomeruli primarily supply blood to structures in the cortical medullary rays. Blood returning from the medullary rays then supplies the structures of the midcortical and juxtamedullary labyrinth, from where it flows into interlobular veins.

The efferent arterioles of juxtamedullary glomeruli turn toward the medulla. They are called descending vasa recta and supply the entire medulla. The descending vasa recta are in tight contact with the ascending vasa recta, which bring back the venous outflow. This close contact again provides the basis for effective oxygen shunting. Because of

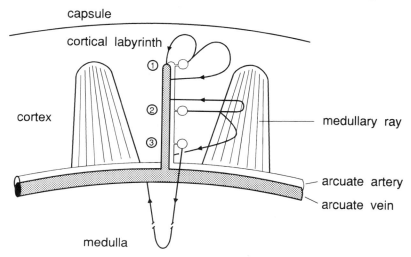

capsule

cortical labyrinth

cortex

medullary ray

arcuate artery

arcuate vein

medulla

Figure 6.4. A schematic drawing of the delivery of blood to the capillary plexus in the cortical labyrinth for superficial (1), midcortical (2), and juxta-medullary (3) nephrons.

the countercurrent mechanism, the oxygen tension in the renal medulla is chronically low (28). Trapping of carbon dioxide as in the cortex, however, has not been observed in the papilla, probably because the rate of carbon dioxide production of the inner medulla is very low in comparison with that of the cortex (29).

The renal vasculature (in particular, the arterial tree down to the glomeruli) has an interesting functional feature. Its resistance increases with the perfusion pressure, thus uncoupling the renal blood flow from the blood pressure. The physiologic relevance of this autoregulation of the renal blood flow is to maintain glomerular filtration independently of the systemic arterial pressure in a range of 80 to 180 mm Hg (Fig 6.2). At low arterial pressures, the autoregulation of the blood flow and glomerular filtration cannot be maintained, resulting in a linear relationship between the renal blood flow and glomerular filtration and the arterial pressure and finally cessation of glomerular filtration. Another unique feature of the renal vasculature is that the resistance of the afferent arterioles is directly related to the concentration of sodium chloride in the tubular fluid at the macula densa. This mechanism, which is termed tubuloglomerular feedback, adapts the glomerular filtration rate and the renal cortical blood flow rate to the sodium reabsorption capacities of the proximal tubule and the thick limb of Henle.

The Renal Interstitium

The volume fraction of the renal interstitium displays a gradient from the cortex to the inner medulla (15). Although the interstitium is rather scanty in the cortex, amounting to about 7 to 9 percent by volume, it can reach about 40 percent at the tip of the papilla. The cell type dominating in the cortex and also in the interstitium of the outer medulla is the fibrocyte. (Capillary endothelial cells are considered part of the vasculature.) In the inner medulla, however, the majority of the interstitial cells are represented by a unique cell type, the lipid-laden interstitial cells. These cells and, in particular, their lipid metabolism are thought to exert a regulatory effect on tubular function in that region.

Local Renal Oxygen Tension and the Localization of Renal Erythropoietin-producing Cells

A human kidney is perfused with a blood flow rate of about 4 ml/g/minute, more than 90 percent of which is distributed to the renal cortex. Under normal conditions, this flow rate corresponds to an oxygen delivery rate of 0.8 ml/g/minute. About 8 percent of the oxygen delivered is consumed by the kidney. The oxygen consumption rates of the different renal zones are markedly different. When related to weight, the oxygen consumption rates of the cortex, outer medulla, and inner medulla have a ratio of 9:6:0.4, respectively.

Summarizing the available data on renal oxygen tensions and taking into account the pre- and postglomerular shunt diffusion of oxygen between interlobular vessels and the vasa recta results in an interesting and unexpected profile of tissue oxygen tensions in the kidney (Fig 6.5). The profile depends on the axis of the section considered. If the section is made along the axis of a medullary ray from the cortex to the papilla, the oxygen tension drops in the superficial cortex to a value of about 10 torr and remains at low values until the tip of the papilla. A similar profile probably exists in most parts of the cortical labyrinth. However, if the section follows the axis of an interlobular artery, which is in the center of a cortical labyrinth region and which continues into a vascular bundle in the medulla, the oxygen tension profile displays a more complex pattern. The highest values of Po_2, similar to systemic arterial oxygen tension, are found in the region of the arcuate arteries at the border between cortex and outer medulla. Because of shunt diffusion between interlobular arteries and veins, oxygen tension drops to about 50 torr in passage to the renal capsule. Shunt diffusion of oxygen between the descending and ascending vasa recta also causes oxygen tension to drop

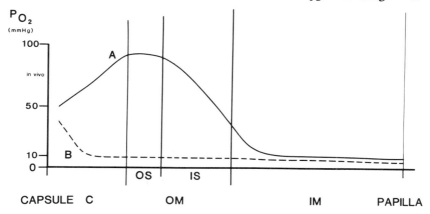

Figure 6.5. Profiles of oxygen tension along an interlobular artery and vascular bundle (A) and along a medullary ray (B). C, cortex; OS, outer stripe of outer medulla; OM, outer medulla; IS, inner stripe of outer medulla; IM, inner medulla. *Source: Adapted from Reference 30*

along the passage through the medulla, reaching the lowest values in the inner medulla (about 12 torr).

The difficulty in localizing the erythropoietin-producing cells by immunohistochemical means necessitated the localization of erythropoietin mRNA by in situ hybridization. Although it is still undetermined whether erythropoietin is produced by tubular or interstitial cells, the more convincing evidence supports the latter interpretation (31,32). The interstitial cells identified as producing erythropoietin are positioned close to the proximal convoluted tubules (33). From circumstantial evidence it was inferred that the erythropoietin-producing cells are either capillary endothelial cells (31,32) or perhaps interstitial fibroblasts (34). In any case, they are clearly restricted to the renal cortex and there to the cortical labyrinths.

Applying graded degrees of anemia, investigators found that the number of erythropoietin-producing cells relates inversely to the hemoglobin concentration (35). Furthermore, evidence was provided that the content of erythropoietin mRNA is rather constant among individual erythropoietin-producing cells, strongly suggesting that the regulation of renal erythropoietin production results from "on-off" regulation rather than from "up-down" regulation of erythropoietin gene transcription. Moreover, the pattern of recruitment of erythropoietin-producing cells is characteristic. At normal or only slightly decreased hemoglobin concentrations, erythropoietin-producing cells are found in the juxtamedullary cortical labyrinths. With increasing stimulation, erythropoietin-producing cells also become recruited in the midcortical region and finally in the superficial cortex (35). There is no recruitment of cells in the medulla or in the cortical medullary rays.

The Renal Oxygen Sensor

The assumption that renal production of erythropoietin is under the control of an intrarenal oxygen-sensing device that measures interstitial Po_2 leads to two obvious questions: Where in the kidney is the oxygen sensor located? How does this type of sensor control the formation of erythropoietin?

Location

The concept of oxygen sensing by erythropoietin-producing cells is supported strongly by the recent finding that two hepatoma cell lines produce erythropoietin when exposed to hypoxia, indicating that oxygen sensing and oxygen production can reside within the same cell (36). For these hepatoma cells, circumstantial evidence suggests that a heme protein that can undergo reversible conformational changes is involved in the oxygen sensing. This concept may also explain how cobalt can exert a stimulatory effect on the formation of erythropoietin; it has been proposed that cobalt replaces the central iron atom and thereby arrests the heme protein in a "deoxy-conformation" (37). If the concept of a heme protein as the oxygen sensor is valid for hepatoma cells, it is reasonable to assume the same for the kidney.

On the other hand, it is not self-evident that oxygen-sensing mechanisms in the liver and kidney are identical. In fact, findings in transgenic mice suggest that renal and hepatic erythropoietin gene transcription may be regulated differently (38). Therefore, in principle it is also conceivable that oxygen sensing in the kidney and erythropoietin production are localized in different but closely positioned cells, such as the proximal tubular cells and their surrounding interstitial cells. In this case, the proximal tubule would be the primary oxygen sensor, which then transfers a diffusible stimulatory signal to the erythropoietin-producing cells.

Inasmuch as an oxygen-consuming process is likely to be involved in the oxygen sensing and as 80 percent of renal oxygen consumption is due to active sodium reabsorption, it seems reasonable to suspect that the tubules act as oxygen sensors. To examine this possibility, investigators studied the effects of site-specific inhibitors of active sodium reabsorption on the production of erythropoietin. The study revealed that effective inhibition of sodium reabsorption in the collecting duct, distal tubule, or thick loop of Henle had no effect on erythropoietin production in response to hypoxic hypoxia or to functional anemia induced by carbon monoxide (39). It is not very likely, therefore, that the oxygen consumption of the distal parts of the nephron is essential for oxygen sensing. By exclusion, one would suspect that the oxygen consumption of the proximal tubule is involved. Although the proximal tubule reabsorbs about 75 percent of the filtered sodium, only one-third of this amount (in particular, sodium bicarbonate) is thought to be actively reabsorbed (24). Although it is difficult to interfere with the active sodium reabsorption in the proximal tubule, acetazolamide inhibits carboanhydrase activity and consequently the reabsorption of sodium bicarbonate (40). In fact, acetazolamide treatment attenuates the oxygen-dependent formation of erythropoietin in parallel with its natriuretic effect (39). This effect is independent of the systemic acidosis resulting from urinary bicarbonate loss. Although direct effects on erythropoietin-producing cells cannot be excluded, the inhibition of erythropoietin formation by acetazolamide seems to support an involvement of the proximal tubule in oxygen sensing. It should also be recalled that the vast majority of erythropoietin-producing interstitial cells have been found in tight contact with proximal tubular cells (33).

Function

If the proximal tubular cells are involved, how do they generate signals triggering erythropoietin gene expression in the interstitial cells? Principally, such signals may be related to the normal metabolism of tubular cells or may emerge from a restriction of energy metabolism due to an insufficient supply of oxygen. Regarding the first possibility, it has been pointed out that many oxygen-dependent enzymes can be found in tubular cells (41). Such enzymes (e.g., oxygenases and oxidases), many of which are heme proteins like the putative oxygen sensor controlling the production of erythropoietin in hepatoma cells (37), may be sensitive indicators of cellular oxygenation, and their allosteric alterations may generate signals.

The second type of signal produced by the proximal tubule could emerge from a restriction in the energy metabolism due to an insufficient supply of oxygen. As mentioned before, the proximal tubular cells are particularly sensitive to restriction of the oxygen supply because they contain two major ATP-consuming processes (namely, sodium/potassium adenosine triphosphatase [ATPase] and gluconeogenesis) and, on the other hand, are unable to generate ATP anaerobically. Because of the subcellular distribution of mitochondria and energy-consuming enzymes, gradients of oxygen and also of ATP exist within cells with high rates of energy consumption (41). As a result of such gradients, oxidative phosphorylation is limited at interstitial P_{O_2} values higher than the K_m for oxygen of mitochondria, which is about 1 torr. Restrictions of ATP generation will manifest themselves first in areas with high ATP consumption. In proximal tubular cells and other nephron segments with active sodium reabsorption, these sites are the basolateral membranes in contact with the interstitium because they bear the sodium/potassium ATPase. Inasmuch as the K_m for ATP of the sodium/potassium ATPase is relatively low (around 1 mM) when compared to the cellular concentration of ATP (around 3–4 mM), it would require a marked energy depletion before the sodium pump becomes impaired.

This is not the case for other ATP-consuming enzymes, such as the acyl coenzyme A synthase, which esterifies free fatty acids into membrane lipids. The K_m for ATP of this enzyme is 4 to 5 mM (42), and, therefore, small decreases in local ATP levels may attenuate the activity of this enzyme, leading to an increase in the cytosolic levels of free fatty acids. An increase in free fatty acids upon insufficient oxygen supply is not restricted to the kidneys but is known for a variety of tissues. Fatty acids give rise to a number of membrane-permeable second messenger molecules, such as prostaglandins, lipoxygenase and epoxygenase products, and leukotrienes. On the basis of indirect evidence, prostaglandins have long been hypothesized as messengers in the oxygen-sensing process (43). However, direct proof of such a role for arachidonic acid or one of its conversion products has thus far not been established.

Because of the intracellular stoichiometry of ATP/adenosine triphosphate (ADP) (which occurs at millimolar concentrations) and adenosine monophosphate (AMP) (which is in the micromolar range under normal conditions), it is expected that even small decreases in local ATP levels can lead to relatively large increases in AMP levels. The basolateral membrane of proximal tubular cells is permeable for phosphates, and one can expect a release of AMP into the interstitium in relation to the decrease in ATP levels. Extracellular AMP is presumably very unstable because of the degradation to adenosine by the 5-ectonucleotidase in the peritubular space (44). In fact, renal interstitial levels of adenosine increase in response to increased tubular work or to decreased oxygen supply (45,46). A possible second messenger role for adenosine in the oxygen sensing of erythropoietin control has been hypothesized (47), but thus far has not convincingly been demonstrated.

Whether interstitial or tubular cells are the principal oxygen sensors, it is necessary that the interstitial Po_2 around proximal tubular cells in the cortical labyrinth drop to critically low values capable of inducing the formation of erythropoietin. Considering the exponential fashion of the recruitment of erythropoietin-producing cells, it is also necessary that the cortical areas that reach this critical oxygen tension increase inversely in relation to the hemoglobin concentration and to the arterial oxygen tension. Finally, an explanation must be found for how the areas reaching the critical Po_2 are distributed in the same pattern as for the recruitment of erythropoietin-producing cells, namely, with a gradient from the inner to the outer cortex.

At present, the critical Po_2 for triggering erythropoietin gene expression is unknown. If the renal erythropoietin producers behave like hepatoma cells (HepG2 or Hep3B), significant erythropoietin production would be expected at Po_2 values lower than 15 torr (36). Can the interstitial Po_2 in the cortical labyrinth reach such low oxygen tensions? The oxygen tension profile indicates that such low oxygen tensions can occur in the renal cortex even under "normoxic" conditions. Because of the special pattern of blood distribution to the juxtamedullary, midcortical, and superficial areas of the labyrinth, as shown in Figure 6.4, the cortical labyrinth is largely supplied with blood returning from the medullary rays. Taking into account the oxygen profile in the medullary rays (Fig 6.5B), we can estimate that the oxygen tension is lowest in the juxtamedullary region, with an uphill gradient to the superficial cortex. This in fact agrees with the localization and recruitment of erythropoietin-producing cells.

It should be recalled at this point that those low levels of interstitial oxygen tension result from the cortical oxygen consumption and from oxygen shunting. The existence of an oxygen shunt, moreover, seems to provide an amplification mechanism for the decreases in cortical tissue Po_2 in response to anemia. Assuming that the renocortical oxygen consumption is more or less unaltered during anemia, the oxygen tension in the primary capillary effluate leaving the parenchyma will be decreased in comparison to the nonanemic state. This decrease in venous oxygen tension will increase the driving force for oxygen shunting between interlobular arteries and veins and in consequence further lower the arterial oxygen tension of the blood entering the renocortical parenchyma. This hypothesis has in fact been confirmed in recent ex-

medullary   cortical
    ray   glomerulus   labyrinth

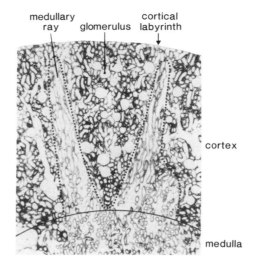

cortex

medulla

Figure 6.6. A photomicrograph of a normal rat cortex stained for 5-ecto-nucleotidase by the indirect immunoperoxidase method (original magnification × 90). Only the cortical labyrinth stains positive for the nucleotidase. *Source: Courtesy of Brigitte Kaissling*

periments, showing that the oxygen tension in superficial glomeruli decreases during anemia (48). This decrease further decreases the interstitial Po_2.

Changes in the interstitial concentrations of adenosine and in pH may also play a role. As mentioned before, the interstitial levels of adenosine depend on the degradation of AMP to adenosine, a reaction that is catalyzed by 5-ectonucleotidase. In this context, it is of interest that the expression of the 5-ectonucleotidase on renal interstitial fibroblasts is confined to the same area where erythropoietin gene expression occurs, i.e., the cortical labyrinth (34) (Fig 6.6). Furthermore, the expression of the enzyme is inversely related to the hemoglobin concentration (49).

In regard to pH, acidosis has long been known to inhibit the formation of erythropoietin (50). This may be caused by a diminished sensitivity of the oxygen sensor (Fig 6.7) (50,51). As already outlined, there is evidence for gradient trapping of carbon dioxide in the renal cortex, with the gradient directed opposite that for the recruitment of erythropoietin-producing cells.

Other factors, especially metabolic hormones, could also play a role in oxygen sensing and the formation of erythropoietin. However, at

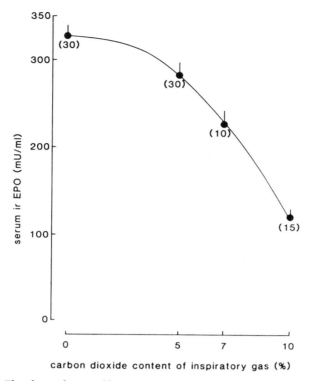

Figure 6.7. The dependency of hypoxia-induced (8 percent oxygen for 3 hours) erythropoietin (EPO) formation in mice on the carbon dioxide concentration in the inspiration atmosphere. *Source: Reference 51*

present we must concede that the concept of a renal oxygen sensor is supported by many hypotheses but few facts.

ACKNOWLEDGMENTS

The authors thank Brigitte Kaissling and Hans-Joachim Schurek for many helpful discussions. The skillful artwork of Christian Gasser is also gratefully acknowledged.

REFERENCES

1. Jelkmann W. Renal erythropoietin: properties and production. Rev Physiol Biochem Pharmacol 1986;104:140–215.

2. Eckardt K-U, Boutellier U, Kurtz A, Koller EA, Bauer C. Rate of erythropoietin formation in humans in response to acute hypobaric hypoxia. J Appl Physiol 1989;66:1785–8.

3. Pagel H, Jelkmann W, Weiss CH. Erythropoietin production in the isolated perfused kidney. Biomed Biochim Acta 1990;42:S271–4.

4. Ratcliffe PJ, Jones RW, Phillips RE, Nicholls LG, Bell JI. Oxygen-dependent modulation of erythropoietin mRNA levels. J Exp Med 1990;172: 657–60.

5. Kurtz A, Eckardt K-U, Tannahill L, Bauer C. Regulation of erythropoietin production. Contrib Nephrol 1988;66:1–16.

6. Lechermann B, Jelkmann W. Erythropoietin production in normoxic and hypoxic rats with increased blood O_2 affinity. Respir Physiol 1985;60:1–8.

7. Erslev AJ, Caro J. Secondary polycythemia: a boon or a burden? Blood Cells 1984;10:177–91.

8. Pagel H, Jelkmann W, Weiss C. A comparison of the effects of renal artery constriction and anemia on the production of erythropoietin. Pflugers Arch 1988;413:62–6.

9. Pagel H, Jelkmann W, Weiss C. O_2-supply to the kidneys and the production of erythropoietin. Respir Physiol 1989;77:111–8.

10. Erslev AJ, Wilson J, Caro J. Erythropoietin titers in anemic, nonuremic patients. J Med 1987;109:429–33.

11. Hansen AJ, Fogh J, Møllgard K, Sørensen SC. Evidence against EPO production by the carotid body. Respir Physiol 1973;18:101–6.

12. Mirand EA, Murphy GP, Bennett TB, Grace JT. Erythropoietin response to repeated hemorrhage in renal allotransplanted, nephrectomized, or intact dogs. Life Sci 1968;7:689–96.

13. Eckardt K-U, Frei U, Kliem V, Bauer C, Koch KM, Kurtz A. Role of excretory graft function for erythropoietin formation after renal transplantation. Eur J Clin Invest 1990;20:564–74.

14. Kirchheim H, Ehmke H, Persson P. Sympathetic modulation of renal hemodynamics, renin release and sodium excretion. Klin Wochenschr 1989; 67:858–64.

15. Kriz W, Kaissling B. Structural organization of the mammalian kidney. In: Seldin DW, Giebisch G, eds. The kidney: physiology and pathophysiology. New York: Raven Press, 1985:265–306.

16. Kaissling B, Kriz W. Structural analysis of the rabbit kidney. Adv Anat Embryol Cell Biol 1979;56:1–123.

17. Klahr S, Hammerman M. Renal metabolism. In: Seldin DW, Giebisch G, eds. The kidney: physiology and pathophysiology. New York: Raven Press, 1985:699–718.

18. Cohen JJ, Kamm DE. Renal metabolism: relation to renal function. In: Brenner BM, Rector FC, eds. The kidney. Philadelphia: WB Saunders, 1981: 144–248.

19. Schmidt U, Guder WG, Schmidt H, Funk B, Paris K, Dubach UC. Metabolism of various portions of the nephron. In: Colloque européen de physiologie rénale. Paris: INSERM, 1974:81–91.

20. Weidemann MJ, Krebs HA. The fuel of respiration of rat kidney cortex. Biochem J 1969;112:149–66.

21. Guder WG, Ross BD. Enzyme distribution along the nephron. Kidney Int 1984;26:101–11.

22. Frömter E, Rumrich G, Ullrich K. Phenomenologic description of Na, Cl,

and HCO$_3$ absorption from proximal tubules of rat kidney. Pflugers Arch 1973;343:189–220.

23. Kiil F. Renal energy metabolism and regulation of sodium reabsorption. Kidney Int 1977;11:153–60.

24. Mathisen O, Montclair T, Kiil F. Oxygen requirement of bicarbonate-dependent sodium reabsorption in the dog kidney. Am J Physiol 1980;238: F175–80.

25. Klein KL, Wang MS, Torikai S, Davidson WD, Kurokawa K. Substrate oxidation by isolated single nephron segments of the rat. Kidney Int 1981; 20:29–35.

26. Kida K, Nakajo S, Kamiya F, Toyama Y, Nishio T, Nakagawa H. Renal net glucose release in vivo and its contribution to blood glucose in rat. J Clin Invest 1978;62:721–6.

27. Schurek HJ, Jost U, Baumgärtl H, Bertram H, Heckmann U. Evidence for a preglomerular oxygen diffusion shunt in rat renal cortex. Am J Physiol 1990;259:F910–F915.

28. Baumgärtl H, Leichtweiss HP, Lübbers DW, Weiss C, Huland H. The oxygen supply of the dog kidney: measurements of intrarenal Po$_2$. Mirovasc Res 1972;4:247–57.

29. DuBose TD, Bidani A. Kinetics of CO$_2$ exchange in the kidney. Annu Rev Physiol 1988;50:653–67.

30. Schurek HJ. Die Nierenmarkhypoxie: ein Schlüssel zum Verständnis des akuten Nierenversagens? Klin Wochenschr 1988;66:828–35.

31. Lacombe C, DaSilva J-L, Bruneval P, et al. Peritubular cells are the site of erythropoietin synthesis in the murine hypoxic kidney. J Clin Invest 1988; 81:620–3.

32. Koury ST, Bondurant MC, Koury MJ. Localization of erythropoietin synthesizing cells in murine kidneys by in situ hybridization. Blood 1988; 71:524–7.

33. Koury ST, Thamer SL, Koury MJ, Bondurant MC. Erythropoietin-producing interstitial cells are primarily found adjacent to proximal tubules in murine kidneys [Abstract]. Blood 1989;74(Suppl. 1):18a.

34. Kurtz A, Eckardt K-U, Neumann R, Kaissling B, Le Hir M, Bauer C. Site of erythropoietin formation. Contrib Nephrol 1989;76:14–23.

35. Koury ST, Koury MJ, Bondurant MC, Caro J, Graber SE. Quantitation of erythropoietin-producing cells in kidneys of mice by in situ hybridization: correlation with hematocrit, renal erythropoietin mRNA, and serum erythropoietin concentration. Blood 1989;74:645–51.

36. Goldberg MA, Glass GA, Cunningham JM, Bunn HF. The regulated expression of erythropoietin by two human hepatoma cell lines. Proc Natl Acad Sci USA 1987;84:7972–6.

37. Goldberg MA, Dunning SP, Bunn HF. Regulation of the erythropoietin gene: evidence that the oxygen sensor is a heme protein. Science 1988; 242:1412–5.

38. Semenza GL, Dureza RC, Traystman MD, Gearhart JD, Antonarakis SE. Human erythropoietin gene expression in transgenic mice: multiple transcription initiation sites and cis-acting regulatory elements. Mol Cell Biol 1990; 10:930–8.

39. Eckardt K-U, Kurtz A, Bauer C. Regulation of erythropoietin formation is related to proximal tubular function. Am J Physiol 1989;256:F942–7.

40. Suki WN, Stinebaugh BJ, Frommer JP, Eknoyan G. Physiology of di-

uretic action. In: Seldin DW, Giebisch G, eds. The kidney: physiology and pathophysiology. New York: Raven Press, 1985:2127–62.

41. Jones DP. Renal metabolism during normoxia, hypoxia, and ischemic injury. Annu Rev Physiol 1986;48:33–50.

42. Walker LA, Frölich JC. Renal prostaglandins and leukotrienes. Rev Physiol Biochem Pharmacol 1987;107:2–72.

43. Fisher JW. Prostaglandins and kidney erythropoietin production. Nephron 1980;25:53–6.

44. Dawson TP, Gandhi R, Le Hir M, Kaissling B. Ecto-5′-nucleotidase: localization in rat kidney by light microscopic histochemical and immunohistochemical methods. J Histochem Cytochem 1989;37:39–47.

45. Osswald H, Hermes HH, Nabakowski G. Role of adenosine in signal transmission of tubuloglomerular feedback. Kidney Int 1982;22(Suppl.): S136–42.

46. Miller WL, Thomas RA, Berne RM, Rubio RR. Adenosine production in the ischemic kidney. Circ Res 1978;43:390.

47. Fisher JW. Pharmacologic modulation of erythropoietin production. Annu Rev Pharmacol Toxicol 1988;28:101–22.

48. Schurek HJ, Johns O. Oszillierende Sauerstoffdrucke in der Nierenrinde. Ausdruck einer Feedback (TGF)—Geregelten Nephronfunktion? [Abstract]. Nieren- und Hochdruck 1990;19:416.

49. Le Hir M, Eckardt K-U, Kaissling B. Anemia induces 5′-nucleotidase in fibroblasts of cortical labyrinth of rat kidney. Renal Physiol Biochem 1989; 12:313–9.

50. Cohen RA, Miller ME, Garcia JF, Moccia G, Cronkite EP. Regulatory mechanism of erythropoietin production: effects of hypoxemia and hypercarbia. Exp Hematol 1981;9:513–21.

51. Eckardt K-U, Kurtz A, Bauer C. Triggering of erythropoietin formation by hypoxia is inhibited by respiratory and metabolic acidosis. Am J Physiol 1990;258:R678–83.

Chapter 7

The Erythroid Response
to Erythropoietin

John W. Adamson

Erythropoietin follows the paradigm of a classic endocrine hormone. It is produced in one organ, the kidney, in response to a recognizable physiologic stimulus, reduced oxygen availability. Erythropoietin then circulates through the blood stream to act on cells in a distant organ, the erythroid marrow. This chapter summarizes the effects of erythropoietin on the erythroid marrow.

The Interaction of Erythropoietin with Target Cells

Erythropoietin acts on its target cells through specific cell surface receptors (1–3). Both the murine (4) and the human (5) erythropoietin receptor genes have now been cloned. As reviewed recently (6), the erythropoietin receptor has considerable homology in several regions with other growth factor receptors, including interleukin 3, granulocyte-macrophage colony-stimulating factor (GM-CSF), interleukin 1β, interleukin 6, and interleukin 4, among others of interest. The erythropoietin receptor lacks a tyrosine kinase binding domain. Also of interest is the suggestion that the erythropoietin receptor gene product is likely to be only part of the receptor complex and that another membrane component (perhaps a naturally occurring but not erythroid-specific membrane protein) may participate in the complex. This model would explain the fact that the erythropoietin receptors on the surface of mammalian cells expressing a transfected erythropoietin receptor gene display two classes of binding sites.

After the binding of erythropoietin to its receptor, the whole complex is probably internalized, initiating the intracellular signal for erythropoietin action (7). Little is known, however, about how the erythropoietin effect is translated. In fact, the precise role of erythropoietin in erythroid cell development is not clear. Is erythropoietin a proliferative signal or a survival factor? Identification of the second messengers in the erythropoietin signal transduction pathway remains elusive. The accurate assessment of erythropoietin signal transduction requires a relatively homogeneous, erythropoietin-responsive population of cells. Several such progenitor cell lines now exist and are being exploited to answer questions of intracellular mechanisms of erythropoietin action. However, most of these cell lines proliferate but do not differentiate further in the presence of erythropoietin. Consequently, it is possible that the differentiation and proliferation signal pathways are different.

Using one such population, spleen cells from mice infected with the anemia-inducing strain of the Friend murine leukemia virus, Koury et al. (8) showed that the cells required erythropoietin to mature into erythrocytes. This group also provided provocative data implicating erythropoietin as a survival factor (9); purified populations of erythropoietin-dependent cells underwent apoptosis (nuclear degeneration) in the absence of erythropoietin. This would be consistent with the proposed mechanism of action of a number of hematopoietic growth factors (10). In the presence of erythropoietin, the cells could survive and carry out their programmed function.

Attempts by others to elucidate the erythropoietin intracellular signal transduction pathway using various sources of erythroid precursors yielded ambiguous results. There have been early reports (11) of rapid phosphorylation of a 43-kd membrane protein in erythroid cells in response to erythropoietin. Studies were conducted with spleen cells from mice with induced hemolytic disease. These early results have not been extended.

The role of calcium in intracellular signaling in response to erythropoietin is unclear. Mladenovic (12) and Miller and co-workers (13,14) provided evidence of an increase in intracellular free calcium in response to erythropoietin. In contrast, others have been unable to confirm those observations (15–17). Linch provided preliminary evidence that G-proteins may be involved in the response to erythropoietin (16), findings different from those of Koury, whose group had reported earlier that the mechanism of action of erythropoietin does not seem to involve phospholipase C or G-proteins directly.

Beckman et al. (18) reported that the action of erythropoietin is mediated by lipoxygenase metabolites in murine fetal liver cells; this finding also remains unconfirmed. Given the availability of recombinant erythropoietin, the cloned erythropoietin receptor gene, and hormone-dependent cell lines, this field should advance rapidly.

The Cellular Anatomy of the Marrow and Its Response to Erythropoietin

Erythropoietin stimulates erythropoiesis through its action on erythropoietin-responsive cells. The cellular anatomy of erythropoiesis was revealed through in vitro studies of progenitor cells in colony-forming assays.

The first erythroid progenitor described was the erythroid colony-forming cell (CFU-E) (19). This progenitor proliferates in semisolid medium only in the presence of erythropoietin. In normal marrow, about 0.1 to 0.2 percent of nucleated cells are CFU-E. These progenitors have limited proliferative potential, probably not more than six or seven cell divisions. Thus, CFU-E-derived colonies generally contain 60 to 120 hemoglobinized cells. Murine erythroid colonies achieve their maximal size after 48 to 72 hours of culture, and then the number of cells declines.

A more primitive erythroid progenitor is the burst-forming unit-erythroid (BFU-E). This progenitor received its name because of the appearance of the colonies ("bursts") that appeared in culture (20). Erythroid bursts contain multiple subcolonies in clusters in semisolid medium. In such cultures, the early divisions of this progenitor are independent of erythropoietin, but final maturation and hemoglobinization of the cells of the burst are erythropoietin-dependent (see below).

In the mouse, phlebotomy, phenylhydrazine-induced anemia, or erythropoietin injection results in an increase in the number of CFU-E in the marrow and spleen (21–25). By comparison, the number of BFU-E in the marrow only transiently increases; it then declines in concert with an increase in the numbers in circulation and in the spleen. In contrast, hypertransfusion-induced polycythemia results in a 70 to 80 percent reduction in the number of CFU-E in marrow and spleen, with little or no change in the number of BFU-E. In this setting, the injection of erythropoietin restores the number of CFU-E within 1 to 2 days. Thus, CFU-E are extremely sensitive to circulating levels of erythropoietin. Hypertransfusion and acute erythropoietic stress have only a transient effect on BFU-E, suggesting that this progenitor is not dependent upon ambient levels of erythropoietin for maintenance of its numbers.

The proliferative rate of CFU-E, as measured by the number of cells in DNA synthesis, is normally high and seems to change only slightly with anemia. There is a transient decline in the proliferative rate of CFU-E with transfusion-induced polycythemia (23,24,26).

The number and cell cycle activity of BFU-E are significantly affected by regulatory factors other than erythropoietin (see below) (23). In regenerating marrow, the recovery in the number of BFU-E and their cell cycle activity increase markedly. Neither the recovery in BFU-E numbers nor their increased cell-cycle activity is suppressed by hypertransfusion. In contrast, the numbers of recovering CFU-E are markedly reduced if the animal undergoes hypertransfusion, confirming the effectiveness of hypertransfusion in reducing erythropoietin stimulation. Consequently, during regenerative stress, the responses of early BFU-E are erythropoietin-independent.

In addition to BFU-E and CFU-E, a third class of erythroid progenitor was identified by Gregory (27). In cultures of murine marrow cells, CFU-E-derived colonies peak in number at 48 to 72 hours, whereas erythroid bursts, which may contain several thousand cells, appear optimally at day 7 or 8. At days 3 to 4 of culture, erythroid colonies of intermediate size, comprising three to eight clusters of hemoglobinized cells, appear. The cell giving rise to these colonies has been named the day 3 or "mature" BFU-E. The size of the colonies, the sensitivity of the progenitor to erythropoietin, and the time of appearance in culture of these colonies suggest that the day 3 BFU-E is intermediate in its state of maturation between CFU-E and the more primitive BFU-E (28).

The response of this more mature class of BFU-E to physiologic manipulation is controversial. Adamson and co-workers reported a 50 percent reduction in day 3 (mature) BFU-E with hypertransfusion (24), whereas Gregory and Eaves reported no effect of hypertransfusion on the numbers of these mature progenitor cells (28). Inasmuch as erythropoietic differentiation most likely occurs on a continuum, observed differences in the response of mature BFU-E to changes in endogenous erythropoietin levels are probably methodologic.

The hierarchy of differentiation of erythroid progenitors and their relationship to pluripotent stem cells were shown by Gregory and Henkelman (29) using an ingenious analysis of correlation first described by Wu et al. (30). This analysis assumes that the degree of relatedness of progenitors is reflected by the correlation of the numbers of different kinds of colony-forming cells to one another in expanding clones. The model is depicted in Figure 7.1. Individual spleen colonies growing in lethally irradiated mice that had received transplants were isolated and

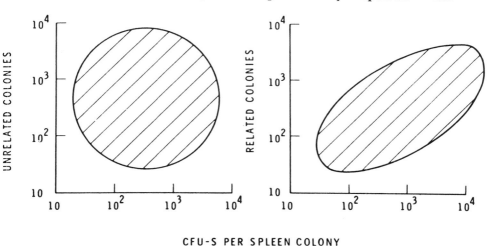

CFU-S PER SPLEEN COLONY

Figure 7.1. The patterns of correlations expected between different kinds of colony-forming cells either related or unrelated numerically to spleen colony-forming units (CFU-S) in expanding clones. For experimental purposes, an expanding clone is a growing spleen colony. The numbers of CFU-S recovered from individual clones are represented on the abscissa. Colony-forming cells that are not closely related to CFU-S or to one another in their stage of differentiation will show no proportionality, whereas the numbers of those that are closely related should be correlated. The diagram on the left is derived when the numbers of CFU-E recovered from individual clones are plotted on the ordinate against the numbers of CFU-S recovered from the same clones; the lack of correlation suggests that CFU-E and CFU-S are not closely related in the differentiation pathway. The diagram on the right results if the numbers of colonies derived from BFU-E are plotted on the ordinate against the numbers of CFU-S. The strong correlation indicates a close relationship between CFU-S and BFU-E in the lineage of differentiation. *Source: Reference 24*

assayed for various colony-forming cells. The progenitors analyzed included the spleen colony-forming cell (CFU-S), the granulocyte-macrophage colony-forming cell (CFU-GM), day 8 (primitive) and day 3 (mature) BFU-E, and CFU-E. In these studies, no relationships between the numbers of CFU-E and CFU-S or CFU-E and CFU-GM were found. This suggested that CFU-E were separated from pluripotent stem cells by several cell divisions and that random or regulatory events weakened or abolished possible correlations. In contrast, a close correlation was found between CFU-S and primitive BFU-E and also between primitive BFU-E and CFU-GM. Weaker correlations were found between day 8 and day 3 BFU-E. The results were compatible with a lineage relationship proceeding from primitive BFU-E to day 3 BFU-E and then to CFU-E. Significantly, these correlations held regardless of whether the mature cells in the original spleen colony were predominantly erythroid or granulocytic. Thus, it appeared that early restriction of differentiation events occurred either in a random fashion or in a manner independent of later regulatory events. This model—the stochastic model of stem cell differentiation—has found considerable experimental support in the studies of Ogawa and co-workers (31–33).

Human erythroid progenitors have also been described, and they are analogous to those found in the mouse (34). In human marrow cell cultures that contain erythropoietin, colonies of 8 to 64 hemoglobinized cells arise from CFU-E by 5 to 7 days. By 12 to 14 days, colonies of 3 to 8 well-hemoglobinized subunits appear, derived from mature BFU-E. Finally, macroscopic bursts containing up to 10^4 cells and originating from primitive BFU-E are seen in culture after 16 to 21 days in the presence of erythropoietin and appropriate growth factors or conditioned medium. Although the colony-forming cells themselves are not morphologically identifiable, each class of progenitor can be partially separated by physical and functional properties (35). As in the mouse, human progenitors of increasing maturity are more likely to be in the DNA-synthetic phase of the cell cycle, are larger when analyzed by velocity sedimentation, can be separated by panning or cell sorting with selected antibodies (36,37), and show increased sensitivity to erythropoietin.

Erythroid colony-forming cells are also found in human fetal liver (38), umbilical cord blood (39), and peripheral blood (40,41). Normally, however, circulating progenitors in both mice and humans are limited to BFU-E, and CFU-E are not found (42). Human circulating BFU-E are CD34-positive and CD33-negative (43). They are easily accessible, more homogeneous in many of their properties, and more amenable to quantitation than their marrow counterparts. The relationship of these progenitors to those in the marrow and the mechanism that permits their circulation are unknown; however, increased circulating numbers and an increased fraction in DNA synthesis are seen when erythropoietin (44) or a variety of other hematopoietic growth factors (45) are administered to humans.

The Effect of Other Hematopoietic Growth Factors on Erythropoiesis

Evidence that early erythropoiesis may be regulated by factors other than erythropoietin is derived from the observation that BFU-E are virtually unaffected by changes in erythropoietin levels in vivo (23,46). A number of early studies in vitro supported this hypothesis: (*a*) BFU-E will not grow optimally in all sera (47); (*b*) erythropoietin can be added late to cultures without impairing burst growth (48,49); and (*c*) medium conditioned by leukocytes enhances burst growth (50). The factors in conditioned media and in selected sera are referred to as having burst-promoting activity. In the absence of burst-promoting activity, despite the presence of erythropoietin, large bursts will not form.

Several growth factors with burst-promoting activity have now been isolated and their genes cloned. Among these are granulocyte-macrophage colony-stimulating factor (GM-CSF) (51), interleukin 3 (52), interleukin 4 (53), and interleukin 6 (54). At least some of these factors, particularly interleukin 4 and interleukin 6, affect erythroid burst growth indirectly, most likely through accessory cells (55,56).

Accessory cells are probably critical to the regulation of early hematopoiesis, including erythropoiesis. As an example, GM-CSF is produced by activated connective tissue cells, such as fibroblasts, endothelial cells, smooth muscle cells, and macrophages (57–59). All of these cells are candidate marrow stromal cells. Therefore, they are anatomically positioned to be able to influence early hematopoiesis. Similarly, interleukin 6 is produced by activated fibroblasts and endothelial cells (60). Interleukin 3, which has potent burst-promoting activity, is produced by activated T-helper lymphocytes (61).

Other Humoral Factors

In vitro, several other hormones, including β-adrenergic agonists, thyroid hormone, growth hormone, and androgenic and nonandrogenic steroids, enhance the cloning efficiency of CFU-E (62,63). Certain hormones seem to work by different mechanisms because some target cell populations can be separated by physical means (64–66). These hormones are unable to stimulate erythroid growth in the absence of erythropoietin; rather, they seem to augment the effect of erythropoietin. Whether this enhanced colony growth represents recruitment of earlier classes of colony-forming cells or an increased sensitivity of the target-responsive cell to erythropoietin is not known. Such increased sensitivity could be caused by changes in the numbers of erythropoietin receptors, their affinity for erythropoietin, or both.

The physiologic significance of such modulating factors is not known, but their importance in certain clinical states suggests that they may have in vivo relevance by influencing primary regulatory events in hematopoiesis.

The Effects of Erythropoietin on Hemoglobin Synthesis

In addition to its effects on cell proliferation, erythropoietin, under selected experimental conditions, affects the globin gene program expressed. Normally, small amounts (0.2 to 0.8 percent) of fetal hemoglobin continue to be produced in adults, where it is restricted to a small proportion (0.3 percent) of the circulating red cells, called F cells (67). F cells, which contain approximately 10 to 25 percent hemoglobin F, are increased in certain diseases, in accelerated erythropoiesis, and in the first trimester of pregnancy (68,69).

Papayannopoulou et al. (70) were the first to recognize that relatively high levels of hemoglobin F were synthesized in cultures of adult human marrow cells; these levels were much higher than the levels measured in vivo in the individual from whom the marrow cells had been obtained. These workers demonstrated that the distribution of hemoglobin F synthesis in vitro was extremely heterogeneous among colonies. This same group showed that the frequency of F-positive clones among CFU-E-derived colonies was low, closer to the values obtained in vivo, whereas the frequency of F-positive clones from erythroid bursts was up to five times higher (71). These and other studies (72–75) indicate that hemoglobin F programming is dependent upon the level of differentiation of the progenitor. When hemoglobin F in the colonies of erythroid bursts is analyzed, both adult and fetal hemoglobin are synthesized (75,76). These data imply that changes in hemoglobin F synthesis are consequential to BFU-E division and can be influenced in vitro.

Studies of the actual amounts of fetal and adult hemoglobin synthesized over time showed that, as the erythroid burst becomes more hemoglobinized, the relative rate of hemoglobin F synthesis declines (77–79). Therefore, it also seems that the ability to express hemoglobin F decreases with erythroid maturation.

Most of these observations were made in cultures of adult cells. Similar studies with fetal blood, neonatal blood, or fetal liver show that hemoglobin F is synthesized in vitro at levels similar to the levels seen in the erythrocytes of the fetus at that particular stage of development (80–82). Colonies grown from cord blood show levels of hemoglobin F synthesis intermediate between fetal and adult values. Thus, there is direct correlation between the amount of hemoglobin F synthesized by fetal erythroid progenitor cells and the levels of hemoglobin F found in the erythrocytes at that stage.

There also is reasonable evidence that environmental (extracellular) influences affect hemoglobin F production. In one study, transplantation of cells from the late fetal period into adult animals resulted in hemoglobin A production, although the fetal cells may already have been undergoing the switch to the adult program (83). Preliminary in vitro experiments demonstrated that the addition of irradiated adult cells to cord blood mononuclear cells increased the amount of hemoglobin A synthesized (84). Whether this was due to recruitment of earlier progenitors of the A type, an increase in size of the already-switching burst, or true acceleration of the fetal to adult switch was not clear.

The effect of known humoral hematopoietic regulators on hemoglobin F synthesis has also been studied. Erythropoietin itself does not seem to activate hemoglobin F synthesis in culture (69,82,85–87). Differences in the measured amounts of hemoglobin F synthesized in the presence of high concentrations of erythropoietin are probably due either to the acceleration of maturation (84) or the recruitment of earlier progenitors by the hormone (71). If a source of burst-promoting activity is added, the number of hemoglobin F-containing bursts is increased while the number of F-negative bursts remains constant. This is consistent with the view that more primitive progenitors, when induced to proliferate in vitro, are more likely to express hemoglobin F.

More precise studies under serum-deprived conditions indicate that factor(s) present in serum can affect the level of hemoglobin F synthesized in culture. Thus, under defined conditions but in the presence of interleukin 3, GM-CSF, and erythropoietin, erythroid bursts form which have normal (<1.0 percent) hemoglobin F levels (88,89). Serum-deprived conditions with different concentrations of interleukin 3 and GM-CSF probably do not affect hemoglobin F synthesis, although this is disputed (90). Consequently, studies of hemoglobin F synthesis in serum-deprived cultures provide an opportunity to assess the effects of regulatory factors that can affect the globin gene program.

Based on in vitro observations, in vivo studies of high-dose pulse-administered erythropoietin showed a sharp increase in hemoglobin F synthesis in primates (91,92). This result is believed to be due to a direct effect of erythropoietin not on the globin gene program but, rather, on altered erythroid kinetics. The interest in this phenomenon and the reason that it is being researched vigorously lie in the possible use of erythropoietin, either alone or in combination with other agents, to promote hemoglobin F synthesis and the accumulation of F-containing cells in patients with hemoglobinopathies.

The results of the primate studies raised the hope that pulsed, high doses of erythropoietin might stimulate hemoglobin F synthesis in patients with sickle cell anemia. The results in baboons are encouraging, but the early results in patients with sickle cell anemia have been less impressive (93). However, it is possible that the combination of erythropoietin and other agents may augment hemoglobin F synthesis in patients with sickle cell anemia (94,95). One such agent is hydroxyurea. This drug is a cell cycle-active agent that interferes with DNA synthesis and augments hemoglobin F production in experimental animals. Recent studies used hydroxyurea and erythropoietin to raise hemoglobin F levels in patients with sickle cell disease. Although the first published clinical trial was disappointing (96), more recent studies, admittedly in small numbers of patients, seem more promising (97). Consequently, continued study is warranted to determine whether erythropoietin therapy, in conjunction with other agents, will be useful in augmenting hemoglobin F synthesis in patients with hemoglobinopathies, thereby ameliorating the consequences of these disorders.

REFERENCES

1. Sawyer ST, Krantz SB, Luna J. Identification of the receptor for erythropoietin by cross-linking to Friend virus-infected erythroid cells. Proc Natl Acad Sci USA 1987;84:3690–4.

2. Tojo A, Fukamachi H, Kasuga M, Urabe A, Takaku F. Identification of erythropoietin receptors on fetal liver erythroid cells. Biochem Biophys Res Commun 1987;148:443–8.

3. Broudy VC, Lin N, Egrie J, Weiss T, Papayannopoulou T, Adamson JW. Identification of the receptor for erythropoietin on human and murine erythroleukemia cells and modulation by phorbol ester and dimethyl sulfoxide. Proc Natl Acad Sci USA 1988;85:6513–7.

4. D'Andrea AD, Lodish HF, Wong GG. Expression cloning of the murine erythropoietin receptor. Cell 1989;57:277–85.

5. Winkelmann JC, Penny LA, Deaven LL, Forget BG, Jenkins RB. The gene for the human erythropoietin receptor: analysis of the coding sequence and assignment to chromosome 19p. Blood 1990;76:24–30.

6. D'Andrea AD, Zon LI. Erythropoietin receptor. Subunit structure and activation. J Clin Invest 1990;86:681–7.

7. Sawyer ST, Krantz SB, Goldwasser E. Binding and receptor-mediated endocytosis of erythropoietin in Friend virus-infected erythroid cells. J Biol Chem 1987;262:5554–62.

8. Koury MJ, Sawyer ST, Bondurant MC. Splenic erythroblasts in anemia-inducing Friend disease: a source of cells for studies of erythropoietin-mediated differentiation. J Cell Physiol 1984;121:526–32.

9. Koury MJ, Bondurant MC. Erythropoietin retards DNA breakdown and prevents programmed death in erythroid progenitor cells. Science 1990;248:378–81.

10. Williams GT, Smith CA, Spooncer E, et al. Haemopoietic colony stimulating factors promote cell survival by suppressing apoptosis. Nature 1990;343:76–9.

11. Choi H-S, Wojchowski DM, Sytkowski AJ. Erythropoietin rapidly alters phosphorylation of pp43, an erythroid membrane protein. J Biol Chem 1987;262:2933–6.

12. Mladenovic J, Kay NE. Erythropoietin induces rapid increases in intracellular free calcium in human bone marrow cells. J Lab Clin Med 1988;112:23–7.

13. Miller BA, Scaduto RC Jr, Tillotson DL, Botti JJ, Cheung JY. Erythropoietin stimulates a rise in intracellular free calcium in single early human erythroid precursors. J Clin Invest 1988;82:309–15.

14. Miller BA, Cheung JY, Tillotson DL, Hope SM, Scaduto RC Jr. Erythropoietin stimulates a rise in intracellular-free calcium concentration in single BFU-E derived erythroblasts at specific stages of differentiation. Blood 1989;73:1188–94.

15. Thompson LP, Sawyer ST, Blackmore PF, Krantz SB. A search for the second messenger of erythropoietin [Abstract]. FASEB J 1988;2:A813.

16. Linch DC, Jones HM, Tidman N, Roberts PJ. The effects of erythropoietin on primitive human erythroid cells [Abstract]. Blood 1987;70:177a.

17. Imagawa S, Smith BR, Palmer-Crocker R, Bunn HF. The effect of recombinant erythropoietin on intracellular free calcium in erythropoietin responsive cells. Blood 1989;73:1452–7.

18. Beckman BS, Mason-Garcia M, Nystuen L, King L, Fisher JW. The action of erythropoietin is mediated by lipoxygenase metabolites in murine fetal liver cells. Biochem Biophys Res Commun 1987;147:392–8.

19. Stephenson JR, Axelrad AA, McLeod DC, et al. Induction of colonies of hemoglobin-synthesizing cells by erythropoietin in vitro. Proc Natl Acad Sci USA 1971;68:1542–6.

20. Axelrad AA, McLeod DL, Shreeve MM, et al. Properties of cells that produce erythrocytic colonies in vitro. In: Robinson WA, ed. Hemopoiesis in Culture. Washington, D.C.: Second International Workshop, 1973:226–34; DHEW publication no. 74-205.

21. Gregory CS, Tepperman AD, McCulloch EA, et al. Erythropoietic progenitors capable of colony formation in culture: response of normal and genetically anemic W/W^v mice to manipulations of the erythron. J Cell Physiol 1974;84:1–12.

22. Hara H, Ogawa M. Erythropoietic precursors in mice with phenylhydrazine-induced anemia. Am J Hematol 1976;1:453–8.

23. Iscove NN. The role of erythropoietin in regulation of population size and cell cycling of early and late erythroid precursors in mouse bone marrow. Cell Tissue Kinet 1977;10:323–34.

24. Adamson JW, Torok-Storb B, Lin N. Analysis of erythropoiesis by erythroid colony formation in culture. Blood Cells 1978;4:89–103.

25. Peschle C, Cillo C, Rappaport IA, et al. Early fluctuations of BFU-E pool size after transfusion or erythropoietin treatment. Exp Hematol 1979;7:87–93.

26. Peschle C, Cillo C, Migliaccio G, et al. Fluctuations in BFU-E and CFU-E cycling after erythroid perturbations: correlation with variations of pool size. Exp Hematol 1980;8:96–102.

27. Gregory CJ. Erythropoietin sensitivity as a differentiation marker in the hemopoietic system: studies of three erythropoietic colony responses in culture. J Cell Physiol 1976;89:289–302.

28. Gregory CJ, Eaves AC. Three stages of erythropoietic progenitor cell differentiation distinguished by a number of physical and biologic properties. Blood 1978;51:527–37.

29. Gregory CJ, Henkelman RM. Relationships between early hemopoietic progenitor cells determined by correlation analysis of their numbers in individual spleen colonies. In: Baum SJ, Ledney GD, eds. Experimental hematology today. New York: Springer-Verlag, 1977;93–101.

30. Wu AM, Siminovitch L, Till JE, et al. Evidence for a relationship between mouse hemopoietic stem cells and cells forming colonies in culture. Proc Natl Acad Sci USA 1968;59:1209–15.

31. Ogawa M, Porter PN, Nakahata T. Renewal and commitment to differentiation of hemopoietic stem cells: an interpretive review. Blood 1983;61:823–9.

32. Suda T, Suda J, Ogawa M. Single cell origin of mouse hemopoietic colonies expressing multiple lineages in variable combinations. Proc Natl Acad Sci USA 1983;80:6689–93.

33. Suda J, Suda T, Ogawa M. Analysis of differentiation of mouse hemopoietic stem cells in culture by sequential replating of paired progenitors. Blood 1984;64:393–9.

34. Gregory CJ, Eaves AC. Human marrow cells capable of erythropoietic differentiation in vitro: definition of three erythroid colony responses. Blood 1977;49:855–64.

35. Ogawa M, MacEachern MD, Avila L. Human marrow erythropoiesis in culture: II. Heterogeneity in the morphology, time course of colony formation and sedimentation velocities of the colony-forming cells. Am J Hematol 1977;3:29–39.

36. Yokochi T, Brice M, Rabinovitch PS, et al. Monoclonal antibodies detecting antigenic determinants with restricted expression on erythroid cells: from the erythroid committed progenitor level to the mature erythroblast. Blood 1984;63:1376–84.

37. Das Gupta A, Samoszuk MK, Papayannopoulou T, Stamatoyannopoulos G. SFL 23.6: a monoclonal antibody reactive with CFU-E, erythroblasts, and erythrocytes. Blood 1985;66:522–6.

38. Hassan MW, Lutton JD, Levere RD, et al. In vitro culture of erythroid colonies from human fetal liver and umbilical cord blood. Br J Haematol 1979;41:477–84.

39. Ogawa M, MacEachern MD, Wilson JM, et al. Erythropoietic precursors in human umbilical cord blood. Blood 1976;48:980–6.

40. Clarke BJ, Housman D. Characterization of an erythroid precursor cell of high proliferative capacity in normal human peripheral blood. Proc Natl Acad Sci USA 1977;74:1105–9.

41. Ogawa M, Gruish OC, O'Dell RF, et al. Circulating erythropoietic pre-

cursors assessed in culture: characterization in normal men and patients with hemoglobinopathies. Blood 1977;50:1081–92.

42. Nathan DG, Chess L, Hillman DG, et al. Human erythroid burst-forming unit: T-cell requirement for proliferation in vitro. J Exp Med 1978;147: 324–39.

43. Sieff CA, Emerson SG, Mufson A, et al. Dependence of highly enriched human bone marrow progenitors on hemopoietic growth factors and their response to recombinant erythropoietin. J Clin Invest 1986;77:74–81.

44. Dessypris EN, Graber SE, Krantz SB, Stone WJ. Effects of recombinant erythropoietin on the concentration and cycling status of human marrow hematopoietic progenitor cells in vivo. Blood 1988;72:2060–2.

45. Miles SA, Mitsuyasu RT, Lee K, et al. Recombinant human granulocyte colony-stimulating factor increases circulating burst forming unit-erythron and red blood cell production in patients with severe human immunodeficiency virus infection. Blood 1990;75:2137–42.

46. Hara H, Ogawa M. Erythropoietic precursors in mice under erythropoietic stimulation and suppression. Exp Hematol 1977;5:141–8.

47. Iscove NN, Guilbert LJ. Erythropoietin-independence of early erythropoiesis and a two-regulator model of proliferative control in the hemopoietic system. In: Murphy MJ, Peschle C, eds. In vitro Aspects of Erythropoiesis. New York: Springer-Verlag, 1978:3–7.

48. Iscove NN. Erythropoietin independent stimulation of early erythropoiesis in adult marrow cultures by conditioned media from lectin stimulated mouse spleen cells. In: Golde DW, Cline MJ, Metcalf D, eds. Hemopoietic Cell Differentiation. New York: Academic Press, 1978:37–52. (ICN-UCLA Symposia on Molecular and Cellular Biology; vol 10.)

49. Tsang RW, Aye MT. Evidence of proliferation of early erythroid progenitors in the absence of added erythropoietin. Exp Hematol 1979;7:383–8.

50. Aye MT. Erythroid colony formation in cultures of human marrow: effect of leukocyte conditioned media. J Cell Physiol 1977;91:69–78.

51. Kaushansky K, O'Hara PJ, Berkner K, Segal GM, Hagen FS, Adamson JW. Genomic cloning, characterization and expression of human granulocyte/macrophage colony stimulating factor. Proc Natl Acad Sci USA 1986;83: 3101–5.

52. Sieff CA, Niemeyer CM, Nathan D, et al. Stimulation of human hematopoietic colony formation by recombinant gibbon multicolony-stimulating factor or interleukin 3. J Clin Invest 1987;80:818–23.

53. Peschel C, Paul WE, Ohara J, Green I. Effects of B cell stimulatory factor-1/interleukin 4 on hematopoietic progenitor cells. Blood 1987;70:254–63.

54. Gardner JD, Liechty KW, Christensen RD. Effects of interleukin-6 on fetal hematopoietic progenitors. Blood 1990;75:2150–5.

55. Migliaccio AR, Migliaccio G, Shimada Y, Adamson JW. Direct effects of IL-4 on the in vitro differentiation and proliferation of hematopoietic progenitor cells. Biotechnol Therapeutics (in press).

56. Migliaccio G, Migliaccio AR, Adamson JW. In vitro differentiation and proliferation of human hematopoietic progenitors: the effects of interleukins 1 and 6 are indirectly mediated by production of granulocyte/macrophage colony-stimulating factor and interleukin 3. Exp Hematol (in press).

57. Broudy VC, Kaushansky K, Segal GM, Harlan JM, Adamson JW. Tumor necrosis factor type alpha stimulates human endothelial cells to produce gran-

ulocyte/macrophage colony-stimulating factor. Proc Natl Acad Sci USA 1986;
83:7467–71.

58. Broudy VC, Kaushansky K, Harlan JM, Adamson JW. Interleukin-1
stimulates human endothelial cells to produce granulocyte-macrophage colony-
stimulating factor and granulocyte colony-stimulating factor. J Immunol 1987;
37:464–8.

59. Kaushansky K, Lin N, Adamson JW. Interleukin-1 stimulates fibroblasts
to synthesize granulocyte/macrophage and granulocyte colony-stimulating factors. Mechanism for the hematopoietic response to inflammation. J Clin Invest
1988;81:92–7.

60. Kishimoto T. The biology of interleukin-6. Blood 1989;74:1–10.

61. Morris CF, Young IG, Hapel AJ. Molecular and cellular biology of in-
terleukin-3. In: Dexter TM, Garland JM, Testa NG, eds. Colony-stimulating factors: molecular and cellular biology. New York: Marcel Dekker, 1990:177–214.

62. Adamson JW. Pharmacological stimulation of marrow function. Clin
Haematol 1978;7:555–69.

63. Golde DW, Cline MJ. Hormonal interactions with hematopoietic cells in
vitro. Transplant Proc 1978;10:95–7.

64. Singer JW, Adamson JW. Steroids and hematopoiesis. I. The effect of
steroids on in vitro erythroid colony growth: evidence for different target cells
for different classes of steroids. J Cell Physiol 1976;88:135–44.

65. Brown JE, Adamson JW. Modulation of in vitro erythropoiesis: the influence of β-adrenergic agonists on erythroid colony formation. J Clin Invest
1977;60:70–7.

66. Popovic WJ, Brown JE, Adamson JW. The influence of thyroid hormones
on in vitro erythropoiesis. J Clin Invest 1977;60:907–13.

67. Boyer SH, Belding EK, Margolet L, et al. Fetal hemoglobin restriction to
a few erythrocytes (F cells) in normal human adults. Science 1975;188:
361–3.

68. Wood WG, Stamatoyannopoulos G, Lim G, et al. F cells in the adult:
normal values and levels in individuals with hereditary and acquired elevations
of HbF. Blood 1975;46:671–82.

69. Nathan DG, Alter BG. F cell regulation. Ann NY Acad Sci 1980;
344:219–32.

70. Papayannopoulou T, Brice M, Stamatoyannopoulos G. Stimulation of fetal hemoglobin synthesis in bone marrow cultures from adult individuals. Proc
Natl Acad Sci USA 1976;73:2033–7.

71. Papayannopoulou T, Brice M, Stamatoyannopoulos G. Hemoglobin F
synthesis in vitro: evidence for control at the level of primitive erythroid stem
cells. Proc Natl Acad Sci USA 1977;74:2923–7.

72. Kidoguchi K, Ogawa M, Karam JD, et al. Augmentation of fetal hemoglobin (HbF) synthesis in culture by human erythropoietic precursors in the
marrow and peripheral blood: studies in sickle cell anemia and nonhemoglo-
binopathic adults. Blood 1978;52:1115–24.

73. Clarke BJ, Nathan DG, Alter BP, et al. Hemoglobin synthesis in human
BFU-E and CFU-E-derived erythroid colonies. Blood 1979;54:805–17.

74. Vainchenkar W, Testa U, Hinard N, et al. Hemoglobin synthesis in 7-day
and 14-day-old erythroid colonies from the bone marrow of normal individuals.
Hemoglobin 1980;4:53–67.

75. Kidoguchi K, Ogawa M, Karam JD. Hemoglobin biosynthesis in indi-

vidual erythropoietic bursts in culture: studies of adult peripheral blood. J Clin Invest 1979;63:804–6.

76. Peschle C, Migliaccio G, Caelli A, et al. Hemoglobin synthesis in individual bursts from normal adult blood: all bursts and subcolonies synthesize G_γ and A_γ globin chains. Blood 1980;56:218–26.

77. Papayannopoulou T, Kalmantis T, Stamatoyannopoulos G. Cellular regulation of hemoglobin switching: evidence of inverse relationship between fetal hemoglobin synthesis and degree of maturity of human erythroid cells. Proc Natl Acad Sci USA 1979;76:6420–4.

78. Chui DHK, Wong SC, Enkin MW, et al. Proportion of fetal hemoglobin synthesis decreases during erythroid cell maturation. Proc Natl Acad Sci USA 1980;77:2757–61.

79. Papayannopoulou T, Kurachi S, Brice M, et al. Asynchronous synthesis of HbF and HbA during erythroblast maturation. II. Studies of G_γ and A_γ and β chain synthesis in individual erythroid clones from neonatal and adult BFU-E cultures. Blood 1981;57:531–6.

80. Stamatoyannopoulos G, Rosenblum B, Papayannopoulou T, et al. HbF and HbA production in erythroid cultures from human fetuses and neonates. Blood 1979;54:440–50.

81. Hassan MW, Ibrahim A, Rieder RF, et al. Synthesis of HbA and HbF in erythroid colonies cultured from human fetal liver and umbilical cord blood. Blood 1979;54:1140–51.

82. Beuzard Y, Vainchenkar W, Testa U, et al. Fetal to adult hemoglobin switch in cultures of early erythroid precursors from human fetuses and neonates. Am J Hematol 1979;7:207–18.

83. Zanjani ED, McGlave PB, Bhakthavasthsalan A, et al. Sheep fetal hematopoietic cells produce adult hemoglobin when transplanted in adult animals. Nature 1989;280:495–7.

84. Vainchenkar W, Testa U, Dubart A, et al. Acceleration of the hemoglobin switch in cultures of neonate erythroid precursors by adult cells. Blood 1980;56:541–7.

85. Papayannopoulou T, Nakamoto B, Buckley J, et al. Erythroid progenitors circulating in the blood of adult individuals produce fetal hemoglobin in culture. Science 1978;199:1349–50.

86. Fauser AA, Messner HA. Fetal hemoglobin in mixed hemopoietic colonies (CFU-GEMM), erythroid bursts (BFU-E), and erythroid colonies (CFU-E): assessment by radioimmune assay and immunofluorescence. Blood 1979;54:1384–94.

87. Vainchenkar W, Dubart A, Bouguet J, et al. Fetal hemoglobin synthesis in cultures of early erythroid precursors (BFU-E) from the blood of normal adults. J Cell Physiol 1980;102:297–303.

88. Fujimori Y, Ogawa M, Clark SC, Dover GJ. Serum-free culture of enriched hematopoietic progenitors reflects physiologic levels of fetal hemoglobin biosynthesis. Blood 1990;75:1718–22.

89. Migliaccio AR, Migliaccio G, Brice M, et al. Influence of recombinant hematopoietins and of fetal bovine serum on the globin synthetic pattern of human BFUe. Blood 1990;76:1150–7.

90. Gabbianelli M, Pelosi E, Bassano E, et al. Granulocyte-macrophage colony-stimulating factor reactivates fetal hemoglobin synthesis in erythroblast clones from normal adults. Blood 1989;74:2657–67.

91. DeSimone J, Biel SI, Heller P. Stimulation of fetal hemoglobin synthesis

in the baboon by hemolysis and hypoxia. Proc Natl Acad Sci USA 1978; 75:2937–40.

92. Al-Khatti A, Veith RW, Papayannopoulou T, Fritsch EF, et al. Stimulation of fetal hemoglobin synthesis by erythropoietin in baboons. N Engl J Med 1987;317:415–20.

93. Al-Khatti A, Umemura T, Clow J, et al. Erythropoietin stimulates F-reticulocyte formation in sickle cell anemia. Trans Assoc Am Physicians 1988; 101:54–61.

94. Charache S, Dover GJ, Moyer MA, Moore JW. Hydroxyurea-induced augmentation of fetal hemoglobin production in patients with sickle cell anemia. Blood 1987;69:109–16.

95. Al-Khatti A, Papayannopoulou T, Knitter G, Fritsch EF, Stamatoyannopoulos G. Cooperative enhancement of F-cell formation in baboons treated with erythropoietin and hydroxyurea. Blood 1988;72:817–9.

96. Goldberg MA, Brugnara C, Dover GJ, et al. Treatment of sickle cell anemia with hydroxyurea and erythropoietin. N Engl J Med 1990;323:366–72.

97. Rodgers GP, Uyesaka N, Dover GJ, et al. Hydroxyurea therapy in sickle cell disease: effects of dose schedule and recombinant erythropoietin on hematological and rheological parameters [Abstract]. Blood 1990;76(Suppl 1): 74a.

Chapter 8

The Physiology and Biochemistry
of Erythropoietin Receptors

Stephen T. Sawyer

Erythropoietin is required by developing erythroid progenitor and precursor cells. If the hormone is absent, these cells die in vitro and presumably also in vivo. Under normal conditions, erythropoietin in the circulation (10 to 30 mU/ml) modulates erythropoiesis such that a stable hematocrit is maintained. However, the number of erythrocytes produced in normal erythropoiesis is much less than possible, and the loss of blood or hypoxia can induce up to a 1000-fold increase in the mRNA encoding erythropoietin in the kidney and a corresponding increase in the serum levels of the hormone. This increase in circulating erythropoietin is quickly followed by an increase in the numbers of erythroid progenitor and precursor cells in the marrow and of reticulocytes and erythrocytes in the circulation. The regulation of erythropoietin production is probably directly connected to the level of O_2 in the kidney, and erythropoietin directs erythropoiesis by the direct interaction of the hormone with receptors on the surface of erythroid progenitor and precursor cells. These represent the primary events in the control of erythropoiesis.

Although receptors for erythropoietin have been thought to exist for a number of years, the direct demonstration of cell surface receptors is a relatively recent event (1). Proteolytic digestion of marrow cells and inhibition of protein synthesis eliminated the response to erythropoietin, but upon recovery of protein synthesis the response to erythropoietin returned (2). This result was consistent with the destruction and resynthesis of surface receptors for erythropoietin but could have reflected proteolytic damage to any number of different cell surface components. Direct demonstration of cell surface erythropoietin receptors was only possible when both biologically active radiolabeled hormone and a relatively pure population of erythroid cells that responded to the hormone were obtained.

In the hematology research laboratory at Vanderbilt, a model cell system for erythropoietin-dependent erythroid maturation using the anemia strain of Friend virus (FVA) evolved over a number of years. Infection of mouse bone marrow cells with FVA gave rise to large colonies or bursts of erythroid precursor cells that required erythropoietin for further maturation. With only a dissecting microscope, these bursts of erythroid cells were plucked from cultures in a labor-intensive procedure, which required the identification of nonhemoglobinized erythroid bursts among a background of similar-sized colonies of other hematopoietic cells (3,4). However, this procedure was abandoned when it was realized that the same erythropoietin-responsive erythroid cells were the predominant cell type in the spleens of mice infected with FVA during the initial phase of the disease. Immature erythroid cells (FVA cells) were then purified from the spleens of mice infected with FVA using unity gravity sedimentation in gradients of serum albumin (5,6). These cells were the first used to demonstrate receptors for erythropoietin.

In 1981, Goldwasser reported that iodination of erythropoietin either directly by iodination of tyrosine residues or indirectly by cross-linking of iodinated compounds through NH_2-terminal or amino side chains (Bolton-Hunter method) resulted in complete loss of biologic activity (7). Consequently, a fluorescent conjugate of erythropoietin was prepared and was found to label 1 to 2 percent of bone marrow cells from anemic mice and rats (8). This result was not a conclusive demonstration of receptors, however, because the fluorescent cells could not be determined to be erythroid. Erythropoietin was tritiated by oxidation of the carbohydrate moiety of erythropoietin and subsequent reduction with tritiated borohydride, which resulted in [³H]erythropoietin with five ³H atoms per erythropoietin molecule and full biologic activity. This material was used to demonstrate specific binding of [³H]erythropoietin to the pure population of erythropoietin-responsive FVA cells (1). Unfortunately, the specific activity was so low that extremely high cell numbers in very small volumes were required to detect binding of [³H]erythropoietin. This resulted in the aggregation of cells such that the number of binding sites was underestimated, the binding parameters were incorrectly measured, and the binding affinity measured was 10- to 60-fold less than subsequent experiments demonstrated.

Iodinated human urinary erythropoietin (^{125}I-erythropoietin), which had been reported to be devoid of biologic activity (7), was found to bind to the FVA cells. Upon further investigation, we found that pure recombinant erythropoietin (Amgen) could be iodinated and still retain full biologic activity. Under no condition tested was the binding of biologically inactive erythropoietin observed. Purified urinary erythropoietin could also be iodinated and still retain greater than 90 percent of biologic activity when assayed in the in vitro FVA cell assay. Urinary [³H]erythropoietin, erythropoietin metabolically labeled with sulfur 35 obtained from Amgen, and erythropoietin labeled with iodine 125 prepared from Amgen recombinant human erythropoietin gave similar numbers of binding sites and binding affinities when the binding was simultaneously tested on FVA cells. Self-displacement analysis showed that ^{125}I-erythropoietin binds to receptors with the same affinity as native erythropoietin.

The Quantitation of Receptors

In contrast to the first report of [³H]erythropoietin binding to FVA cells, ^{125}I-erythropoietin binding to the surface of FVA cells at 0°C showed a biphasic Scatchard plot that suggested the existence of two classes of erythropoietin receptors differing in affinity for the hormone. FVA cells have approximately 1000 receptors for erythropoietin, of which 300 to 400 have a higher affinity for erythropoietin (K_d of 80 to 100 pM), whereas the remaining receptors have a lower affinity (K_d of 0.6 to 1.0 nM) (9). Nonlinear Scatchard plots of this type can be due to negative cooperativity; however, experiments in this laboratory showed that bound ^{125}I-erythropoietin is released from FVA cells at the same rate in the presence and absence of unlabeled erythropoietin, indicating no negative cooperativity.

Binding of ^{125}I-erythropoietin to Friend murine erythroleukemia cells, clone 745, was investigated as a control. Binding was not expected as these cells are totally unresponsive to erythropoietin; however, almost as many receptors were found on these cells as on the FVA cells. Interestingly, these cells expressed only the lower-affinity erythropoietin receptors (K_d of 500 to 1000 pM) (9). Mayeux et al. also reported that clone 745 murine erythroleukemia cells had 500 surface receptors with an affinity of 490 pM (10), whereas Sasaki et al. reported that 745A murine erythroleukemia cells had 100 receptors with a binding constant of 210 pM (11). Because the murine erythroleukemia cells, which have only low-affinity receptors, are totally unresponsive to erythropoietin and because of the predominance of high-affinity receptors occupied on FVA cells at the concentration of erythropoietin which gives the maximal biologic activity, we proposed that the interaction of erythropoietin with the high-affinity receptors is necessary for the full biologic effect of the hormone. When a complementary deoxyribonucleic acid (cDNA) clone encoding an erythropoietin receptor, derived from mRNA of clone 745 murine erythroleukemia cells, was expressed in Cos cells, both high- and low-affinity receptors were expressed (12). This probably indicates a physiologic rather than a genetic basis for two classes of erythropoietin receptors, although further work is necessary to resolve this question.

Erythroid cells that respond to erythropoietin by full differentiation and that show the two classes of erythropoietin receptors include fetal mouse liver cells (13,14), mouse colony-forming units-erythroid (CFU-E) induced by thiamphenicol treatment (15), and human CFU-E derived in vitro from circulating burst-forming units-erythroid (BFU-E) (16), as well as FVA cells. In addition, some cell lines that are partially responsive to erythropoietin also have high- and low-affinity receptors: TSA8 cells have high-affinity receptors of K_d 250 pM and low-affinity receptors of K_d 6nM (17) and JK1 human erythroleukemia cells have high-affinity receptors of K_d 60 pM and low-affinity receptors of K_d 400 pM (18). In addition, some unresponsive cells have high- and low-affinity receptors for erythropoietin (19).

Regenerating mouse CFU-E cells were initially reported to express only receptors for erythropoietin of the lower-affinity type. This was due to the occupancy of the high-affinity receptors with erythropoietin when the cells were recovered from a mouse with elevated erythropoietin (15). Endogenous erythropoietin occupying high-affinity receptors may account for the conflicting observations of only a single class of erythropoietin receptors in fetal mouse liver cells, fetal human liver cells, anemic mouse spleen cells, and fetal rat liver cells because these cells are explanted from sources having high levels of erythropoiesis and therefore significant levels of erythropoietin. Contributing to this problem of endogenous erythropoietin being bound to the cell surface are the observations in FVA cells, mouse CFU-E (15), and human CFU-E that high-affinity receptors are rapidly downregulated after exposure to erythropoietin for as short a period as 2 hours and that only low-affinity receptors are expressed during the maturation to reticulocytes. Therefore, erythroid cells explanted from tissues rich in erythropoietin may express only low-affinity receptors because the high-affinity receptors were downregulated before the cells were harvested or because the cells may be erythroblasts that have lost high-affinity receptors.

The number of receptors and the affinities of the receptors for erythropoietin vary widely in different laboratories measuring the binding of ^{125}I-erythropoietin to the same cells. A single class of receptors was found in FVA cells (11,20), fetal mouse liver cells, and TSA8 cells (11), yet other studies found two classes of high- and low-affinity receptors in these same cells (9,13,14). Technical reasons may explain these discrepancies. With few exceptions, binding studies for a short period (30 to 90 minutes) on intact cells at 37°C in which endocytosis was inhibited by azide or other poisons and for 2 to 4 hours at 20 to 15°C to prevent endocytosis showed a single class of binding sites for erythropoietin; however, binding studies at 0 to 4°C for extended periods (18 to 24 hours) demonstrated both high- and low-affinity receptors for erythropoietin. The reasons for this are unclear, and conditions appropriate for the measurement of the binding of erythropoietin are not certain. In all cases an altered cellular environment is generated. In this laboratory, the 0° to 4°C condition was chosen because FVA cells can survive overnight at this temperature without appreciable loss of viability, whereas incubation at 10° to 15°C results in cell death. Metabolic poisons certainly prevent endocytosis of erythropoietin at 37°C but may also affect other events that might maintain receptors in a high-affinity form.

Disparities between numbers of receptors and binding affinities between different laboratories may also be due to differences in the specific activity of the erythropoietin used. For example, a fivefold difference in the specific activity of erythropoietin has been used in calculations of the number of binding sites for erythropoietin—50,000 (1) to 250,000 units/mg (15).

Recent studies in this laboratory indicate that limited proteolysis of the surface of mouse and human erythroid cells by chymopapain can convert lower-affinity receptors into higher-affinity receptors for erythropoietin. This result suggests that steric interference in the access of erythropoietin to some receptors but not others may result in apparently lower affinity receptors. This idea is also consistent with the observations that deglycosylated erythropoietin binds to receptors with higher affinity than does normal erythropoietin (21) and that the dissociation of ^{125}I-erythropoietin bound to cells fails to identify two distinct affinity receptors (S. T. Sawyer, unpublished results). The observation that both high- and low-affinity receptors are expressed on cells transfected with a cDNA derived from a murine erythroleukemia cell which expresses only low-affinity receptors also suggests that a topographical variation in the location on the cell surface might result in receptors with apparent differences in the binding affinity for erythropoietin. However, additional work is required to resolve the molecular reason for two different binding affinities for erythropoietin.

Low-affinity receptors for erythropoietin are of significance in the response of cells to erythropoietin. This is the case for FVA cells, mouse CFU-E, and human CFU-E, which quickly downregulate high-affinity receptors but still require erythropoietin for development when only the low-affinity receptors are expressed. The effect of erythropoietin through the low-affinity receptors is also shown in the HCD33 and HCD57 cells, which are totally dependent on erythropoietin for survival and proliferation yet express only low-affinity receptors (22). Similarly in DA1, IC2, and FDCP2 cells, which have only the low-affinity receptor, erythropoietin can substitute for the requirement of other hematologic factors (23,24).

The Correlation of Receptor Expression with Responsiveness

The number of receptors for erythropoietin on the surface of erythroid precursor cells most likely parallels the responsiveness of the cells to erythropoietin. CFU-E or cells at the proerythroblast stage of development apparently have the greatest number of receptors (approximately 1000 receptors/cell), and the number of receptors drops substantially as the cells mature to erythroblasts and mature erythroblasts while becoming less dependent on erythropoietin at each successive stage. In the FVA cell system, the total number of receptors drops to half when the cells become basophilic erythroblasts after culture for 24 hours. At this stage, these basophilic FVA erythroblasts are no longer dependent on erythropoietin for maturation (25). Erythropoietin receptors are rapidly lost during the next 24 hours of culture as the basophilic FVA erythroblasts mature to reticulocytes, which have no receptors. These results were also found in regenerating mouse CFU-E (15) and human CFU-E (26). All of these findings in cell systems generally agree with the finding of Fraser et al., who used autoradiography of bound ^{125}I-erythropoietin to estimate the relative distributions of receptors among erythroid cells at different stages of maturation in cells from the spleens of anemic mice and normal human bone marrow (27).

It is not known how the number of receptors for erythropoietin changes when the earliest erythroid progenitors differentiate into CFU-E and proerythroblasts. However, a study by Sawada and co-workers indicated very low numbers of erythropoietin receptors on purified BFU-E and an increase in receptor number as these BFU-E matured to CFU-E in culture (28). The low number of receptors for erythropoietin on cell lines which are multipotent (such as DA1, IC2, and FDCP2) reinforce the idea that the earliest erythroid cells have low number of receptors. The finding that some murine erythroleukemia cells increase the number of receptors when induced by chemicals has been interpreted as showing the shift of an earlier progenitor to a more mature erythroid stage (29,30).

A recent study found that erythropoietin receptors on hamster yolk sac erythroid cells varied 20-fold between the 8th and 13th days of gestation, reaching a maximum of 700 receptors/cell on the 10th day of gestation. Surprisingly, a single class of erythropoietin receptors was detected on each day, but the binding affinity varied 40-fold from 10 pM on day 8 to 376 pM on day 13 (31). This finding is remarkable in that a molecular mechanism for changing the binding affinity of a receptor on a cell through a continuum of different affinities is unprecedented. Although the authors suggested the above possibility, the more likely explanation is that the earliest cells have very-high-affinity receptors and that this population of cells is diluted with another population of erythroid cells of normal binding affinity (K_d of 500 pM) in the following days.

There is some evidence that a subpopulation of FVA cells has very-high-affinity receptors for erythropoietin similar in binding affinity to the value of 10 pM described for day 8 yolk sac erythroid cells. Autoradiography of ^{125}I-erythropoietin bound to FVA cells at a saturating concentration reveals a relatively homogeneous population of cells containing bound ^{125}I-erythropoietin. Reducing the concentration of ^{125}I-erythropoietin to a point where mostly high-affinity receptors are occupied also shows a fairly homogeneous distribution of grains among the cells. However, reducing the concentration of ^{125}I-erythropoietin to physiologic levels of 10 to 50 mU/ml shows that a minor population of cells (10 percent or less) has a moderate grain count, whereas the majority of cells have no grains (unpublished data). The number of these cells labeled with ^{125}I-erythropoietin correlates with the number of FVA cells that differentiate at suboptimal levels of the hormone. It is not certain whether these cells are unique because they have only a high-affinity-receptor or because they have an elevated number of receptors. Because of the low frequency of these cells, binding studies of the whole cell population do not detect these high-affinity receptors for erythropoietin. Proteolytic digestion of the cell surface can shift the binding constant of ^{125}I-erythropoietin to as low as 9 pM. This is in the range of the physiologic concentration of erythropoietin (30 mU/ml = 8 pM) and may be the maximal affinity of the receptor for erythropoietin. It will be of great interest to learn how the affinity of the erythropoietin receptor is modulated on the molecular level. Moreover, resolving the problem of how a minor subpopulation of erythroid cells expresses the receptor with a maximal affinity for the hormone while the remaining cells have receptors with binding constants that are 10- to 100-fold higher (less able to bind erythropoietin) will be of great importance to understanding how erythropoietin regulates erythropoiesis.

Direct studies of human erythroid cells may reveal the involvement of erythropoietin receptors in the pathologic state. Sawada and co-workers developed a method for purifying burst-forming units-erythroid from human blood (16,26,28). BFU-E can then be cultured in vitro in the presence of erythropoietin to give rise to a sufficient number of colony-forming units-erythroid so that binding studies can be performed with ^{125}I-erythropoietin directly. As mentioned previously, these CFU-E have high- and low-affinity receptors for erythropoietin similar to receptors in other cell types (16) and the BFU-E have very low levels of receptors as judged by autoradiography of bound ^{125}I-erythropoietin (26). (BFU-E are purified in insufficient numbers for direct experiments.) These cells can be procured from individuals who have hematopoietic disorders to see if the receptors for erythropoietin are altered in these disease states. Thus far, the receptors for erythropoietin on CFU-E from patients with polycythemia vera have been studied. Although a hypersensitivity of these cells to erythropoietin has been proposed, the CFU-E from polycythemia vera had normal numbers of receptors; surprisingly, however, the high-affinity receptors were absent (32).

Receptors for erythropoietin are found predominantly on mature erythroid progenitor cells and early precursor cells; however, receptors have also been identified on mouse megakaryocytes (33) and in placenta from rodents (34). The first finding is consistent with the reported effects of erythropoietin on the numbers of megakaryocytes that develop in cultures of murine bone marrow (35). However, the effect is mostly restricted to the megakaryocytes as erythropoietin has only a slight if any effect on the number of platelets in vivo.

Receptors for erythropoietin in the placentas of mice were identified as a result of the finding that ^{125}I-erythropoietin could pass from the maternal circulation to the fetus (36). The transfer experiment was conducted when the mRNA coding for erythropoietin could not be identified in the mouse fetal liver or other fetal tissue. The transplacental transfer of erythropoietin suggests that the low-affinity receptors for erythropoietin in the placenta are the mediators of this transport, but this is not yet proved.

The Endocytosis of Erythropoietin and Metabolism of the Receptor

Binding of ^{125}I-erythropoietin to FVA cells was observed to be twofold greater at 37°C than at 0°C. Because this is typical for ligands that are internalized by receptor-mediated endocytosis, this possibility was pursued. Removal of surface-bound erythropoietin by a high-salt, pH 2.5 wash or by digestion with proteases demonstrated endocytosis of erythropoietin within 1 minute of adding ^{125}I-erythropoietin to the cells. In a time course study, surface-bound erythropoietin first accumulated and then declined as radioactivity in the cell interior became greater than that at the surface. ^{125}I-Erythropoietin was bound to the surface at 0°C, and the distribution of radioactivity among the cell surface, the cell interior, and the medium was examined at intervals after the FVA cells were washed and then warmed to 37°C. Surface-bound ^{125}I-erythropoietin declined as radioactivity accumulated inside the cell. After 30 minutes, the radioactivity inside the cell declined as radioactivity was secreted into the medium. Analysis of the medium revealed that the majority of radioactivity was [^{125}I]iodotyrosine, which was the product of the degradation of ^{125}I-erythropoietin within the cell. Inhibition of lysosomal function with NH_4Cl and chloroquine greatly reduced the degradation of internalized ^{125}I-erythropoietin, which suggested the degradation of erythropoietin in lysosomes after endocytosis. All of the above-discussed studies in FVA cells (9) were repeated in human CFU-E by Sawada et al. (16). Subsequent reports documented the internalization of [^{35}S]erythropoietin in erythroid cells from the spleens of anemic mice (21) and demonstrated internalization of ^{125}I-erythropoietin in TSA8 murine erythroleukemia cells and fetal mouse liver cells (17). Mufson and Gesner reported that ^{125}I-erythropoietin bound to the receptor for erythropoietin but that the ^{125}I-erythropoietin was not endocytosed (21); however, this is completely contradictory to the other reports using ^{125}I-erythropoietin as well as to our studies showing that ^{125}I-erythropoietin, [^{3}H]erythropoietin, and [^{35}S]erythropoietin were equally endocytosed.

The fate of the receptor for erythropoietin after the receptor-mediated endocytosis of ^{125}I-erythropoietin into the cell is not known. By analogy to the metabolism of other growth factors and hormones, the erythropoietin receptor will probably follow one or both of two pathways within the cell. In the first pathway, the receptor and hormone are both degraded in the lysosomes after endocytosis into the cell. This is the fate of the epidermal growth factor receptor (37). In the second pathway, the receptor can recycle to the surface to bind another ligand after the initial endocytosis of the receptor-ligand complex. In the case of the transferrin receptor, the ligand and receptor both are recycled back to the surface of the cell after the internalization of the receptor and the iron-loaded transferrin complex (37). Insulin and low-density lipoprotein are degraded when endocytosed, but the receptors are recycled to the cell surface (37). The acidic nature of endosomes typically results in dissociation of peptide hormones and growth factors from the receptors. Thus, the receptor can recycle when the ligand is degraded in the lysosomes. Because bound erythropoietin is released from the receptor at a pH equal to or less than 4.0, it is possible that the fates of erythropoietin and the receptor diverge after internalization into an acidic endosome, with the receptor recycling to the surface even though the erythropoietin is degraded.

In the case of receptors that are degraded after endocytosis, such as the receptor for epidermal growth factor, the number of surface receptors is downregulated to a much lower (10 to 20 percent of initial) steady state level. An equilibrium is reached between new syntheses of receptors and degradation after treatment of the cells with the growth factor. When FVA cells (9), fetal mouse liver cells (21), or TSA8 cells were exposed to ^{125}I-erythropoietin (17), the ^{125}I-erythropoietin that bound to the surface of the cells increased during the first 30 minutes and then fell to 75 to 50 percent of the maximum by 2 hours. These experiments are inconclusive because the downregulation is small; in the case of FVA and fetal mouse liver cells, erythroid maturation could account for the loss of receptors. In the case of FVA cells, mouse regenerating CFU-E, and fetal mouse liver cells, downregulation of high-affinity receptors occurs to a greater extent than that of low-affinity receptors for erythropoietin. Because the low-affinity receptors are endocytosed equally well as the high-affinity receptors (34), these studies suggest the possibility of recycling of low-affinity receptors and the degradation of high-affinity receptors.

Recent experiments in our laboratory show evidence of erythropoietin receptor degradation as the mechanism of downregulation of the receptor in HCD33 and HCD57 cells exposed to erythropoietin (22). These cells have only the lower-affinity receptors for erythropoietin but require erythropoietin for survival and proliferation. HCD33 and HCD57 cells do not differentiate in response to erythropoietin. When these cells are taken from cultures that contain erythropoietin, they have 400 to 600 receptors for erythropoietin per cell. However, the receptor number increases 5- to 10-fold when erythropoietin is removed from the culture. Upon subsequent reculture in the presence of ^{125}I-erythropoietin, the receptor number is downregulated to 10 to 20 percent by 24 hours in culture. The recovery of erythropoietin receptors after the downregulation requires protein synthesis. This result is consistent with the downregulation of erythropoietin receptors through degradation and the subsequent upregulation of receptors when erythropoietin is removed from the environment through synthesis of new receptors.

The Structure of the Receptor

Chemical cross-linking of ^{125}I-erythropoietin bound to plasma membranes from FVA cells identified two proteins as the receptor for erythropoietin (38). These two ^{125}I-erythropoietin cross-linked proteins are bands of 140 and 125 kd molecular mass on polyacrylamide gel electrophoresis in the presence of sodium dodecyl sulfate (SDS-PAGE). Subtraction of the molecular mass of erythropoietin in this SDS-PAGE system (40 kd) from the molecular mass of the cross-linked protein results in the apparent molecular mass of 100 and 85 kd for the receptor proteins. Our recent results with a radiolabeled, photoactivatable, cleavable cross-linker attached to erythropoietin showed that the true molecular masses of these two proteins are 105 and 90 kd (39). This experiment involved the transfer of the radiolabeled, photoactive group to the receptor proteins followed by the cleavage of the cross-linker molecule so that erythropoietin was no longer cross-linked to the radiolabeled receptor. Therefore, the initial cross-linking studies with bifunctional cross-linkers gave a very close estimation of the molecular mass of the erythropoietin receptor.

The two receptor proteins labeled by cross-linking to ^{125}I-erythropoietin are not disulfide-bridged subunits of a larger receptor complex. Some workers reported that these subunits are connected by disulfide bridges such that the receptor is so large a molecule that it does not enter the gel in SDS-PAGE (11,18,20,40). However, a number of reports show no disulfide bridging of these subunits (15,29,34,38,41–43). The observation of a high-molecular-weight receptor composed of disulfide-bridged subunits seems to be an artifact of incomplete solubilization of the cross-linked membranes such that free ^{125}I-erythropoietin and cross-linked ^{125}I-erythropoietin are trapped at the top of the stacking gel and running gel (41).

Subsequent to our report of the structure of the receptor for erythropoietin in FVA cells as proteins of 100 and 85 kd (38), others reported a similar structure in fetal mouse liver erythroid cells and cell lines. Todokoro et al. reported the structure of the receptor in SKT6 cells as proteins of 119, 94, and 63 kd (42), with only the 63-kd protein in T3C1, K-1, GM86 (murine erythroleukemia clone 745), and 707 cells, which are not responsive to erythropoietin (43). These authors claimed that the lack of erythropoietin responsiveness in these cells was due to a mutant erythropoietin receptor; however, erythropoietin receptors on murine eurythroleukemia cells, clone 745, in our laboratory have the identical cross-linked structure as FVA cells (i.e., 100- and 85-kd proteins) (34). Broudy et al. (29) and Tojo et al. (30) also published the same structure for the erythropoietin receptor in murine erythroleukemia cells not responsive to erythropoietin. Mayeux et al. reported the structure of the erythropoietin receptor as proteins of 94 and 78 kd in rat fetal liver erythroid cells (40), whereas we found the 100- and 85-kd proteins in rat placenta (and mouse placenta) (34). The receptor of a normal human CFU-E was identified as proteins of 100 and 90 kd (34), which is in close agreement with the report of Hitomi et al. of the receptor in JK1 human erythroleukemia cells (18). In contrast to all of these studies, Pekonen et al. found two proteins of 86- and 41-kd molecular mass cross-linked to ^{125}I-erythropoietin human fetal tissue (44). In view of the sensitivity of the erythropoietin receptor to endogenous proteinase activity (41) and the generation of lower-molecular-mass proteolytic fragments of the cross-linked receptors when rigorous steps are not taken to control proteinase activity, the erythropoietin receptor is likely to exist as two proteins of approximately 105- and 90-kd molecular mass in all tissues. Reports of lower-molecular-mass erythropoietin receptors are most likely artifacts due to endogenous proteinase activities.

Proteolytic peptide mapping by the Cleveland method showed that the 105-kd protein and the 90-kd protein of the erythropoietin receptor have a similar if not identical amino acid sequence (41). Differential processing or post-translational modification by the cell may result in the expression of these two proteins from a common gene. Alternatively, the 90-kd protein may be a laboratory artifact that results from the cleavage of the 100-kd receptor during the binding and cross-linking of ^{125}I-erythropoietin.

D'Andrea, Wong, and Lodish cloned a cDNA presumably encoding the erythropoietin receptor from an expression library of murine erythroleukemia cells (clone 745) (12). Positive clones were identified by the presence of functional receptors for ^{125}I-erythropoietin on Cos cell transfectants. When the cDNA was sequenced, a protein of 507 amino acids was deduced; it had a single membrane-spanning region characteristic of transmembrane proteins. As described earlier, the Cos cells expressing the cloned receptor exhibited high- and low-affinity classes of receptors, whereas the murine erythroleukemia cell had only lower-affinity receptors. Surprisingly, when the ^{125}I-erythropoietin bound to Cos cell transfectants was cross-linked to the expressed receptors, proteins of 66 and 105 kd were identified as the binding proteins.

Work by D'Andrea and co-workers and also experiments in our laboratory with antibodies to synthetic peptides selected from the inferred sequence of the cloned receptor show that a 66-kd protein exists in transfected cells, FVA cells, and other erythroid cells. However, no 105-kd protein was detected by these antireceptor antisera. In the report by D'Andrea and co-workers, the 105-kd receptor was speculated to be either a highly glycosylated form of the 66-kd receptor or the multiple cross-linking of two receptor proteins and erythropoietin by the bifunctional cross-linkers (12).

In FVA cells Hosoi et al., using a monofunctional, photoactivatable, cleavable cross-linking derivative of erythropoietin (Denny-Jaffe erythropoietin), demonstrated that 105- and 90-kd proteins bind erythropoietin on the cell membrane. The monofunctional cross-linker labeled the exact same 140- and 125-kd bands as those complexed when bifunctional cross-linkers were used. Furthermore, the cleavage of the iodinated, cleavable cross-linked erythropoietin-receptor complex with sodium dithionite resulted in ligand-free labeled proteins of 105- and 90-kd molecular mass (39). These results prove that cross-linking artifacts do not explain the relationship of the 105- and 90-kd proteins, identified on virtually every erythroid cell, with the cloned 66-kd receptor. Indeed, the antipeptide antibodies detected a 66-kd protein by Western blotting and immunoprecipitation which was also shown by cross-linking in Cos cell transfectants; however, it is not understood why the 66-kd protein is present in cells where only the 105- and/or 90-kd proteins are detected by cross-linking.

Although the 66-kd protein seems to be a glycosylated form of the 55-kd peptide inferred from the cDNA sequence, there is no evidence that the 105- and 90-kd proteins are more highly glycosylated species of the cloned erythropoietin receptor. Indeed, digestion of the cross-linked erythropoietin receptor-^{125}I-erythropoietin complex with mixtures of N- and O-glycanases and reductive alkaline hydrolysis failed to detect a significant level of carbohydrate (N- or O-linked) on the 105- and 90-kd receptor proteins even though the carbohydrate on erythropoietin was completely removed (45,46). The finding of only one potential site for N-linked glycosylation on the extracellular domain of the cloned receptor (12) is more in line with glycosylation on the order of the 66-kd protein (11-kd carbohydrate) than with that necessary to convert the 55-kd peptide to 105 kd.

The coexpression of the 105- and 66-kd receptors on Cos cell transfectants suggests but does not prove that the 105-kd protein is derived from the cloned receptor. The following origins of the 105-kd protein are possible: (a) The cloned receptor protein is somehow post-translationally modified to the larger form (apparently by means other than extensive glycosylation and disulfide bridges). (b) The 105-kd protein is constitutively expressed in the Cos cells and forms a complex with the 66-kd receptor protein. (c) The 105-kd receptor protein is induced in Cos cells transfected with the cDNA encoding the 66-kd receptor such that both proteins are expressed. Additional work is required to resolve these questions.

The cloned erythropoietin receptor, 66-kd protein, belongs to a family of growth factor receptors which includes the interleukin 2 receptor β chain (p70), the interleukin 4 receptor, and the interleukin 6 receptor, as well as receptors for prolactin and growth hormone (47,48). Recent reports also include the granulocyte-macrophage colony-simulating factor (GM-CSF) receptor (49) and the interleukin 3 and interleukin 7 receptors (50,51) in this family. The high-affinity form of the interleukin 2 receptor is a heterodimer of α and β chains which can bind interleukin 2 separately, however, with much less affinity than the heterodimer (52). Several subunits of the interleukin 3 receptor have also been proposed, and the receptor for interleukin 6 seems to interact with a 130-kd signal transduction protein (53). This precedent increases the likelihood that the 105- and 90-kd proteins cross-linked to ^{125}I-erythropoietin may be additional proteins not related in amino acid sequence to the 66-kd receptor that has been cloned.

In addition to the similarity of the GM-CSF receptor to the receptor for erythropoietin in predicted amino acid sequence, these receptors are similar in the twofold discrepancy between the predicted molecular weight of the GM-CSF receptor from the cloned cDNA (43 kd) and the molecular weight estimated by chemical cross-linking (85 kd) (49).

The interleukin 6 receptor is a moderately glycosylated protein (30-kd carbohydrate, 50-kd peptide with 5 sites for N-glycosylation) (53). More extensive glycosylation may explain the discrepancy in the size predicted from the cDNA compared to the size of the mature receptor proteins for GM-CSF (49) and erythropoietin (12) and to a lesser extent in the interleukin 2 β chain (70 kd compared to the cDNA prediction of 58 kd) (52), interleukin 3 receptor (105 to 140 kd compared to the cDNA prediction of 95 kd) (50), and interleukin 4 receptor (140 kd compared to the cDNA prediction of 85 kd) (48). However, this possibility is more likely in the GM-CSF receptor, interleukin 2 β chain, and interleukin 4 receptor because there are 11, 5, and 5 possible sites, respectively, for N-glycosylation in the extracellular domain of these proteins compared to 1 site in the receptor for erythropoietin and two sites in the interleukin 3 receptor. As neither the GM-CSF nor the erythropoietin receptors contain disulfide-linked subunits, the cross-linking may be identifying another protein in a complex with either of these receptors, as occurs for the interleukin 2 receptor, or alternatively a non-typically post-translationally modified form of the receptor.

Antibodies directed against synthetic peptides that correspond to predicted sequences from the cloned receptor for erythropoietin interact with a 66-kd protein in a number of erythroid cells, but there is no reactivity to proteins in the range of 100-kd, supporting the idea of separate proteins. D'Andrea suggested that these antipeptide antibodies can immunoprecipitate both the 66- and the 105-kd proteins cross-linked to ^{125}I-erythropoietin. However, it is not known whether the antibody interacted with the 105-kd protein directly or with the 66-kd protein complexed to the 105-kd protein. Experiments are under way to resolve these conflicting experimental results.

In summary, erythropoietin interacts with proteins of 105 and 90 kd on erythroid cells. Cross-linking artifacts do not explain the relationship of the 105- and 90-kd proteins cross-linked to ^{125}I-erythropoietin in erythroid cells with the 66-kd protein that is the product of the cDNA identified as the receptor for erythropoietin by expression cloning. At present, it is possible that the 66-kd receptor protein is modified to become a 105-kd protein or that the erythropoietin receptor is a complex of subunits such that an unrelated 105-kd protein (and/or 90-kd proteins) exist in a complex with the 66-kd protein.

ACKNOWLEDGMENTS

This work supported by National Institutes of Health grants DK-39781 and DK-1555. I thank Mary Jane Rich for typing this manuscript. The author is a scholar of the Leukemia Society of America.

REFERENCES

1. Krantz SB, Goldwasser E. Specific binding of erythropoietin to spleen cells infected with the anemia strain of Friend virus. Proc Natl Acad Sci USA 1984;81:7574–8.
2. Chang SC-S, Sikkema D, Goldwasser E. Evidence for an erythropoietin receptor protein on rat bone marrow cells. Biochem Biophys Res Commun 1974;57:399–405.
3. Koury MJ, Bondurant MC, Duncan DT, Krantz SB, Hankins WD. Specific differentiation events induced by erythropoietin in cells infected in vitro with the anemia strain of Friend virus. Proc Natl Acad Sci USA 1982;71:635–9.
4. Bondurant M, Koury M, Krantz S, Blevins T, Duncan D. Isolation of erythropoietin-sensitive cells from Friend virus-infected marrow cultures: characterization of the erythropoietin response. Blood 1983;61:751–8.
5. Koury MJ, Sawyer ST, Bondurant MC. Splenic erythroblasts in anemia-inducing Friend disease: a source of cells for studies of erythropoietin-mediated differentiation. J Cell Physiol 1984;121:526–32.
6. Sawyer ST, Koury MJ, Bondurant MC. Large scale procurement of erythropoietin-responsive erythroid cells. Methods Enzymol 1987;147:340–7.
7. Goldwasser E. Erythropoietin and red cell differentiation. In: Cunningham D, Goldwasser E, Watson J, Fox DF, eds. Control of cellular division and development, part A. New York: AR Liss, 1981:487–94.
8. Weiss TL, Kung CKH, Goldwasser E. Quantitation of erythropoietin binding to bone marrow cells. J Cell Biochem 1985;27:57–65.
9. Sawyer ST, Krantz SB, Goldwasser E. Binding and receptor-mediated endocytosis of erythropoietin in Friend virus infected erythroid cells. J Biol Chem 1987;262:5554–62.
10. Mayeux P, Billat C, Jacquot R. Murine erythroleukemia cells (Friend cells) possess high-affinity binding sites for erythropoietin. FEBS Lett 1987;211:229–33.
11. Sasaki R, Yanagawa S, Hitomi K, Chiba H. Characterization of erythropoietin receptor of murine erythroid cells. Eur J Biochem 1987;168:43–8.
12. D'Andrea AD, Lodish HF, Wong G. Expression cloning of the murine erythropoietin receptor. Cell 1989;57:277–85.
13. Fukamachi H, Saito T, Tojo A, Kitamura T, Urabe A, Takaku F. Binding of erythropoietin to CFU-E derived from fetal mouse liver cells. Exp Hematol 1987;15:833–7.
14. Tojo A, Fukamachi H, Kasuga M, Urabe A, Takaku F. Identification of erythropoietin receptors on fetal liver erythroid cells. Biochem Biophys Res Commun 1987;148:433–48.
15. Landschulz KT, Noyes AN, Rogers O, Boyer SH. Erythropoietin receptors on murine colony-forming units: natural history. Blood 1989;73:1476–86.
16. Sawada K, Krantz SB, Sawyer ST, Civin CI. Quantitation of specific binding of erythropoietin to human erythroid colony-forming cells. J Cell Physiol 1988;137:337–45.
17. Fukamachi H, Tojo A, Saito T, et al. Internalization of radioiodinated erythropoietin and the ligand-induced modulation of its receptor in murine erythroleukemia cells. Int J Cell Cloning 1987;5:299–319.
18. Hitomi K, Fujita K, Sasaki R, et al. Erythropoietin receptor of a human

leukemic cell line with erythroid characteristics. Biochem Biophys Res Commun 1988;154:902–9.

19. Hitomi K, Masuda S, Ito K, Ueda M, Sasaki R. Solubilization and characterization of erythropoietin receptors from transplantable mouse erythroblastic leukemic cells. Biochem Biophys Res Commun 1989;160:1140–8.

20. McCaffery PJ, Fraser JK, Lin F-K, Berridge MV. Subunit structure of the erythropoietin receptor. J Biol Chem 1989;264:10507–12.

21. Mufson RA, Gesner TG. Binding and internalization of recombinant human erythropoietin in murine erythroid precursor cells. Blood 1987;69: 1485–90.

22. Sawyer ST, Hankins WD. Metabolism of erythropoietin in erythropoietin-dependent cell lines [Abstract]. Blood 1988;72:440.

23. Sakaguchi M, Koishihara Y, Tsuda H, et al. The expression of functional erythropoietin receptors on an interleukin-3 dependent cell line. Biochem Biophys Res Commun 1987;146:7–12.

24. Tsao CJ, Tojo A, Fukamachi H, Kitamura T, Saito T, Urabe A. Expression of the functional erythropoietin receptors on interleukin 3-dependent murine cell lines. J Immunol 1988;140:89–93.

25. Koury MJ, Bondurant MC. Maintenance by erythropoietin on viability and maturation of murine erythroid precursor cells. J Cell Physiol 1988; 137:65–74.

26. Sawada K, Krantz SB, Kans JS, et al. Purification of human erythroid colony-forming units and demonstration of specific binding of erythropoietin. J Clin Invest 1987;80:357–66.

27. Fraser JK, Lin FK, Berridge MV. Expression of high affinity receptors on human bone marrow and HEL cells. Exp Hematol 1988;16:836–42.

28. Sawada K, Krantz SB, Dai C-H, et al. Purification of human blood burst-forming units-erythroid and demonstration of the evolution of erythropoietin receptors. J Cell Physiol 1990;142:219–30.

29. Broudy VC, Lin N, Egrie J, et al. Identification of the receptor for erythropoietin on human and murine erythroleukemia cells and modulation by phorbol ester and dimethyl sulfoxide. Proc Natl Acad Sci USA 1988;85:6513–7.

30. Tojo A, Kukamachi H, Saito T, Kasuga M, Urabe A, Takaku F. Induction of the receptor for erythropoietin in MEL cells after DMSO treatment. Cancer Res 1988;48:1818–22.

31. Boussios T, Bertles JF, Goldwasser E. Erythropoietin receptor characteristics during the ontogeny of hamster yolk sac erythroid cells. J Biol Chem 1989;264:16017–21.

32. Means RT, Krantz SB, Sawyer ST, Gilbert HS. Erythropoietin receptors in polycythemia vera. J Clin Invest 1989;84:1340–4.

33. Fraser JK, Tan AS, Lin FK, Berridge MV. Expression of specific high affinity binding sites for erythropoietin on rat and mouse megakaryocytes. Exp Hematol 1989;17:10–6.

34. Sawyer ST, Krantz SB, Sawada K-I. Receptors for erythropoietin in mouse and human erythroid cells and placenta. Blood 1989;74:103–9.

35. Berridge MV, Fraser JK, Carter JM, Lin FK. Effects of recombinant human erythropoietin on megakaryocytes and on platelet production in the rat. Blood 1988;72:970–7.

36. Koury MJ, Bondurant MC, Graber SE, Sawyer ST. Erythropoietin mes-

senger RNA levels in developing mice and transfer of ^{125}I-erythropoietin by the placenta. J Clin Invest 1988;82:154–9.

37. Goldstein JL, Brown MS, Anderson RGW, Russell DW, Schneider WJ. Receptor-mediated endocytosis. Ann Rev Cell Biol 1985;1:1–39.

38. Sawyer ST, Krantz SB, Luna J. Identification of the receptor for erythropoietin in spleen cells infected with the anemia strain of Friend virus. Proc Natl Acad Sci USA 1987;84:3690–4.

39. Hosoi T, Sawyer ST, Krantz SB. Identification of erythropoietin receptor in a ligand-free form with ^{125}I-labeled, photoreactive, cleavable cross-linker (Denny-Jaffe reagent). Biochemistry 1991;30:329–35.

40. Mayeux P, Billat C, Jacquot R. The erythropoietin receptor of rat erythroid progenitor cells. J Biol Chem 1987;262:13985–90.

41. Sawyer ST. The two proteins of the erythropoietin receptor are structurally similar. J Biol Chem 1989;264:13343–7.

42. Todokoro K, Kanazawa S, Amanuma H, Ikawa Y. Specific binding of erythropoietin to its receptor on responsive mouse erythroleukemia cells. Proc Natl Acad Sci USA 1987;84:4126–30.

43. Todokoro K, Kanazawa S, Amanuma H, Ikawa Y. Characterization of erythropoietin receptor on erythropoietin-unresponsive mouse erythroleukemia cells. Biochim Biophys Acta 1988;943:326–30.

44. Pekonen F, Rosenlof K, Rutanen E-M, Fyhrquist F. Erythropoietin binding sites in human foetal tissues. Acta Endocrinol (Copenh) 1987;116:561–7.

45. Hosoi T, Sawyer ST, Krantz SB. The receptor for erythropoietin lacks detectable glycosylation [Abstract]. Exp Hematol 1988;16:118.

46. Mayeux P, Casadevall N, Muller O, Lacombe C. Glycosylation of the murine erythropoietin receptor. FEBS Lett 1990;269:167–70.

47. Bazan JF. A novel family of growth factor receptors: a common binding domain in the growth hormone, prolactin, erythropoietin, and IL-6 receptors, and IL-2 receptor β-chain. Biochem Biophys Res Commun 1989;164:788–95.

48. Mosley B, Bachman MP, March CJ, et al. The murine interleukin-4 receptor: molecular cloning and characterization of secreted and membrane bound forms. Cell 1989;59:335–48.

49. Gearing DP, King JA, Gough M, Nicola NA. Expression cloning of a receptor for granulocyte-macrophage colony-stimulating factor. EMBO J 1989;8:3667–76.

50. Itoh N, Yonehara S, Schreurs J, et al. Cloning of an interleukin-3 receptor gene, a member of a distinct receptor gene family. Science 1990;247:324–7.

51. Goodwin RG, Friend D, Ziegler SF, et al. Cloning of the human and murine interleukin-7 receptors: demonstration of a soluble form and homology to a new receptor superfamily. Cell 1990;60:941–51.

52. Hatakeyama M, Tsudo M, Minamoto S, et al. Interleukin-2 receptor β chain gene: generation of three receptor forms by clone human α and β chain cDNA's. Science 1989;244:551–6.

53. Taga T, Hibi M, Hirata Y, et al. Interleukin-6 triggers the association of its receptor with a possible signal transducer, gp 130. Cell 1989;58:573–81.

Chapter 9

The Molecular Biology of
Erythropoietin Receptors

Gordon G. Wong, Simon S. Jones,
and Alan D. D'Andrea

To understand the factors and mechanisms that regulate the formation of red cells requires an understanding not only of erythropoietin
but also of its cognate receptors. In vivo, erythropoietin directs erythropoietic stem cells to proliferate and differentiate. Erythroid progenitor
cells are found only in hematopoietic compartments such as the spleen
and bone marrow and are present at low frequency (1 per 10^4 to 10^5
cells) (1). The development of these cells into mature erythrocytes is
regulated predominantly by erythropoietin, secreted by the kidney in
response to varying oxygen tension within the blood. The concentration
of erythropoietin in the intact animal and within the hematopoietic
compartments is exceedingly low compared to the typical concentrations of circulating hormones (2). When there are low concentrations
of a regulatory protein, one would expect the responsive cells to have
a large number of high-affinity cell surface receptor complexes to ensure signal detection. However, erythropoietin-responsive cells have a
relatively low number of erythropoietin-binding sites (100 to 1000 sites
per cell) (3–13) and are likely to require even fewer actual molecules
of erythropoietin to complex with the receptor to trigger a biologic response. Therefore, our understanding of the biology and biochemistry
of erythropoietin and of the interaction with the erythropoietin receptor
has until recently been limited by the experimental inaccessibility of
pure target cell populations, as well as by a dearth of pure erythropoietin and erythropoietin receptor protein.

Despite these technical problems, it has been possible to surmise the
following points. First, there seem to be two classes of erythropoietin

133

receptor-binding complexes, defined by their affinities for erythropoietin: high (20 to 100 pM) and low (300 to 700 pM) erythropoietin-
binding affinity (3–8,13). Second, there are two classes of erythropoietic progenitor cells: cells with both high- and low-affinity erythropoietin-binding sites (3–6) and cells with just low-affinity binding
sites (7,8,11,13). Third, the erythropoietin receptor complex, irrespective of the cell type or binding affinity, consists of two protein species
with molecular masses of 85 and 100 kd (4,6,8,12,13). Finally, cross-
linking studies with radioiodinated erythropoietin suggested that the
85 and 105 kd proteins seem to have amino acids in common (14).
These observations, however important in themselves, do not lead to a
mechanism of action for erythropoietin or to an understanding of signal
transduction by erythropoietin-receptor protein complex.

The Strategy for Isolating the Genes That Encode the Erythropoietin Receptor Protein

The lack of erythropoietin receptor protein prohibited any complementary ribonucleic acid (cDNA) gene isolation strategies based on a
structural route such as protein amino acid sequence or by an anti-
erythropoietin receptor antibody. As an alternative, we exploited the
ability of Cos cells, SV40-transformed African green monkey kidney
cells, to express functional heterologous gene products from cloned
cDNA genes.

The theories and methods of this heterologous expression-function
cDNA gene isolation strategy and its application to genes encoding secreted proteins, receptors, and DNA-binding proteins were reviewed
(15). In brief, the experimental strategy is to convert a mRNA source
encoding the gene product into cDNA. The cDNA is cloned into a bacterial plasmid vector to generate a library of genes. The bacterial plasmid
vector used contains all necessary functional elements for the transcription and translation of the cloned cDNA gene in mammalian cells. When
this recombinant cDNA plasmid is introduced by transfection into the
appropriate mammalian host cell, the promoter and expression elements flanking the cDNA gene direct the heterologous expression of the
gene to yield the putative protein of interest. The heterologously expressed protein can be characterized and identified by biochemical
structure (e.g., reactivity with an antibody), biologic function (e.g., mitogenic activity in a growth factor assay), or biochemical function (e.g.,
the ability to bind a specific ligand). This method has been used to iso-

late the genes for numerous hematopoietic regulatory proteins, receptors, and DNA-binding proteins (15).

In this experimental strategy, we assumed the following: (a) the erythropoietin-receptor complex consists of at least one protein that, by itself, can be targeted to the cell surface and can bind erythropoietin; (b) the binding affinity for erythropoietin of such a protein is equivalent to the native receptor (e.g., in the nanomolar range); (c) the erythropoietin-binding protein is encoded by a single mRNA; and (d) the mRNA can be heterologously expressed in Cos cells to yield functional erythropoietin-binding protein.

The Murine Erythropoietin Receptor Gene

The likelihood of isolating an erythropoietin receptor cDNA gene by the heterologous expression-function cDNA gene-cloning strategy is dependent on both the experimental methods and the frequency of the relevant gene within the cDNA library. The frequency of any particular cDNA gene, and presumably the frequency of the mRNA encoding a particular protein, is generally proportional to its concentration. Although primary sources of erythropoietin-responsive cells and, hence, erythropoietin receptor mRNA are accessible, it is technically difficult to generate sufficiently pure populations of the erythropoietin-responsive cells needed to ensure that the frequency of the putative erythropoietin receptor mRNA and hence cDNA gene is within the limits of the detection system.

To avoid the technical difficulties of purifying primary populations of erythropoietin-responsive cells, we chose an in vitro cultured murine erythroleukemia cell line, derived from the transformation of erythroblasts by the Friend virus complex (16,17), as the source of erythropoietin receptor protein mRNA. Binding experiments with iodinated recombinant human erythropoietin showed that murine erythroleukemia cells were found to have about 800 to 1000 erythropoietin-binding sites per cell, with an affinity of K_d 240 pM (18). This result was consistent with that found for erythroblasts isolated from murine spleen and bone marrow (4,6,8,10). Paradoxically, although murine erythroleukemia cells bind erythropoietin, they are not physiologically responsive to erythropoietin (16,17) and thus may have an aberrant erythropoietin receptor protein complex.

mRNA was isolated from murine erythroleukemia cells, converted into cDNA, and cloned into the mammalian expression vector pXM (18) to generate a bacterial plasmid library of about 800,000 recombinants.

Within this population of cDNA genes are, presumably, the cDNA genes that encode complete and functional erythropoietin-binding protein. The recombinant plasmids were organized into sets or pools of 1000 individual plasmids introduced into a mammalian host cell and were tested for their ability to direct the Cos cell expression of a cell surface protein that bound radioiodinated erythropoietin with nanomolar affinities.

From an analysis of 200 sets of recombinant cDNA plasmids, two sets were found to yield, on transfection, Cos cells that bound erythropoietin. Within each set we presumed that a single recombinant plasmid encoded the erythropoietin-binding protein, and so each set of recombinant plasmids was subdivided and analyzed. With each successive partition of the recombinant plasmids into sets with fewer members, there was a concomitant increase in the amount of erythropoietin bound by Cos cells transfected with the relevant set. Eventually, a single recombinant plasmid was isolated from each set (clone 141 and clone 190).

Functional Analysis of Putative Erythropoietin Receptor cDNA Clones 141 and 190

Cos cells transfected with clone 141, clone 190, or carrier DNA were tested for binding of radioiodinated erythropoietin at various concentrations at 4°C. Cos cells transfected with either clone 141 or 190 bound about 40 times the amount of radioiodinated erythropoietin bound by Cos cells transfected with carrier DNA. The Cos cell-bound erythropoietin could be competitively displaced by unlabeled recombinant human erythropoietin but was unaffected by other growth factors such as insulin, transferrin, and interleukin 3. Scatchard plots of specific erythropoietin binding to Cos cells transfected with either clone yielded similar curves. Analysis of these plots indicated the presence of about 200,000 binding sites per Cos cell, with about 14 percent of the erythropoietin binding sites having an affinity of 30 pM and the remainder having an affinity of 210 pM.

Previous reports indicated that some murine erythroleukemia cell lines (19–21) and primary erythropoietic stem cell populations (3–11) have both low- and high-affinity erythropoietin receptors, although it is unclear whether both classes of receptor exist on the same cell or whether they reflect two cell populations. Paradoxically, specific erythropoietin binding experiments with the variant of the murine erythroleukemia cell line from which the cDNA clones were derived revealed only a single low-affinity (K_d of 240 pM) set of binding sites. We cannot discount, however, that there may be a small population of high-affinity receptors on murine erythroleukemia cells which, because of their low absolute number per cell, would elude detection. Therefore, although we can reconcile the binding affinities of heterologously expressed erythropoietin receptor protein with that of primary erythropoietin-responsive cells, we cannot, from this first analysis, explain how two different binding affinities can arise from a single gene.

Molecular Analysis of Putative Erythropoietin Receptor Gene Clones 141 and 190

The cDNA genes specific to each plasmid, clones 141 and 190, were excised and analyzed by restriction enzyme digestion. Clone 141 and clone 190 contained DNA fragments of 1.9 and 1.8 kilobasepairs, respectively, and yielded similar restriction enzyme maps. The nucleotide sequences of both clones were determined and were similar (18). A close inspection of the nucleic acid sequence of clone 141 revealed an internal 2-base pair deletion when compared to clone 190. Subsequent analysis of the genomic DNA sequence of clones 141 and 190 suggested that the 2-base pair deletion in clone 141 was a cloning artifact. The sequence of the cDNA gene contained in clone 190 is shown in Figure 9.1.

The 1713-nucleotide sequence of clone 190 has a single open reading frame of 507 amino acids with a 161-nucleotide 3'-noncoding region. From clone 141, which contained a longer 5'-noncoding region, no consensus sequence for translation initiation was found in the 5'-non-coding region. There are three in-frame stop codons 5' to the first methionine of the 507-amino acid open reading frame.

From inspection of the predicted 507-amino acid structure and analysis with the Kyte-Doolittle 1982 hydrophobicity and hydrophilicity algorithm (22), we deduced that the amino-terminal 23 amino acids following the first methionine are typical of leader sequences for secreted proteins. The predicted amino-terminal amino acid of the mature protein is alanine. In addition, a hydrophobic stretch of 23 amino acids was predicted for amino acids 250 to 272. The data suggested that clones 141 and 190 encode a single type I transmembrane protein with amino acids 1 to 249 in the extracellular space and amino acids 273 to 507 on the cytoplasmic side of the membrane.

Further inspection of the 507-amino acid reading frame revealed two potential sites for N-linked glycosylation, one extracellular and one in-

```
          -20                  0                   20                  40
TGAGCTTCCTGAAGCTAGGGCTGCATCATGGACAAACTCAGGGTGCCCCTCTGGCCTCGGGTAGGCCCCC          15
                           M   D   K   L   R   V   P   L   W   P   R   V   G   P   L

                 60                  ↓       80                  100
TCTGTCTCCTACTTGCTGGGGCAGCCTGGGCACCTTCACCCAGCCTCCCGGACCCCAAGTTTGAGAGCAA          38
  C   L   L   A   G   A   A   W   A   P   S   P   S   L   P   D   P   K   F   E   S   K

          120                 140                 160                 180
AGCGGCCCTGCTGGCATCCCGGGGCTCCGAAGAACTTCTGTGCTTCACCCAACGCTTGGAAGACTTGGTG          61
  A   A   L   L   A   S   R   G   S   E   E   L   L   C   F   T   Q   R   L   E   D   L   V

                 200                 220        _____        240
TGTTTCTGGGAGGAAGCGGCGAGCTCCGGGATGGACTTCAACTACAGCTTCTCATACCAGCTCGAGGGTG          85
  C   F   W   E   E   A   A   S   S   G   M   D   F   N   Y   S   F   S   Y   Q   L   E   G   E

          260                 280                 300                 320
AGTCACGAAAGTCATGTAGCCTGCACCAGGCTCCCACCGTCCGCGGCTCCGTGCGTTTCTGGTGTTCACT          108
  S   R   K   S   C   S   L   H   Q   A   P   T   V   R   G   S   V   R   F   W   C   S   L

                 340                 360                 380
GCCAACAGCGGACACATCGAGTTTTGTGCCGCTGGAGCTGCAGGTGACGGAGGCGTCCGGTTCTCCTCGC          131
  P   T   A   D   T   S   S   F   V   P   L   E   L   Q   V   T   E   A   S   G   S   P   R

          400                 420                 440                 460
TATCACCGCATCATCCATATCAATGAAGTAGTGCTCCTGGACGCCCCCGCGGGGCTGCTGGCGCGCCGGG          155
  Y   H   R   I   I   H   I   N   E   V   V   L   L   D   A   P   A   G   L   L   A   R   R   A

                 480                 500                 520
CAGAAGAGGGCAGCCACGTGGTGCTGCGCTGGCTGCCACCTCCTGGAGCACCTATGACCACCCACATCCG          178
  E   E   G   S   H   V   V   L   R   W   L   P   P   P   G   A   P   M   T   T   H   I   R

          540                 560                 580                 600
ATATGAAGTGGACGTGTCGGCAGGCAACCGGGCAGGAGGGGACACAAAGGGTGGAGGTCCTGGAAGGCCGC          201
  Y   E   V   D   V   S   A   G   N   R   A   G   G   T   Q   R   V   E   V   L   E   G   R

                 620                 640                 660
ACTGAGTGTGTTCTGAGCAACCTGCGGGGGCGGGACGCGCTACACCTTCGCTGTTCGAGCGCGCATGGCCG          225
  T   E   C   V   L   S   N   L   R   G   G   T   R   Y   T   F   A   V   R   A   R   M   A   E

          680                 700                 720                 740
AGCCGAGCTTCAGCGGATTCTGGAGTGCCTGGTCTGAGCCCGCGTCACTACTGACCGCTAGCGACCTGGA          248
  P   S   F   S   G   F   W   S   A   W   S   E   P   A   S   L   L   T   A   S   D   L   D

          760                 780                 800
CCCTCTCATCTTGACGCTGTCTCTCATTCTGGTCCTCATCTCGCTGTTGCTGACGGTTCTGGCCCTGCTG          271
  P   L   I   L   T   L   S   L   I   L   V   L   I   S   L   L   L   T   V   L   A   L   L

          820                 840                 860                 880
TCCCACCGCCGGACTCTGCAGCAGAAGATCTGGCCTGGCATCCCAAGCCCAGAGAGCGAGTTTGAGGGTC          295
  S   H   R   R   T   L   Q   Q   K   I   W   P   G   I   P   S   P   E   S   E   F   E   G   L
```

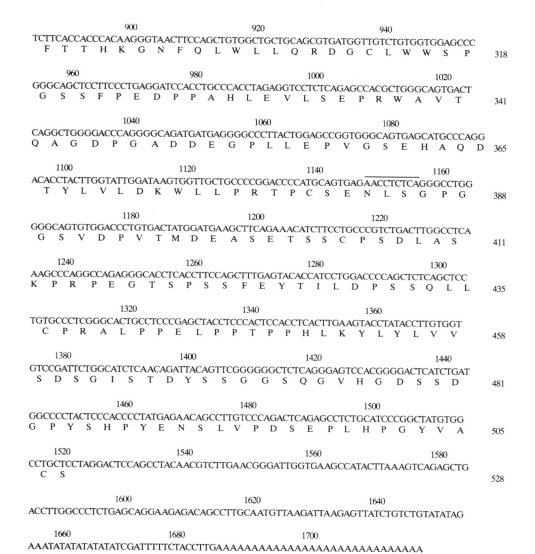

```
                900                920                     940
TCTTCACCACCCACAAGGGTAACTTCCAGCTGTGGCTGCTGCAGCGTGATGGTTGTCTGTGGTGGAGCCC
  F   T   T   H   K   G   N   F   Q   L   W   L   L   Q   R   D   G   C   L   W   W   S   P      318

       960                980                1000                 1020
GGGCAGCTCCTTCCCTGAGGATCCACCTGCCCACCTAGAGGTCCTCTCAGAGCCACGCTGGGCAGTGACT
  G   S   S   F   P   E   D   P   P   A   H   L   E   V   L   S   E   P   R   W   A   V   T      341

              1040                1060                1080
CAGGCTGGGGACCCAGGGGCAGATGATGAGGGGCCCTTACTGGAGCCGGTGGGCAGTGAGCATGCCCAGG
  Q   A   G   D   P   G   A   D   D   E   G   P   L   L   E   P   V   G   S   E   H   A   Q   D   365

      1100                1120                1140  _____ 1160
ACACCTACTTGGTATTGGATAAGTGGTTGCTGCCCCGGACCCCATGCAGTGAGAACCTCTCAGGGCCTGG
  T   Y   L   V   L   D   K   W   L   L   P   R   T   P   C   S   E   N   L   S   G   P   G      388

              1180                1200                1220
GGGCAGTGTGGACCCTGTGACTATGGATGAAGCTTCAGAAACATCTTCCTGCCCGTCTGACTTGGCCTCA
  G   S   V   D   P   V   T   M   D   E   A   S   E   T   S   S   C   P   S   D   L   A   S      411

      1240                1260                1280                1300
AAGCCCAGGCCAGAGGGCACCTCACCTTCCAGCTTTGAGTACACCATCCTGGACCCCAGCTCTCAGCTCC
  K   P   R   P   E   G   T   S   P   S   S   F   E   Y   T   I   L   D   P   S   S   Q   L   L   435

      1320                1340                1360
TGTGCCCTCGGGCACTGCCTCCCGAGCTACCTCCCACTCCACCTCACTTGAAGTACCTATACCTTGTGGT
  C   R   A   L   P   P   E   L   P   P   T   P   P   H   L   K   Y   L   Y   L   V   V      458

      1380                1400                1420                1440
GTCCGATTCTGGCATCTCAACAGATTACAGTTCGGGGGGCTCTCAGGGAGTCCACGGGGACTCATCTGAT
  S   D   S   G   I   S   T   D   Y   S   S   G   G   S   Q   G   V   H   G   D   S   S   D      481

              1460                1480                1500
GGCCCCTACTCCCACCCCTATGAGAACAGCCTTGTCCCAGACTCAGAGCCTCTGCATCCCGGCTATGTGG
  G   P   Y   S   H   P   Y   E   N   S   L   V   P   D   S   E   P   L   H   P   G   Y   V   A   505

      1520                1540                1560                1580
CCTGCTCCTAGGACTCCAGCCTACAACGTCTTGAACGGGATTGGTGAAGCCATACTTAAAGTCAGAGCTG
  C   S                                                                                   528

              1600                1620                1640
ACCTTGGCCCTCTGAGCAGGAAGAGACAGCCTTGCAATGTTAAGATTAAGAGTTATCTGTCTGTATATAG

      1660                1680                1700
AAATATATATATATATCGATTTTTCTACCTTGAAAAAAAAAAAAAAAAAAAAAAAAAAAAAAAAAA
```

Figure 9.1. The structure of the murine erythropoietin receptor. The putative mature amino terminus at residue 25 is indicated by an arrow. The sites of potential N-linked glycosylation are overlined. The putative transmembrane domain is underlined.

tracellular. In both the extracellular and the intracellular domain are a substantial number of serine (61) and threonine (24) residues that are potential sites for O-linked glycosylation and phosphorylation and also a significant number of aspartic acid, glutamic acid, and proline residues. The importance of the acidic amino acid residues is not immediately apparent, although the proline residues will certainly contribute to both the three-dimensional geometry and the apparent molecular weight of the putative erythropoietin receptor protein. The expected molecular mass of this putative erythropoietin receptor protein backbone is 55 kd.

From the predicted amino acid sequence of clones 141 and 190, no obvious protein domains can be assigned to either the role of ligand binding (e.g., immunoglobulin-type variable region) (23) or signal transduction (e.g., there is no protein kinase domain) (24). However, clone 141, which contained the two-base pair deletion within the putative intracellular domain, did not show any detectable differences in binding affinities for erythropoietin when compared to clone 190. Further biochemical characterization of the putative erythropoietin binding proteins encoded by clones 141 and 190 follows.

The Molecular Weight of Heterologously Expressed Murine Erythropoietin Receptor Protein

With unlimited resources, the ideal experimental route would be to isolate the erythropoietin-binding protein, heterologously expressed by Cos cells transfected with clone 190, and determine its amino acid structure. However, this is still a formidable task even with such an enriched receptor protein source. In addition, there would still be the formal requirement of purifying the erythropoietin-binding protein from the native source, murine erythroleukemia cells, to verify that structural identity was consistent with functional identity. Consequently, we elected to use an antibody specific for the putative erythropoietin receptor protein to address the above questions.

An antibody was generated to a synthetic peptide constructed from the first 14 amino acids of the predicted mature erythropoietin receptor protein (25). This antibody was used to immunoprecipitate the putative receptor from Cos cells transfected with clone 190 DNA or no DNA and murine erythroleukemia cells. Sodium dodecyl sulfate-polyacrylamide gel electrophoresis of the immunoprecipitated products revealed a single protein band of 66 kd from Cos cells transfected with clone 190 and from murine erythroleukemia cells. No immunoprecipitable material was detected in the mock DNA-transfected Cos cells. This result suggests that clone 190 directed the expression of a cell membrane surface protein that is consistent with the predicted amino acid sequence and that is antigenically similar to a cell surface protein expressed by murine erythroleukemia cells, the original source of clones 141 and 190.

The Molecular Weight of the Erythropoietin-binding Protein Complex Heterologously Expressed by Clone 190-transfected Cos Cells

The previous section described our determination of the molecular weight of the putative erythropoietin receptor protein encoded by clone 190 and expressed by murine erythroleukemia cells; however, this determination does not describe the specific structure of the receptor complex on binding erythropoietin. Previous cross-linking experiments with radiolabeled erythropoietin found a significantly higher-molecular-weight erythropoietin receptor (4,6,8,12,13,26,27) than that determined by the above immunoprecipitation experiment. We sought to reconcile these differences by a similar determination.

The molecular weight of the Cos cell-expressed erythropoietin-binding protein was determined by treating Cos cells, bound with radio-iodinated erythropoietin, with disuccinimidyl suberate (18). By this treatment the bound erythropoietin was chemically linked to its respective binding protein. The cross-linked products were specifically immunoprecipitated with an antibody to the putative erythropoietin receptor protein encoded by clone 190 and analyzed by sodium dodecyl sulfate-polyacrylamide gel electrophoresis.

Two major protein bands of equivalent abundance with apparent molecular masses of 100 and 140 kd were observed. Both protein bands seem to contain a peptide antigen similar to the first 10 amino acids of the putative erythropoietin receptor protein encoded by clone 190.

A presumed molecular mass of 35 kd for radioiodinated erythropoietin would indicate molecular masses of 65 and 105 kd for the putative murine erythropoietin receptor proteins. A molecular mass of 65 kd is consistent with that predicted from the putative erythropoietin receptor protein sequence including possible N- and O-linked carbohydrate.

In theory, the larger molecular mass of 105 kd can be accounted for by more extensive glycosylation, the binding of an additional erythropoietin molecule, or an additional membrane protein that is complexed with the putative murine erythropoietin receptor.

The following observations suggest that the heterologous murine erythropoietin receptor protein was complexed to a specific endogenous Cos cell membrane-associated protein. First, immunoprecipitated Cos cell-expressed murine erythropoietin receptor protein appears as a single band of 66 kd on sodium dodecyl sulfate-polyacrylamide gel analysis. Second, the higher-molecular-weight protein band revealed by cross-linking appears very tight and therefore suggests specificity, as opposed to a diffuse band expected if the erythropoietin receptor protein was complexed nonspecifically with a random and heterogeneous population of cell membrane-associated proteins. Third, the higher-molecular-weight erythropoietin receptor complex is revealed by cross-linking receptor-bound radioiodinated erythropoietin, suggesting that the associated protein is part of a biologically relevant erythropoietin receptor. Finally, as is described below, the isolated erythropoietin receptor gene is, by structural homologies, a member of a family of hematopoietin receptors. One characteristic of some members of this receptor family is the multisubunit nature of the complete receptor complex. It remains to be determined whether the two different classes of erythropoietin cross-proteins on Cos cells expressing the receptor are functionally related to the classes of erythropoietin binding sites based on affinity.

The Human Erythropoietin Receptor Gene

With the murine erythropoietin receptor gene, we sought to isolate the human homologue and, by comparing and contrasting, continue our efforts to understand both the structure and the regulation of the erythropoietin-receptor complex.

Numerous erythroleukemia cell lines and human tissues were analyzed for erythropoietin receptor-related mRNA expression by standard RNA blot analysis using the murine erythropoietin receptor cDNA gene as a probe. Two RNA sources, the human erythroleukemia cell line OCIM1 (28) and human fetal liver, were found to be candidate sources for erythropoietin receptor-related mRNA. Human fetal liver was the preferred source of RNA for cDNA gene library construction; however, because of its limited availability we opted to use readily available RNA from OCIM1 cells. We constructed a cDNA library in the bacterial plasmid pMT21 of about 180,000 independent clones (29). This cDNA library was screened by standard techniques, under stringent conditions, for clones containing DNA sequences homologous to the murine erythropoietin receptor cDNA gene. Numerous clones were isolated, characterized, and found by DNA sequencing to be similar or overlapping. From the DNA sequence of the overlapping clones, a composite sequence for the human homologue of the erythropoietin receptor was assembled (Fig 9.2).

As in the situation for the murine erythropoietin receptor cDNA gene, we were concerned that the OCIM1 cell line may be expressing an aberrant erythropoietin receptor mRNA. A "wild-type" human erythropoietin receptor cDNA sequence was determined from human fetal liver (29) by application of polymerase chain reaction technology (30).

From the composite putative human erythropoietin receptor cDNA sequence (hEPO-R), as shown in Figure 9.2, oligonucleotides were designed to amplify and construct additional human erythropoietin receptor clones. A number of human fetal liver clones were sequenced and found to match the sequence depicted in Figure 9.2.

The nucleotide sequence of hEPO-R contains a single open reading frame of 1524 nucleotides encoding a 508-amino acid protein with a calculated molecular mass of 55 kd. Both the cDNA and the protein sequence of the putative human receptor were 82 percent, similar to the corresponding mEPO-R sequences (Fig 9.3). This similarity is predictable from the cross-reactivity of human erythropoietin on murine erythroid progenitor cells. The main structural features of the human and murine receptors are conserved between species, except for an amino acid insertion in the region of amino acids 71 to 76 and the absence of an N-linked glycosylation site in the cytoplasmic domain for hEPO-R (Fig 9.3).

The Genomic Structure of the Human Erythropoietin Receptor Gene

The commitment of immature hemopoietic cells to the erythroid lineage, characterized by the acquisition of sensitivity to erythropoietin, is the crucial event in the development of mature erythrocytes. Therefore, it is important to understand the temporal regulation of expression of the erythropoietin receptor gene; for this, the genomic sequence for the receptor is required.

Eight hundred thousand recombinant phages from a human placental genomic library (λFIX II placenta, Stratagene Cloning Systems) were screened by standard techniques, using the murine erythropoietin receptor cDNA gene as the probe, under stringent conditions. Several clones were isolated. One of these was subcloned, and fragments cov-

```
      -100                    -80                     -60                      -40
TCAGCTGCGTCCGGCGGAGGCAGCTGCTGACCCAGCTGTGGACTGTGCCGGGGGCGGGGGACGGAGGGGC

            -20                     0                       20
AGGAGCCCTGGGCTCCCCGTGGCGGGGGCTGTATCATGGACCACCTCGGGGCGTCCCTCTGGCCCCAGGT
                                    M   D   H   L   G   A   S   L   W   P   Q   V      12

         40                      60            ↓         80                      100
CGGCTCCCTTTGTCTCCTGCTCGCTGGGGCCGCCTGGGCGCCCCCGCCTAACCTCCCGGACCCCAAGTTC
 G   S   L   C   L   L   L   A   G   A   A   W   A   P   P   P   N   L   P   D   P   K   F     35

            ▽  120                      140                     160
GAGAGCAAAGCGGCCTTGCTGGCGGCCCGGGGGGCCCGAAGAGCTTCTGTGCTTCACCGAGCGGTTGGAGG
 E   S   K   A   A   L   L   A   A   R   G   P   E   E   L   L   C   F   T   E   R   L   E   D    59

     180                     200                      220                      240
ACTTGGTGTGTTTCTGGGAGGAAGCGGCGAGCGCTGGGGTGGGCCCGGGCAACTACAGCTTCTCCTACCA
 L   V   C   F   W   E   E   A   A   S   A   G   V   G   P   G   N   Y   S   F   S   Y   Q      82

         ▽   260                      280                     300
GCTCGAGGATGAGCCCATGGAAGCTGTGTCGCCTGCACCAGGCTCCCACGGCTCGTGGTGCGGTGCGCTTC
 L   E   D   E   P   W   K   L   C   R   L   H   Q   A   P   T   A   R   G   A   V   R   F    105

     320                     340                      360                      380
TGGTGTTCGCTGCCTACAGCCGACACGTCGAGCTTCGTGCCCCTAGAGTTGCGCGTCACAGCAGCCTCCG
 W   C   S   L   P   T   A   D   T   S   S   F   V   P   L   E   L   R   V   T   A   A   S   G   129

                 400                     420         ▽          440
GCGCTCCGCGATATCACCGTGTCATCCACATCAATGAAGTAGTGCTCCTAGACGCCCCGTGGGGCTGGT
 A   P   R   Y   H   R   V   I   H   I   N   E   V   V   L   L   D   A   P   V   G   L   V   152

     460                     480                      500                      520
GGCGCGGTTGGCTGACGAGAGCGGCCACGTAGTGTTGCGCTGGCTCCCGCCGCCTGAGACACCCATGACG
 A   R   L   A   D   E   S   G   H   V   V   L   R   W   L   P   P   P   E   T   P   M   T   175

                 540                     560                      580         ▽
TCTCACATCCGCTACGAGGTGGACGTCTCGGCCGGCAACGGCGCAGGGAGCGTACAGAGGGTGGAGATCC
 S   H   I   R   Y   E   V   D   V   S   A   G   N   G   A   G   S   V   Q   R   V   E   I   L   199

     600                     620                      640                      660
TGGAGGGCCGCACCGAGTGTGTGCTGAGCAACCTGCGGGGCCGGACGCGCTACACCTTCGCCGTCCGCGC
 E   G   R   T   E   C   V   L   S   N   L   R   G   R   T   R   Y   T   F   A   V   R   A   222

                 680                     700                      720
GCGTATGGCTGAGCCGAGCTTCGGCGGCTTCTGGAGCGCCTGGTCGGAGCCTGTGTCGCTGCTGACGCCT
 R   M   A   E   P   S   F   G   G   F   W   S   A   W   S   E   P   V   S   L   L   T   P   245

     740         ▽           760                      780                      800
AGCGACCTGGACCCCCTCATCCTGACGCTCTCCCTCATCCTCGTGGTCATCCTGGTGCTGCTGACCGTGC
 S   D   L   D   P   L   I   L   T   L   S   L   I   L   V   V   I   L   V   L   L   T   V   L   269

                 820         ▽           840                      860
TCGCGCTGCTCTCCCACCGCCGGGCTCTGAAGCAGAAGATCTGGCCTGGCATCCCGAGCCCAGAGAGCGA
 A   L   L   S   H   R   R   A   L   K   Q   K   I   W   P   G   I   P   S   P   E   S   E   292
```

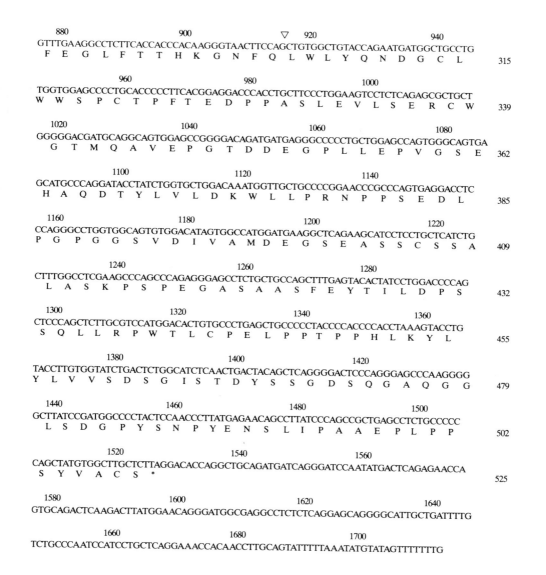

```
        880              900              ▽  920                       940
GTTTGAAGGCCTCTTCACCACCCACAAGGGTAACTTCCAGCTGTGGCTGTACCAGAATGATGGCTGCCTG
 F  E  G  L  F  T  T  H  K  G  N  F  Q  L  W  L  Y  Q  N  D  G  C  L    315

              960              980              1000
TGGTGGAGCCCCTGCACCCCCTTCACGGAGGACCCACCTGCTTCCCTGGAAGTCCTCTCAGAGCGCTGCT
 W  W  S  P  C  T  P  F  T  E  D  P  P  A  S  L  E  V  L  S  E  R  C  W  339

    1020             1040                1060                1080
GGGGGACGATGCAGGCAGTGGAGCCGGGGACAGATGATGAGGGCCCCCTGCTGGAGCCAGTGGGCAGTGA
  G  T  M  Q  A  V  E  P  G  T  D  D  E  G  P  L  L  E  P  V  G  S  E    362

          1100             1120             1140
GCATGCCCAGGATACCTATCTGGTGCTGGACAAATGGTTGCTGCCCCGGAACCCGCCCAGTGAGGACCTC
 H  A  Q  D  T  Y  L  V  L  D  K  W  L  L  P  R  N  P  P  S  E  D  L     385

      1160             1180             1200             1220
CCAGGGCCTGGTGGCAGTGTGGACATAGTGGCCATGGATGAAGGCTCAGAAGCATCCTCCTGCTCATCTG
 P  G  P  G  G  S  V  D  I  V  A  M  D  E  G  S  E  A  S  S  C  S  S  A  409

          1240             1260             1280
CTTTGGCCTCGAAGCCCAGCCCAGAGGGGAGCCTCTGCTGCCAGCTTTGAGTACACTATCCTGGACCCCAG
 L  A  S  K  P  S  P  E  G  A  S  A  A  S  F  E  Y  T  I  L  D  P  S    432

    1300             1320             1340             1360
CTCCCAGCTCTTGCGTCCATGGACACTGTGCCCTGAGCTGCCCCCTACCCCACCCCACCTAAAGTACCTG
 S  Q  L  L  R  P  W  T  L  C  P  E  L  P  P  T  P  P  H  L  K  Y  L    455

          1380             1400             1420
TACCTTGTGGTATCTGACTCTGGCATCTCAACTGACTACAGCTCAGGGGACTCCCAGGGAGCCCAAGGGG
 Y  L  V  V  S  D  S  G  I  S  T  D  Y  S  S  G  D  S  Q  G  A  Q  G  G 479

    1440             1460             1480             1500
GCTTATCCGATGGCCCCTACTCCAACCCTTATGAGAACAGCCTTATCCCAGCCGCTGAGCCTCTGCCCCC
  L  S  D  G  P  Y  S  N  P  Y  E  N  S  L  I  P  A  A  E  P  L  P  P   502

          1520             1540             1560
CAGCTATGTGGCTTGCTCTTAGGACACCAGGCTGCAGATGATCAGGGATCCAATATGACTCAGAGAACCA
 S  Y  V  A  C  S  *                                                    525

    1580             1600             1620             1640
GTGCAGACTCAAGACTTATGGAACAGGGATGGCGAGGCCTCTCTCAGGAGCAGGGGCATTGCTGATTTTG

          1660             1680             1700
TCTGCCCAATCCATCCTGCTCAGGAAACCACAACCTTGCAGTATTTTTAAATATGTATAGTTTTTTTG
```

Figure 9.2. The structure of the human erythropoietin receptor. The putative mature amino terminus at residue 25 is indicated by an arrow. The site of potential N-linked glycosylation is overlined. The putative transmembrane domain is underlined. Open triangles indicate intron-extron junctions.

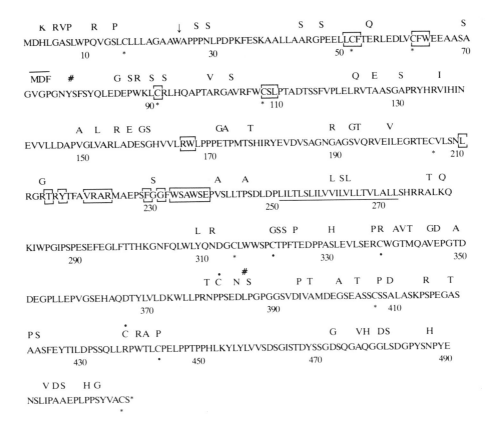

Figure 9.3. A comparison of the predicted amino acid sequence of the human erythropoietin receptor with that of the murine erythropoietin receptor. The human receptor sequence is denoted by the contiguous amino acid sequence in single-letter code, and differences from the murine receptor are indicated above the human sequence. Asterisks indicate conserved cysteine residues; closed circles indicate nonconserved cysteine residues. The transmembrane domain is underlined. The region of the single amino acid insertion in the human receptor is overlined. The number signs (#) indicate sites of N-linked glycosylation. Conserved sequences with other hematopoietic growth factor receptors are boxed. The putative mature amino terminus is indicated by an arrow.

ering the entire coding region, introns, and flanking noncoding sequences were isolated.

The gene seems to be approximately 6 kilobasepairs in length, and the coding sequence is essentially identical to that of the human erythropoietin receptor cDNA from fetal liver and OCIM1 cells. The extracellular domain is encoded by five exons (Fig 9.2), and the transmembrane domain is almost exactly demarcated by the sixth exon. The cytoplasmic domain is defined by two exons: exon 7, a relatively small exon encoding 12 percent of the intracellular region, and exon 8, the largest exon in the gene, which covers the remainder of the protein sequence. The exon-intron boundaries for the human receptor are conserved with those delineated in the recently cloned genomic sequence of the murine erythropoietin receptor (31).

Of particular interest is the 5' noncoding region, which would be expected to contain regulatory sequences controlling transcription. The first 700 base pairs of this region are shown in Figure 9.4. There seems to be no canonical CAAT or TATA sequences within this sequence. However, there is one potential Sp1 binding site (CCGCCC) (32), a site for the erythroid-specific transcription factor GF-1 (TTATCT) (33,34), and, much further upstream, a structural, possibly functional, motif (CACCC) found in the promoter regions of globin genes (35).

Further studies are in progress to define these and other functional elements within the promoter region, such as the transcriptional start site, and the relevance of the sequence motifs to the regulation and erythroid-specific expression of the human erythropoietin receptor.

The Heterologous Expression and Characterization of the Human Erythropoietin Receptor

The hEPO-R cDNA was cloned into a mammalian gene expression plasmid containing the necessary transcription and translation elements and was transfected into Cos cells. Transfected Cos cell membranes were lysed and treated with the antibody specific to the murine erythropoietin receptor protein (25). From sodium dodecyl sulfate-polyacrylamide gel electrophoresis, a protein of an apparent molecular mass of 66 kd was detected (29). Treatment with either endoglycosidase H or N-glycosidase F, which remove N-linked high mannose and complex carbohydrate, respectively, reduced the apparent molecular mass to about 60 kd. This result is consistent with the expected molecular mass of 55 kd for the hEPO-R protein with a single N-linked glycosylation site and possibly containing O-linked carbohydrate. We next

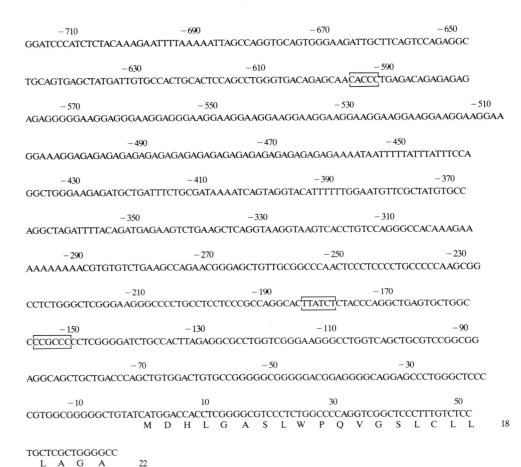

Figure 9.4. The sequence of 5' noncoding region and part of exon 1 from the human erythropoietin receptor genomic clone. The protein sequence is indicated by the single-letter amino acid code. Potential regulatory elements are boxed.

sought to determine the molecular weight of the Cos cell-expressed human erythropoietin receptor complex that bound erythropoietin.

Cos cells expressing the human erythropoietin receptor protein were incubated with radioiodinated erythropoietin and then treated with the cross-linking reagent, disuccinimidyl suberate. The cross-linked products were analyzed by sodium dodecyl sulfate-polyacrylamide gel electrophoresis and autoradiography. Two protein bands of apparent molecular masses of 105 and 140 kd were detected (29). If we assume a molecular mass of 35 kd for the radioiodinated erythropoietin, we can deduce molecular masses of 65 and 105 kd for the erythropoietin receptor-binding complex. This result is similar to that found for the Cos cell-expressed murine erythropoietin receptor protein. The host cell Cos is of primate origin; therefore, we can, in light of these results, exclude the possibility that the cross-linking results are the consequence of subtle differences between murine and primate erythropoietin receptor proteins. Additional studies are in progress to characterize the human erythropoietin receptor protein.

The Murine and Human Erythropoietin Receptor cDNA Genes Encode Proteins That Can Transduce a Mitogenic Signal

After the binding of erythropoietin, the complete erythropoietin receptor complex would be expected to transduce the appropriate physiologic signal. The experiments described thus far have shown that the isolated putative erythropoietin receptor cDNA does encode a type I transmembrane protein similar in both structure and biochemical function to the erythropoietin receptor found in murine erythroleukemia cells. However, murine erythroleukemia and OCIM1 cells, unlike primary erythroblasts, are not dependent on erythropoietin for growth or differentiation (16,17,28). This apparent erythropoietin independence could be an inherent aberration in the erythropoietin receptor protein or a consequence of the cell line's transformed phenotype. A comparison of the genomic erythropoietin receptor gene sequences isolated from wild-type BALB/c mice to clone 190 showed that the murine erythroleukemia cell-derived erythropoietin receptor gene had no apparent differences in the coding sequence. However, this analysis does not eliminate the possibility of an alteration in the processing of the erythropoietin receptor mRNA transcript in murine erythroleukemia cells as compared to normal erythroblasts. These alternative hypotheses could be tested by expressing the erythropoietin receptor protein in a context where the signal transduction mechanism could be directly tested.

Various transformed hematopoietic cell lines (e.g., leukemias and lymphomas) whose growth is strictly dependent on specific hematopoietic growth factors may be the appropriate experimental system in which to study signal transduction. The growth factor specificity of particular cell lines was hypothesized to be a consequence of the repertoire of growth factor receptors expressed by that cell. In addition, disparate growth factor receptors were known, in some cells, to share common postreceptor signal transduction pathways (36). Therefore, it was conceivable that particular factor-dependent cell lines could assume a new growth factor responsiveness merely by the expression of a heterologous growth factor receptor. For instance, consider the murine myeloid leukemia cell line, 32D (37), which is strictly dependent on murine interleukin 3 for survival. In the absence of interleukin 3, 32D cells will die within 24 to 48 hours (38), while another hematopoietin such as macrophage colony-stimulating factor (M-CSF) is ineffective in supporting 32D cell growth. However, the nonresponsiveness of 32D cells may be due merely to the absence of M-CSF receptors on the cell surface. In support of this, it has been shown that recombinant 32D cells that express heterologous epidermal growth factor receptors and thereby become mitogenically responsive to epidermal growth factor can be constructed (36).

In an analogous experiment, we tested erythropoietin receptor function by transfecting clone 190, the murine erythroleukemia cell-derived erythropoietin receptor gene, into the interleukin 3-dependent murine B-cell lymphoma line Ba/F3 (39,40). Ba/F3 cells are strictly dependent on interleukin 3 for growth and do not respond to or bind erythropoietin. This cell line can be made dependent on interleukin 2, however, by transfection of the human *IL-2R*β (p70–75) gene, even though there is endogenous expression of the murine *IL-2R*α subunit (41). Ba/F3 cells expressing the heterologous "murine erythroleukemia" erythropoietin receptor were isolated and found to bind erythropoietin. These erythropoietin receptor-expressing Ba/F3 cells retained their dependence for interleukin 3 and were now found to respond mitogenically to erythropoietin (25). This result showed that the erythropoietin receptor cDNA gene derived from murine erythroleukemia cells was capable of both binding erythropoietin and transducing a mitogenic signal. Therefore, the apparent nonresponsiveness of murine erythroleukemia cells may be due to mechanisms exclusive of the erythropoietin receptor.

The human erythropoietin receptor gene, when introduced into Ba/

F3 cells, behaved in an analogous fashion and was able to confer on Ba/F3 cells dependence on erythropoietin (29). This result demonstrated not only the functional integrity of the heterologously expressed human erythropoietin receptor protein but also the close functional similarity in signal transduction mechanisms between mouse (Ba/F3) and human erythropoietin-responsive cells.

A Comparison of the Erythropoietin Receptor to the Hematopoietin Receptor Super Family

One of the most interesting consequences of the cloning of the murine and human erythropoietin receptors is the discovery that they belong to a novel family of receptors (42–46), designated the hematopoietin receptor super family. This family currently includes several cytokine receptors; receptors for interleukin 2β (47), interleukin 3 (48), interleukin 4 (42,49–51), interleukin 6 (52), interleukin 7 (43); granulocyte-macrophage colony-stimulating factor (GM-CSF) (53); and granulocyte colony-stimulating factor (G-CSF) (54), as well as the receptors for growth hormone and prolactin (55–57).

As outlined by others (42–46), and shown in Figure 9.3 for the murine and human erythropoietin receptors, the family has several distinguishing features in the extracellular domain, notably a Gly-X-Trp-Ser-X-Trp-Ser-X-Pro motif close to the putative transmembrane domain and two pairs of conserved cysteine residues, as well as other conserved residues within subgroups of the family (54). There seems to be no specific sequence similarity in the cytoplasmic domains of the receptor family and no homology with protein kinases or sequences commonly found at sites of tyrosine phosphorylation. Indeed, the actual size of the domain is quite variable and some receptors seem to have a naturally occurring soluble form of the membrane-bound receptor (43,50). Even so, there are similarities in amino acid content between the cytoplasmic domain of the erythropoietin receptors and some (interleukin 2β, interleukin 3, interleukin 4, and interleukin 7 [42,43,47–51,54]) but not all (interleukin 6 and GM-CSF [52,53]) members of the family—for instance, the high content of proline, serine/threonine (potential sites for phosphorylation), and acidic amino acids.

How can these structural parallels be reconciled between receptors whose cognate ligands can have a narrow or wide range of different yet overlapping effects and, in particular, are these observations relevant to understanding the mechanism of action of the erythropoietin-receptor complex? Several lines of speculation can be considered. First, as discussed by others (45), the gross structure of the receptor and the ligand is probably conserved while the specificity is generated in the particular amino acid contacts, as has been recently demonstrated for the growth hormone-prolactin combination (58). From this supposition, erythropoietin would be expected to consist of an antiparallel, four-helix bundle based on the crystal structure of growth hormone (59) and interleukin 2 (60).

Second, the conserved structural motifs in the extracellular domain and similar amino acid content in the cytoplasmic domain may indicate common mechanisms of signal transduction. For instance, interleukin 2R consists of two subunits, if not additional units (61), and it has been demonstrated that the Ser-Thr-rich region is essential for signal transduction (41). Interleukin 6 triggers the association of its receptor with a membrane glycoprotein, gp130, in a human myeloma cell line, U266 (62). On some hemopoietic cells, however, binding of radiolabeled GM-CSF to the GM-CSF receptor can be completed not only by GM-CSF but also by interleukin 3 (63–66). Also, as is discussed below, the envelope glycoprotein, gp55, of the Friend virus complex can associate with the erythropoietin receptor and provide the necessary mitogenic signal for cell growth in the absence of erythropoietin.

Finally, the restricted or pleiotropic effects of different cytokines can be explained by a shared mechanism of action through cell-specific receptor subunits, which may interact with a specific or a number of different "primary" cytokine receptors. These subunits, as well as the receptors themselves, would be expected to be developmentally regulated and induced by initial binding of a particular cytokine to the "primary" receptor.

The Erythropoietin Receptor May Be a Complex of Proteins

The murine erythroleukemia cell line used in erythropoietin receptor characterization and as a source for the erythropoietin receptor gene arose by the transformation of an erythropoietic progenitor cell by the Friend virus complex (16,17). The Friend virus complex is composed of both the Friend spleen focus-forming virus (SFFV), a defective C-type virus, and the Friend murine leukemia helper virus (67–70). The SFFV virus, the causative agent in Friend erythroleukemia, encodes a membrane glycoprotein, gp55, found in both the cell membrane and the endoplasmic reticulum (71–73) which is essential for the induction of leukemia in vivo (74–78) and transformation in vitro (71,74).

Among the many hypotheses for Friend virus action has been the speculation that the gp55 glycoprotein was mimicking the action of the erythropoietin receptor and transducing a mitogenic signal or that the gp55 protein itself was interacting with the native erythropoietin receptor to bypass the need for erythropoietin to induce a mitogenic signal (79).

With the availability of antibodies specific to gp55 or to the murine erythropoietin receptor, this latter hypothesis can be simply tested. With the use of retroviral expression vectors, fibroblast cells were constructed to express either or both gp55 glycoprotein and the murine erythropoietin receptor (25). The specificity of each of the antibodies was verified by the demonstration that anti-gp55 antibodies would only immunoprecipitate glycoprotein from fibroblasts expressing gp55 and did not react with fibroblast that expressed only the murine erythropoietin receptor. The contrary experiment with the anti-erythropoietin receptor antibodies also gave the expected results. For fibroblasts expressing both gp55 and the murine erythropoietin receptor, however, anti-gp55 antibodies would immunoprecipitate both gp55 glycoprotein and the murine erythropoietin receptor. A similar result was obtained by treatment with the anti-murine erythropoietin receptor antibodies (25). This result suggested that there was a tight association between the Friend virus glycoprotein gp55 and the erythropoietin receptor.

A similar experimental analysis on radiolabeled MEL cell proteins showed an association between the intracellular form of gp55 and the erythropoietin receptor. These data suggest that a multisubunit structure is the predominant erythropoietin-binding complex in murine erythroleukemia cells with a low-affinity binding constant of 240 pM. In addition, the apparent low-affinity erythropoietin binding constant may be due to the competition between erythropoietin and gp55 for the same binding site or indirectly due to modulation of the erythropoietin binding site by gp55. In contrast, single-unit or homodimeric erythropoietin-receptor complexes, observed in transfected Cos cells, would be hypothesized to have the higher picomolar binding affinity for erythropoietin.

Cross-linking experiments with radioiodinated erythropoietin bound to murine erythroleukemia cells revealed a complex of 145 kd (18) that is consistent with a complex of the erythropoietin-receptor protein with gp55 and erythropoietin, in addition to a complex of 100 kd, presumably the erythropoietin receptor and erythropoietin. The existence of the two types of complex could be an experimental artifact, or it could actually reflect the existence of two different populations of erythropoietin-binding complexes. It is more likely to be a consequence of the experimental methods used because the concentration of gp55 protein in murine erythroleukemia cells is probably in excess of the number of erythropoietin receptor proteins and therefore sufficient to complex with all of the available erythropoietin receptor protein. In addition, there is no correlation of the relative abundance of the two different-sized complexes with a physical property such as erythropoietin-binding affinity.

Finally, there is an additional experiment that lends support to the hypothesis that the gp55 interacts with the erythropoietin receptor protein at the native erythropoietin-binding sites. Ba/F3 cells, which are interleukin 3-dependent for growth, can also be converted to erythropoietin dependency by transfection with a retrovirus encoding the erythropoietin receptor (25), thus demonstrating that the cloned murine erythropoietin receptor is capable of biologic function. These same erythropoietin-dependent Ba/F3 cells can be converted to erythropoietin independency by transfection with a retrovirus encoding the Friend virus gp55 glycoprotein (25). This result in combination with the above observation suggests that there may exist cell membrane surface proteins, such as the Friend virus gp55, which can tightly associate with the erythropoietin receptor and transduce a mitogenic signal. This model would also explain that the apparent binding affinity of the murine erythroleukemia erythropoietin binding complex was due to the competition of gp55 and erythropoietin for the same binding site on the erythropoietin receptor protein. We can speculate that the induction of erythroleukemia by the Friend virus is due to the constitutive nature of the signal from an erythropoietin receptor saturated by gp55 protein or possibly that there is a subtle difference in the nature of the signal transduced by an erythropoietin receptor complexed with gp55 as opposed to erythropoietin.

In a similar analysis of the murine erythropoietin receptor heterologously expressed by Cos cells, two different-sized erythropoietin binding complexes were detected by cross-linking experiments (18). The relative abundances of both sized complexes were equivalent. In light of the above experiments revealing tight association of gp55 protein with the erythropoietin receptor in murine erythroleukemia cells and its respective erythropoietin-binding affinity, we propose that the 240 pM erythropoietin-binding affinity complex detected in Cos cells was due to the association of an endogenous Cos cell membrane protein with the murine erythropoietin receptor protein. Again, the equivalent relative abundance of both sized complexes is believed to be a consequence of the experimental method. This hypothesis would predict that erythropoietin receptor protein in the absence of any associated proteins would have binding affinities for erythropoietin in the 30-pM range.

Conclusion

The murine and human erythropoietin receptor cDNA genes encode 507- and 508-amino acid polypeptides, respectively, which have an overall structural homology of about 82 percent. Both polypeptides seem to have a 24-amino acid secretory leader sequence preceding a typical type I transmembrane protein, with the extracellular and cytoplasmic domains being approximately the same size. The predicted molecular mass of both the murine and the human erythropoietin receptor is about 55 kd.

Heterologous expression of either murine or human erythropoietin receptor genes in the SV40-transformed primate cell line, Cos, results in the generation of a cell membrane-associated protein with an apparent molecular mass of 66 kd. These proteins can be specifically immunoprecipitated with an antibody generated to a tetradecapeptide derived from the first 14 amino acids of the putative mature erythropoietin receptor protein. The difference in molecular weight between that observed and that predicted could be accounted for by N- and O-linked glycosylation. In the mouse erythropoietin receptor there are two potential sites for N-linked glycosylation, one extracellular and one intracellular. In the human erythropoietin receptor there is only a single extracellular site for N-linked glycosylation. Both murine and human forms of the erythropoietin receptor protein have a high frequency of serine and threonine residues, which are potential sites of O-linked glycosylation and phosphorylation.

Cos cells transfected with either the murine or the human erythropoietin receptor cDNA genes specifically bind erythropoietin. Scatchard analysis of Cos cells transfected with the murine erythropoietin receptor gene show about 200,000 erythropoietin binding sites per Cos cell. These binding sites are distributed into two binding affinities; 14 percent of the binding sites have a high (30 pM) affinity and 86 percent have a low (240 pM) affinity for erythropoietin.

Cos cells expressing either the murine or human erythropoietin receptor proteins were found to have erythropoietin-binding complexes with apparent molecular weights of 65 and 105 kd. The lower-molecular-weight complex is consistent with the predicted molecular mass for either the human or the murine erythropoietin receptor protein. The larger-molecular-weight complex could be due to the association of a second molecule of erythropoietin or an endogenous Cos cell protein.

Li et al. (25) demonstrated by antibody immunoprecipitation experiments that there is a tight association between gp55, the Friend virus envelope glycoprotein, and the murine erythropoietin receptor protein. Murine erythroleukemia cells have both a 65- and a 105-kd erythropoietin binding complex, although it remains to be proven that the 105-kd complex arises from an association of gp55 and the erythropoietin receptor. It is possible that the 105-kd complex, in murine erythroleukemia cells, is due to the association of the erythropoietin receptor with a protein other than gp55, such as an accessory signal transduction protein common to both murine erythroleukemia and Cos cells. Nevertheless, both murine and human erythropoietin receptor cDNA clones encode proteins capable of both binding erythropoietin and transducing a mitogenic signal.

The heterologous expression of either the murine or the human erythropoietin receptor protein in the interleukin 3-dependent murine B-cell lymphoma Ba/F3 renders these cells dependent on erythropoietin, whereas coexpression of the Friend virus gp55 protein with the erythropoietin receptor allows the cells to become independent of either erythropoietin or interleukin 3 for growth. An analogous process may be occurring in murine erythroleukemia cells, which are independent of erythropoietin for growth.

Now, for the first time, it is possible to examine the nature and mechanism of action of the erythropoietin receptor complex in erythro- and megakaryopoiesis, as well as the significance of the tight association between Friend virus gp55 protein and the erythropoietin receptor.

REFERENCES

1. Goldwasser E, Krantz SB, Wang FF. Erythropoietin and erythroid differentiation. In: Ford RJ, Maizel AL, eds. Mediation in cell growth and differentiation. New York: Raven Press, 1985;103–7.

2. Koettler HP, Goldwasser E. Erythropoietin radioimmunoassay in evaluating patients with polycythemia. Ann Intern Med 1981;97:44–7.

3. Fukamachi H, Saito T, Tojo A, Kitamura T, Urabe A, Takaku F. Binding of erythropoietin to CFU-E derived from fetal mouse liver cells. Exp Hematol 1987;15:833–7.

4. Krantz SB, Sawyer ST, Sawada K-I. Purification of erythroid progenitor

cells and characterization of erythropoietin receptors. Br J Cancer 1988;58:31–5.

5. Hoshino S, Teramura M, Takahashi M, et al. Expression and characterization of erythropoietin receptors on normal human bone marrow cells. Int J Cell Cloning 1989;7:156–67.

6. Landschulz KT, Noyes AN, Rogers O, Boyer SH. Erythropoietin receptors on murine erythroid colony-forming units: natural history. Blood 1989;73:1476–86.

7. Fraser JK, Tan AS, Lin F-K, Berridge MV. Expression of specific high-affinity binding sites for erythropoietin on rat and mouse megakaryocytes. Exp Hematol 1989;17:10–6.

8. Sawyer ST, Krantz SB, Sawada K-J. Receptors for erythropoietin in mouse and human erythroid cells and placenta. Blood 1989;74:103–9.

9. Sawada K-J, Krantz SB, Dai C-H, et al. Purification of human blood burst-forming units-erythroid and demonstration of the evolution of erythropoietin receptors. J Cell Physiol 1990;142:219–30.

10. Mufson RA, Gesner TG. Binding and internalization of recombinant human erythropoietin in murine erythroid precursor cells. Blood 1987;69:1485–90.

11. Fraser JK, Lin F-K, Berridge MV. Expression of high affinity receptors for erythropoietin in human bone marrow cells and on the human erythroleukemic cell line, HEL. Exp Hematol 1988;16:836–42.

12. Tojo A, Fukamachi H, Kasuga M, Urabe A, Takaku F. Identification of erythropoietin receptors on fetal liver erythroid cells. Biochem Biophys Res Commun 1987;148:443–8.

13. Means RT Jr, Krantz SB, Sawyer ST, Gilbert HS. Erythropoietin receptors in polycythemia vera. J Clin Invest 1989;84:1340–4.

14. Sawyer ST. The two proteins of the erythropoietin receptor are structurally similar. J Biol Chem 1989;264:13343–7.

15. Wong GG. The isolation and identification of cDNA genes by their heterologous expression and function. In: Setlow J, ed. Genetic engineering: principles and methods, vol 12. New York: Plenum, 1990:44–7.

16. Sawyer ST, Krantz SB, Goldwasser E. Binding and receptor-mediated endocytosis of erythropoietin in Friend virus-infected erythroid cells. J Biol Chem 1987;262:5554–62.

17. Mayeux P, Billat C, Jacquot R. Murine erythroleukaemia cells (Friend cells) possess high-affinity binding sites for erythropoietin. FEBS Lett 1987;211:229–33.

18. D'Andrea AD, Lodish HF, Wong GG. Expression cloning of the murine erythropoietin receptor. Cell 1989;57:277–85.

19. Hitomi K, Fujita K, Sasaki R, et al. Erythropoietin receptor of a human leukemic cell line with erythroid characteristics. Biochem Biophys Res Commun 1988;154:902–9.

20. Kitamura T, Tojo A, Fukamachi H, et al. Characterization of the erythropoietin receptor on a Friend murine erythroleukemic cell clone, TSA8. Acta Haematol Jpn 1988;51:677–85.

21. Kukamachi H, Tojo A, Saito T, et al. Internalization of radioiodinated erythropoietin and the ligand-induced modulation of its receptor in murine erythroleukemia cells. Int J Cell Cloning 1987;5:209–19.

22. Kyte J, Doolittle RF. A simple method for displaying the hydropathic character of a protein. J Mol Biol 1982;157:105–32.

23. Williams AF, Barclay AN. The immunoglobulin superfamily—domains for cell surface recognition. Annu Rev Immunol 1988;6:381–405.

24. Hanks SK, Quinn AM, Hunter T. The protein kinase family: conserved features and deduced phylogeny of the catalytic domains. Science 1988; 241:42–52.

25. Li J-P, D'Andrea AD, Lodish HF, Baltimore D. The Friend spleen focus-forming virus gp55 glycoprotein binds to the erythropoietin receptor and activates cell growth. Nature 1990;343:762–4.

26. Todokoro K, Kanazawa S, Amanuma H, Ikawa Y. Specific binding of erythropoietin to its receptor on responsive mouse erythroleukemia cells. Proc Natl Acad Sci USA 1987;84:4126–30.

27. Hitomi K, Masuda S, Ito K, Ueda M, Samaki R. Solubilization and characterization of erythropoietin receptor from transplantable mouse erythroblastic leukemic cells. Biochem Biophys Res Commun 1989;160:1140–8.

28. Broudy VC, Lin N, Egrie J, et al. Identification of the receptor for erythropoietin on human and murine erythroleukemia cells and modulation by phorbol ester and dimethyl sulfoxide. Proc Natl Acad Sci USA 1988;85: 6513–7.

29. Jones SS, D'Andrea AD, Haines L, Wong GG. Human erythropoietin receptor: cloning, expression and biological characterization. Blood 1990;76: 31–5.

30. Innis MA, Gelfand DH, Sninsky JJ, eds. PCR protocols: a guide to methods and applications. New York: Academic Press, 1989.

31. Youssoufian H, Zon LI, Orkin SH, D'Andrea AD, Lodish HF. Structure and transcription of the mouse erythropoietin receptor gene. Molecular and Cellular Biology 1990;10:3675–82.

32. Dynan WS, Tjian R. Control of eukaryotic messenger RNA synthesis by sequence-specific DNA-binding proteins. Nature 1985;316:774–8.

33. Evans T, Felsenfeld G. The erythroid-specific transcription factor Eryf1: a new finger protein. Cell 1989;58:877–85.

34. Martin DIK, Tsai S-F, Orkin SH. Increased γ-globin expression in a nondeletion HPFH mediated by an erythroid-specific DNA-binding factor. Nature 1989;338:435–8.

35. Mignotte V, Wall L, De Boer E, Grosveld F, Romeo P-H. Two tissue-specific factors bind the erythroid promoter of the human porphobilinogen deaminase gene. Nucleic Acids Res 1989;17:37–54.

36. DiFiore PP, Segatto O, Taylor WG, Aaronson SA, Pierce JH. EGF receptor and erbB-2 tyrosine kinase domains confer cell specificity for mitogenic signaling. Science 1990;248:79–83.

37. Greenberger JS, Eckner RJ, Sakakeeny M, et al. Interleukin 3-dependent hematopoietic progenitor cell lines. Fed Proc 1983;42:2762–71.

38. Hapel AJ, Warren HS, Hume DA. Different colony-stimulating factors are detected by the "interleukin-3"-dependent cell lines FDC-P1 and 32D cl-23. Blood 1984;64:786–90.

39. Mathey-Prevot B, Nabel G, Palacios R, Baltimore D. Abelson virus abrogation of interleukin-3 dependence in a lymphoid cell line. Mol Cell Biol 1986;6:4133–5.

40. Palacios R, Steinmetz M. IL3-dependent mouse clones that express B-220 surface antigen, containing Ig genes in germ-line configuration, and generate B lymphocytes in vivo. Cell 1985;41:727–34.

41. Hatakeyama M, Mori H, Doi T, Taniguchi T. A restricted cytoplasmic

region of IL-2 receptor β chain is essential for growth signal transduction but not for ligand binding and internalization. Cell 1989;59:837–45.

42. Idzerda RL, March CJ, Mosley B, et al. Human interleukin 4 receptor confers biological responsiveness and defines a novel receptor superfamily. J Exp Med 1990;171:861–73.

43. Goodwin RG, Friend D, Ziegler SF, et al. Cloning of the human and murine interleukin-7 receptors: demonstration of a soluble form and homology to a new receptor superfamily. Cell 1990;60:941–51.

44. D'Andrea AD, Fasman GD, Lodish HF. Erythropoietin receptor and interleukin-2 receptor β chain: a new receptor family. Cell 1989;58:1023–4.

45. Bazan FJ. A novel family of growth factor receptors: a common binding domain in the growth hormone, prolactin, erythropoietin and IL-6 receptors, and the p75 IL-2 receptor β-chain. Biochem Biophys Res Commun 1989; 164:788–95.

46. Patthy L. Homology of a domain of the growth hormone/prolactin receptor family with type III modules of fibronectin. Cell 1990;61:13–4.

47. Hatakeyama M, Tsudo M, Minamoto S, et al. Interleukin-2 receptor β chain gene: generation of three receptor forms by cloned human α and β chain cDNA's. Science 1989;244:551–6.

48. Itoh N, Yonehara S, Schreurs J, et al. Cloning of an interleukin-3 receptor gene: a member of a distinct receptor gene family. Science 1989; 247:324–7.

49. Harada N, Castle BE, Gorman DM, et al. Expression cloning of a cDNA encoding the murine interleukin 4 receptor based on ligand binding. Proc Natl Acad Sci USA 1990;87:857–61.

50. Mosley BM, Beckmann P, March CJ, et al. The murine interleukin-4 receptor: molecular cloning and characterization of secreted and membrane bound forms. Cell 1989;59:335–48.

51. Zuber CE, Galizzi J-P, Valle A, Harada N, Howard M, Banchereau J. Interleukin 4 receptors on normal human B lymphocytes: characterization and regulation. Eur J Immunol 1990;20:551–5.

52. Yamasaki K, Taga T, Hirata Y, et al. Cloning and expression of the human interleukin-6 (BSF-2/IFNβ 2) receptor. Science 1988;241:825–8.

53. Gearing DP, King JA, Gough NM, Nicola NA. Expression cloning of a receptor for human granulocyte-macrophage colony-stimulating factor. EMBO J 1989;8:3667–76.

54. Fukunaga R, Ishizaka-Ikeda E, Seto Y, Nagata S. Expression cloning of a receptor for murine granulocyte colony-stimulating factor. Cell 1990;61:341–50.

55. Leung DW, Spencer SA, Cachianes G, et al. Growth hormone receptor and serum binding protein: purification, cloning and expression. Nature 1987; 330:537–43.

56. Boulin J-M, Jolicoeur C, Okamura H, et al. Cloning and expression of the rat prolactin receptor, a member of the growth hormone/prolactin receptor gene family. Cell 1988;53:69–77.

57. Edery M, Jolicoeur C, Levi-Meyrueis C, et al. Identification and sequence analysis of a second form of prolactin receptor by molecular cloning of complementary DNA from rabbit mammary gland. Proc Natl Acad Sci USA 1989;86:2112–6.

58. Cunningham BC, Henner DH, Wells JA. Engineering human prolactin to bind to the human growth hormone receptor. Science 1990;247:1461–5.

59. Abdel-Meguid SS, Shieh H-S, Smith WW, et al. Three-dimensional structure of a genetically engineering variant of porcine growth hormone. Proc Natl Acad Sci USA 1987;84:6434–7.

60. Brandhuber BJ, Boone T, Kenney WC, McKay DB. Three-dimensional structure of interleukin-2. Science 1987;238:1707–9.

61. Saragovi H, Malek TR. Evidence for additional subunits associated to the mouse interleukin 2 receptor p55/p75 complex. Proc Natl Acad Sci USA 1990;87:11–5.

62. Taga T, Hibi M, Hirata Y, et al. Interleukin-6 triggers the association of its receptor with a possible signal transducer, gp130. Cell 1989;58:573–81.

63. Park LS, Friend D, Price V, et al. Heterogeneity in human interleukin-3 receptors. J Biol Chem 1989;264:5420–7.

64. Lopez AF, Eglinton JM, Gillis D, Park LS, Clark S, Vadas MA. Reciprocal inhibition of binding between interleukin 3 and granulocyte-macrophage colony-stimulating factor to human eosinophils. Proc Natl Acad Sci USA 1989;86:7022–6.

65. Budel LM, Elbaz O, Hoogerbrugge H, et al. Common binding structure for granulocyte macrophage colony-stimulating factor and interleukin-3 on human acute myeloid leukemia cells and monocytes. Blood 1990;75:1439–45.

66. Gesner T, Mufson AR, Turner KJ, Clark SC. Identification through chemical cross-linking of distinct granulocyte-macrophage colony-stimulating factor and interleukin-3 receptors on myeloid leukemic cells, KG-1. Blood 1989;74:2652–6.

67. Hankins WD, Kost TA, Koury MJ, Krantz SB. Erythroid bursts produced by Friend leukaemia virus in vitro. Nature 1978;276:506–8.

68. Friend C. Cell-free transmission in adult Swiss mice of a disease having the character of a leukemia. J Exp Med 1956;105:307–18.

69. Hankins DW. Polycythemia- and anemia-inducing erythroleukemia viruses exhibit differential erythroid transforming effects in vitro. 1980;22:693–9.

70. Wolff L, Ruscetti S. Malignant transformation of erythroid cells in vivo by introduction of a nonreplicating retrovirus vector. Science 1985;228:1549–52.

71. Dresler S, Ruta M, Murray MJ, Kabat D. Glycoprotein encoded by the Friend spleen focus-forming virus. J Virol 1979;30:564–75.

72. Ruta M, Clarke S, Boswell B, Kabat D. Heterogeneous metabolism and subcellular localization of a potentially leukemogenic membrane glycoprotein encoded by Friend erythroleukemia virus. J Biol Chem 1982;257:126–34.

73. Ruscetti S, Wolff L. Biological and biochemical differences between variants of spleen focus-forming virus can be localized to a region containing the 3' end of the envelope gene. J Virol 1985;56:717–22.

74. Li J-P, Bestwick RK, Machida C, Kabat D. Role of a membrane glycoprotein in Friend virus erythroleukemia: nucleotide sequences of nonleukemogenic mutant and spontaneous revertant viruses. J Virol 1986;57:534–8.

75. Linemeyer DL, Menke JG, Ruscetti SK, Evans LH, Scolnick EM. Envelope gene sequences which encode the gp52 protein of spleen focus-forming virus are required for the induction of erythroid cell proliferation. J Virol 1982;43:223–33.

76. Ruta M, Bestwick R, Machida C, Kabat D. Loss of leukemogenicity caused by mutations in the membrane glycoprotein structural gene of Friend spleen focus-forming virus. Proc Natl Acad Sci USA 1983;80:4704–8.

77. Linemeyer DL, Ruscetti SK, Scolnick EM, Evans LH, Duesberg PH. Biological activity of the spleen focus-forming virus is encoded by a molecularly cloned subgenomic fragment of spleen focus-forming virus DNA. Proc Natl Acad Sci USA 1981;78:1401–5.

78. Li J-P, Bestwick RK, Spiro C, Kabat D. The membrane glycoprotein of Friend spleen focus-forming virus: evidence that the cell surface component is required for pathogenesis and that it binds to a receptor. J Virol 1987;61:2782–92.

79. Ruscetti SK, Janesch NJ, Chakraborti A, Sawyer ST, Hankins WD. Friend spleen focus-forming virus induces factor independence in an erythropoietin-dependent erythroleukemia cell line. J Virol 1990;63:1057–62.

Chapter 10

The Pharmacokinetics and Metabolism of Erythropoietin

Jerry L. Spivak and P. Mary Cotes

Erythropoietin is unique among the hematopoietic growth factors because it is the only one that behaves like a hormone. Indeed, it was because of this that erythropoietin was the first hematopoietic growth factor to be discovered (1). Produced in the kidneys and to a small extent in the liver, erythropoietin interacts with erythroid progenitor cells in the bone marrow to promote their proliferation, maintain their viability, and facilitate their differentiation into mature erythrocytes (2). The plasma clearance kinetics of the hormone were, therefore, of interest to investigators even before it was completely purified. Early studies using nonhomologous, crude hormone preparations and different types of assays suggested that the plasma clearance of erythropoietin could be described by a two-compartment model with an elimination phase that varied from 1 to 10 hours for exogenously administered, nonhomologous erythropoietin (3–7) and 3 to 10 hours for endogenously produced erythropoietin (4,8). With the development of recombinant erythropoietin and sensitive and reliable immunoassay procedures based on reagents derived from the recombinant protein (9,10), it became possible to define the metabolism and pharmacokinetics of erythropoietin more fully. In this chapter, we review the plasma clearance kinetics of erythropoietin in view of what is known about its biochemistry, physiology, and metabolism.

The Biochemistry of Erythropoietin

Erythropoietin is a M_r 30,400 glycoprotein (11), and carbohydrate residues constitute 39 percent of its mass (12,13). The hormone is highly conserved, and the homology between the human, other primate, and rodent molecules exceeds 80 percent (14,15). This genetic conservation is also reflected in other important ways. For example, erythropoietin has no homology with any known protein (16,17) and its gene has many features compatible with those of a housekeeping gene (14). Indeed, erythropoietin behaves much like a housekeeping protein because its gene is constitutively active (18,19) and the hormone is never absent from the plasma even when there is extreme erythrocytosis not induced by hypoxia (20,21).

The erythropoietin gene encodes for a mature peptide containing 166 residues, three sites for N-glycosylation, and one site for O-glycosylation (16,17). The only native form of erythropoietin purified to date (that from human urine) is a 165-residue peptide, as is the recombinant human erythropoietin produced in Chinese hamster ovary cells (22). Thus, post-translational modification of the protein is minimal. The carbohydrate content of the recombinant human peptide expressed in the Chinese hamster ovary cell line is similar to that of native human urine erythropoietin, but there are differences with respect to the nature of the sialylgalactosyl linkages and the numbers of N-acetyllactosamine repeating units in the carbohydrate side chains (12,23). The glycosylation of erythropoietin in different preparations from a single clone of a mammalian cell line derived from baby hamster cells was similar, but there were differences in the glycosylation patterns of erythropoietin preparations isolated from the urine of different humans (24). The biologic significance of this type of heterogeneity is unknown. The virtually faithful recapitulation of glycosylation in the recombinant protein made in Chinese hamster ovary cells as compared with the native human molecule seems to be due not only to the fact that Chinese hamster ovary cells contain the necessary glycosyltransferases but also to the fact that site-specific glycosylation may be influenced by the peptide structure itself in the regions of the glycosylation sites (23,25). As discussed below, the presence in some recombinant hormone preparations from Chinese hamster ovary cells of multiple N-acetyllactosaminyl repeating units may have implications for the plasma clearance of the hormone.

Oligonucleotide-directed mutagenesis studies indicate that glycosylation is essential for normal intercellular processing and secretion of the hormone. Erythropoietin is glycosylated at asparagines 24, 38, and 83 as well as at serine 126 (16,17). Synthesis and secretion of recombinant hormone molecules lacking glycosylation at asparagine 24 were normal, but absence of glycosylation at asparagine 38 or 83 impaired both synthesis and secretion of the protein, as did the absence of glycosylation at serine 126 (26). Synthesis of totally unglycosylated erythropoietin was even lower than that seen when tunicamycin was used to inhibit glycosylation of the protein (26,27). Partially glycosylated erythropoietin is presumably rapidly degraded in the endoplasmic reticulum because mRNA expression of erythropoietin mutants lacking glycosylation sites is not different than that for normal erythropoietin (26).

Incomplete or absent glycosylation also seems to impair biologic activity (26,28). Thus, absence of glycosylation at asparagine 24 or 38 markedly reduces biologic activity in vitro, as does complete removal of all asparagine-linked sugars (26,28). This apparently is not merely a consequence of aggregation of the protein (13) and suggests that the carbohydrate side chains may be involved in establishing the conformation of the protein. Although desialation of erythropoietin either does not alter or actually enhances its in vitro biologic activity (29–31), oxidation of the exposed galactose residues of asialoerythropoietin destroys its biologic activity in vitro, suggesting that carbohydrate residues may play a role other than that involving protein conformation with respect to the interaction of erythropoietin with its specific receptors (29,31). The carbohydrate residues of the hormone also have a crucial role in maintaining it in the circulation, as is discussed below.

The Physiology of Erythropoietin

Erythropoietin production is, of course, inducible as well as constitutive, and tissue hypoxia provides the signal for gene transcription (32–34). Normally, plasma erythropoietin is maintained at a constant level in each individual which is independent of age or gender but which can vary among different individuals by a factor of 6 (4 to 24 mU/ml) (20). This basal level of circulating erythropoietin is maintained by constitutive production of the hormone within certain peritubular interstitial cells in the inner renal cortex which are in proximity to the proximal tubules (35,36). With tissue hypoxia, erythropoietin production is not increased in these cells, which seem to synthesize the hormone maximally, but rather in new cells that are anatomically close to the constitutively active cells (37). If hypoxia is substantial, cell recruitment of cells synthesizing erythropoietin occurs in an exponential fashion. As tissue oxygen requirements are satisfied, the numbers of erythropoietin-producing cells decrease exponentially (37).

There are no preformed stores of erythropoietin in the kidneys or the liver, and hypoxia invokes de novo synthesis of the hormone, a process that is dependent on both RNA and protein synthesis (32,37,38). Recent studies demonstrated that the mediator for transduction of an hypoxic stimulus is a rapidly turning over heme protein; presumably, changes in the conformation of this protein according to whether it is oxygenated or deoxygenated mediate the expression of erythropoietin mRNA (34). The stability of erythropoietin mRNA is also enhanced during hypoxia (39). Thus, there are two mechanisms for regulating the expression of the erythropoietin gene. Because erythropoietin synthesis seems to be regulated at the level of its gene in response to tissue hypoxia and because the mature peptide is identical to the gene product save for one amino acid, circulating erythropoietin should normally faithfully reflect erythropoietin production and, by extension, tissue oxygenation, which seems to be the case.

Studies of mRNA expression in the kidney and of plasma erythropoietin levels indicate that, in response to hypoxia, there is a prompt (within 1 hour) increase in erythropoietin production. If the hypoxia is extreme, this increase can be continuous, but otherwise it is self-limited as other compensatory mechanisms for hypoxia are invoked (40–43). In the latter instance, after an initial linear increase in plasma erythropoietin, the concentration of erythropoietin tends to become constant and then decline (43). Parallel studies of renal and plasma erythropoietin (32,41) or of renal erythropoietin mRNA and plasma erythropoietin levels (37) indicated that plasma hormone titers faithfully reflect renal erythropoietin production. Once erythropoietin production returns to basal levels, there is an exponential decline in plasma erythropoietin until a new steady state is reached (4,8).

The Pharmacokinetics of Erythropoietin after Intravenous Administration

Animal Studies

Studies of the plasma clearance of erythropoietin in a variety of species including humans used native exogenous (human urine) erythropoietin, endogenous plasma erythropoietin, or recombinant human erythropoietin. Rodents are convenient for detailed metabolic studies because of their small size and ease in manipulation. Early studies using crude nonhomologous erythropoietin preparations provided accurate descriptions of the plasma clearance of erythropoietin, namely, that exogenously administered erythropoietin had a complex plasma clearance that could best be explained by a two-compartment model (Fig 10.1)(3–6). This has proved to be true regardless of whether the source

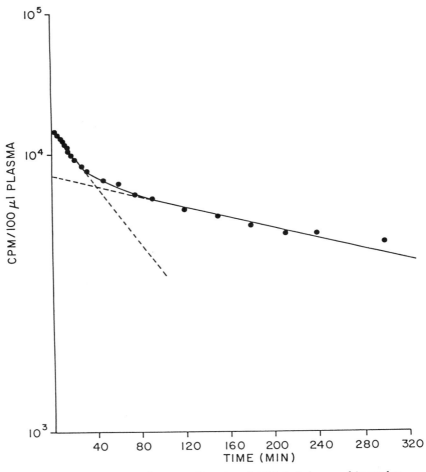

Figure 10.1. The plasma clearance kinetics of ^{125}I-labeled recombinant human erythropoietin given intravenously in the rat. *Source: Reference 44*

of the erythropoietin and the species of the recipient are identical. Table 10.1 describes the plasma clearance of three forms of erythropoietin in the rat (31,43,45). As indicated, the plasma clearance kinetics of iodinated native human urine erythropoietin and iodinated recombinant human erythropoietin were similar and conformed to a two-compartment model (31,45) suggested by earlier studies with impure hormone preparations. Homologous rat plasma erythropoietin behaved in a similar fashion but with an α (distribution) phase that was truncated compared to two of the human erythropoietin preparations, a point to which we will return later (43). In each instance, the immediate volume of distribution after intravenous administration approximated the plasma volume, from which there was additional distribution into the extracellular space. The biphasic clearance of erythropoietin was not a function of its biologic activity because similar plasma clearance kinetics were observed for both inert and biologically active molecules (31,45).

The plasma clearance of exogenous heterologous erythropoietin in the rabbit (6) and the dog (46) also seems to conform to a two-compartment model. As shown in Table 10.2, however, the half-disappearance times differ from those of the rat. The plasma clearance of erythropoietin was also studied in sheep using the homologous plasma hormones, but the data were analyzed only according to a one-compartment model beginning at 1 hour after infusion of the hormone. This type of analysis yielded a half-disappearance time for elimination of 9.1 hours (47). The differences in plasma clearance rates among species, particularly for the elimination phase, are probably not a function of experimental variables; rather, they probably reflect species-specific rates of metabolism for plasma proteins (48). In this regard, it is important to note that the half-disappearance time from the plasma for the elimination of endogenous erythropoietin approximated that of exogenous homologous or heterologous erythropoietin (4,8,49). This suggests that pharmacokinetic measurements made with exogenous erythropoietin are probably physiologically relevant.

Table 10.1. Plasma Clearance of Human Urine Erythropoietin, Recombinant Human Erythropoietin, or Homologous Rat Erythropoietin in the Rat

Erythropoietin Preparation (Ref.)	Recovery, %	Distribution (α) Phase $T_{1/2}$, min	Elimination (β) Phase $T_{1/2}$, min
Human urine (45)	N.D.*	54	204
Recombinant human (31)	88.0 ± 7.5†	53.1 ± 5.6	180.1 ± 16.3
Homologous rat (43)	100	3.6 ± 10.5	86.0 ± 16.0

*N.D., not determined.
†Mean ± SEM.

Table 10.2. Plasma Clearance of Recombinant Human, Crude Human, and Homologous Plasma Erythropoietin in Rabbits, Dogs, and Sheep

Erythropoietin Preparation (Ref.)	Recovery, %	Distribution (α) Phase $T_{1/2}$, min	Elimination (β) Phase $T_{1/2}$, min
Human recombinant in dogs (46)	N.D.*	23.7 ± 5.0†	9.0 ± 0.6
Crude human urine in dogs (46)	N.D.	75.3 ± 21.2	9.0 ± 1.6
Crude human urine in rabbits (6)	N.D.	32.3 ± 8.8	7.8 ± 0.5
Homologous sheep plasma (47)	N.D.	N.D.	9.1 ± 3.9

*N.D., not determined.
†Mean ± SEM.

Human Studies

The plasma clearance of erythropoietin administered intravenously in humans was studied by a variety of investigators, primarily in patients with end-stage renal disease, using recombinant human erythropoietin expressed in Chinese hamster ovary cells. It has been well documented that the clearance of the hormone is not affected by the type of dialysis used (Table 10.3). Although many studies suggest that the plasma clearance of the hormone can be defined by a one-compartment model, others indicate that its plasma clearance is biexponential (Table 10.3). This discrepancy may relate to the quantity of hormone administered because, with the infusion of high concentrations of erythropoietin, it is possible to damp out the initial distribution phase of its plasma clearance. Certainly, the situation is not peculiar to patients with end-stage renal disease. Studies of the pharmacokinetics of erythropoietin in normal individuals suggest that the plasma clearance of the hormone is biexponential when small quantities of erythropoietin are administered (50,51). With large quantities, however, only a monoexponential disappearance curve is obtained (Fig 10.2). In a recent study of normal volunteers given very high doses of erythropoietin (500 to 1000 units/kg), there was a decrease in the rate of plasma clearance of recombinant erythropoietin and in its volume of distribution and its renal clearance (51). The physiologic significance of this is unclear. In patients with chronic renal failure given equivalent doses of erythropoietin, however, neither the plasma clearance nor the volume of distribution of the hormone was tightly linked with the dose of recombinant erythropoietin administered (Table 10.3). Endogenous erythropoietin seems to be

Table 10.3. Plasma Clearance of Recombinant Human Erythropoietin in Humans after Intravenous Administration

Ref.	Volume of Distribution*	Distribution (α) Phase $T_{1/2}$, h	Elimination (β) Phase $T_{1/2}$, h	Comments
(50)	8.9 ± 3.2 litre	0.5 ± 0.1	12.0 ± 5.3	Normal volunteers (300 units/subject)
(51)				Normal volunteers
	90 ml/kg	Present but not measured	4.4 ± 1.1	(10 units/kg)
	60 (40–60) ml/kg	Not present	11.0 ± 0.03	(1000 units/kg)
(52)	5.7% (3.8–7.9) B.W.	0.4 (0.1–4.8)	8.4 (4.8–19)	Predialysis and hemodialysis patients
	4.5% (3.9–6.1) B.W.	0.9 (0.1–2.3)	8.3 (6.6–13)	CAPD patients (100 units/kg)
(53)	75 (63–89) ml/kg	1.8 (0.3–4.8)	8.7 (7.2–11.6)	Hemodialysis patients
	65 (51–82) ml/kg	0.4 (0.02–2.6)	6.8 (3.4–6.9)	After 12 wk of treatment (80 units/kg)
(54)	4.4% ± 2.3 B.W.	N.D.†	8.8 ± 1.8	Hemodialysis patients
	6.7% ± 2.5 B.W.	N.D.	7.7 ± 1.1	After 3 wk of treatment (100 units/kg)
(55)	88 ± 16 ml/kg	2.3 ± 1.2	8.5 ± 1.4	Patients with normal renal function
	65 ± 20 ml/kg	1.9 ± 1.4	8.7 ± 2.1	Hemodialysis patients (150 units/kg)
(56)	5.5% B.W.	N.D.	9.3 ± 3.2	Hemodialysis patients
		N.D.	6.2 ± 1.8	After 2 wk of treatment (15–500 units/kg)
(57)	4.7 ± 1.5 litres	N.D.	5.3 ± 1.3	Hemodialysis patients
	4.2 ± 0.7 litres	N.D.	5.8 ± 1.2	After 8 wk of treatment (24–240 units/kg)
(58)	74 (57–107) ml/kg	N.D.	4.9 (2.3–7.3)	Hemodialysis patients (3–96 units/kg)
	54 (42–70) ml/kg	N.D.	4.2 (3.2–5.2)	After 14–54 wk of treatment (48–192 units/kg)
(59)	33 (21–63) ml/kg	N.D.	8.2 (6.2–10.2)	CAPD patients (120 units/kg)
(44)	—	N.D.	5.1 ± 0.6	CAPD patients
		N.D.	5.6 ± 0.6	After 11–20 week of treatment (100 units/kg)
(60)	4.0 ± 0.39 litres	(0.4)	7.6 ± 1.11 (3.4–12.6)	Predialysis patients
	3.8 ± 0.32 litres	N.D.	4.6 ± 0.28 (3.1–5.4)	After 8 wk of treatment (50–150 units/kg)
(61)	—	N.D.	7.9 ± 0.4	Hemodialysis patients
		N.D.	6.2 ± 0.6	After 6 wk of treatment
		N.D.	5.4 ± 0.9	After 24 wk of treatment
(62)	46 (41–51) ml/kg	N.D.	5.3	Normal volunteers (150 units/kg)
	41 (36–46) ml/kg	N.D.	3.9	After 10 d of q.o.d. therapy

*The variance is provided from the published data as ± SD. or range.
†N.D., not determined.

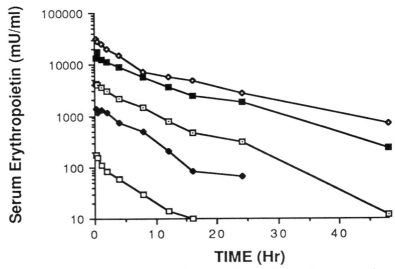

Figure 10.2. The plasma clearance kinetics of recombinant human erythropoietin in normal individuals given different quantities of hormone (10, 50, 150, 500, and 1000 units/kg). The clearance is monoexponential except at the lowest dose, where it is biexponential. *Source: Reference 51*

cleared from the plasma in humans in an exponential fashion. In patients with sickle cell anemia in whom erythropoietin production was suppressed by oxygen administration, the half-disappearance time of endogenous erythropoietin was 1.5 to 3.0 hours (63).

The distribution volume for exogenous erythropoietin varies in different studies (Table 10.3) but seems to be larger than the plasma volume. Differences in the half-disappearance times of the β (elimination) phase of the plasma clearance (Table 10.3) could reflect differences in the recombinant erythropoietin preparations used as well as differences in the metabolism of erythropoietin in the individuals studied. Because circulating erythropoietin levels vary approximately sixfold among normal individuals and the variation is even higher in patients with intrinsic renal disease (64), the latter is not an unlikely supposition. Importantly, some investigators (53–55,60–62) but not others (44,57, 58) observed a slight shortening of the elimination phase of the plasma clearance of erythropoietin after repeated administration of the hormone. As antibodies to recombinant human erythropoietin produced in Chinese hamster ovary cells have never been observed, these data suggested that there was an increase in hormone clearance due to increased utilization by an expanded erythroid progenitor cell pool. As will be discussed below, however, this scenario appears unlikely.

The Pharmacokinetics of Erythropoietin after Subcutaneous or Intraperitoneal Administration

It has been known for many years from small animal studies that erythropoietin is pharmacologically active when administered subcutaneously or by intraperitoneal injection. Indeed, the latter route has been routinely used for convenience in the in vivo mouse bioassay. Recombinant erythropoietin is also pharmacologically active in humans when administered subcutaneously (44,65–67) or via the peritoneum (66), and subcutaneously administered erythropoietin seems equivalent to and perhaps even more effective (in hemodialysis patients, at least) than intravenously administered erythropoietin (66,67). The biologic basis for this seems to be the difference in pharmacokinetics, as shown in Figure 10.3. Although subcutaneously or intraperitoneally administered erythropoietin accumulates in the plasma slowly and to a much lesser extent than a comparable quantity of erythropoietin injected intravenously, the duration of a sustained elevation of plasma erythropoietin above the pretreatment range is much longer for subcutaneously than for intravenously administered erythropoietin. With intraperitoneal administration, plasma accumulation continues long after the erythropoietin has been cleared from the peritoneum, suggesting slow release from another depot such as the lymphatic bed (59,68). Losses of erythropoietin by adsorption on dialysis bags seem to be negligible (44).

Viewed in classic pharmacokinetic terms, the bioavailability of either subcutaneous or intraperitoneal erythropoietin as measured by the area under the curve was approximately 21 to 49 percent (52,53,59) and 2.9 to 6.8 percent (52,53,59), respectively. For the subcutaneously administered hormone, however, the actual effect on the red cell mass was equivalent or even greater than for intravenously administered erythropoietin (66,67). Much larger quantities of the hormone must be administered by the intraperitoneal route for a comparable elevation of circulating erythropoietin (59), suggesting that degradation of erythropoietin is greater in this instance. Thus, classic pharmacokinetic analysis is not useful for predicting the biologic behavior of erythropoietin in vivo, at least when given by the subcutaneous route.

From a biologic perspective, the equipotency of smaller quantities of erythropoietin administered subcutaneously to larger quantities of

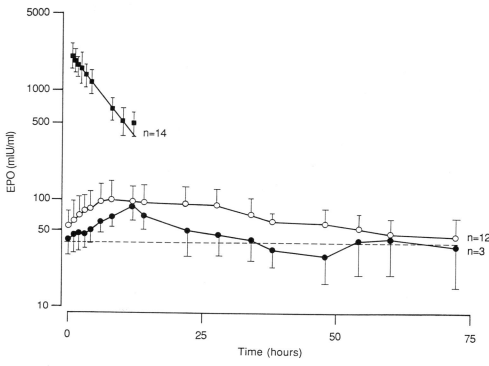

Figure 10.3. The plasma clearance kinetics of recombinant human erythro-poietin (EPO) in patients on continuous ambulatory peritoneal dialysis after administration by different routes. The closed squares indicate the intra-venous route; open circle, subcutaneous; closed circle, intraperitoneal. *Source: Reference 44*

erythropoietin administered intravenously is probably explainable as follows. A bolus intravenous injection of erythropoietin will temporarily saturate tissue receptors while the excess hormone will be eliminated without having any biologic effect. With subcutaneous administration of erythropoietin, the concentration of hormone needed to saturate tis-sue receptors will be present in the plasma continuously because of its slow release from the injection site. An increase in plasma level above normal is likely to be required to sustain an increase in the erythroid progenitor cell pool because erythropoietin acts as a survival factor (69) as well as a mitogen (70). Intermittent bolus intravenous administration of erythropoietin does not result in a sustained increase in plasma erythropoietin, whereas subcutaneous administration is associated with a sustained increase in the plasma erythropoietin level above normal. A constant concentration of erythropoietin in plasma is certainly not a normal phenomenon, even at physiologic levels of the hormone, because there are diurnal changes in plasma erythropoietin (71,72).

The Metabolic Fate of Erythropoietin

Since the discovery of erythropoietin, much effort has been spent in determining how it is metabolized. Early studies focused on the liver, the kidneys, and the bone marrow. Although these studies suggested that the liver has a role in the metabolism of the intact hormone (68,73,74), subsequent studies failed to confirm this (75–77). Because the liver is a site of erythropoietin production (19,78,79), attempts to alter liver function (74) could lead only to ambiguous results; in studies with an isolated perfused liver model, no degradation of the hormone was observed (76,77).

The kidneys have been claimed by some investigators to be a significant site of erythropoietin catabolism (45,46,77,80) in addition to the small proportion of the hormone (usually less than 10 percent) which appears each day in the urine (81). Several laboratories demonstrated a small but significant degradation of erythropoietin by renal tissue (31,45), but other investigators failed to detect a change in the plasma clearance of erythropoietin in anephric animals or humans as compared to its clearance under normal circumstances (43,47,55). Although some of the animal data may be influenced by species' differences, it seems likely that the kidney is not a major site of erythropoietin catabolism or elimination.

Erythropoietin is internalized and degraded by its target cells (82). There has been speculation that the catabolism of the hormone is enhanced when the erythron is increased. Studies in humans and in small animal models have not substantiated this contention (7,83). Thus, the plasma clearance of erythropoietin in mice was identical whether the bone marrow was hypercellular or hypocellular (84,85). This is in keeping with the observation that the circulating erythropoietin level is not different for comparable degrees of anemia in patients with iron deficiency anemia and acquired hemolytic anemia (20). In this regard, it should be noted that erythropoietin production (58) is not influenced by the plasma concentration of the hormone, although its clearance may be (51).

The Role of Carbohydrate Residues in Erythropoietin Metabolism

Erythropoietin is a glycoprotein, and its carbohydrate residues play a significant role with respect to its plasma clearance. Goldwasser and his co-workers were the first to recognize that desialation of erythropoietin did not affect the in vitro activity of the hormone but destroyed its biologic activity in vivo because of rapid removal of the hormone from the circulation (29,86). The importance of the sialic acid residues of erythropoietin is underscored by the observation that their removal is associated with elimination of over 90 percent of the desialated hormone from the circulation within 6 minutes (30,31). The bulk of the hormone is taken up and rapidly degraded by the liver, but an increased proportion is also taken up by the kidneys (31). Oxidation of the penultimate galactose or simultaneous infusion of asialoorosomucoid but not mannose or dextran sulfate prevented rapid loss of the asialoerythropoietin. This indicated that the desialated hormone was being removed from the circulation by hepatic galactose receptors and not by other lectinlike receptors or phagocytosis (31,87). The plasma clearance kinetics of asialogalactoerythropoietin were identical to those of native erythropoietin even though this derivative of the hormone is biologically inactive (31). This suggests that carbohydrate residues may not be the only determinants of the plasma clearance of erythropoietin.

Asialoerythropoietin reaches the bone marrow more quickly than does fully sialated erythropoietin (31). This raises the question of what constitutes the active form of the hormone because it is necessary for erythropoietin to cross the blood-marrow barrier to interact with its progenitor cells. It has been well established that marrow sinus endothelial cells and liver sinus endothelial cells have receptors for galactose (88,89), and this may be the mechanism by which transferrin enters the marrow as well as the liver (90).

With respect to erythropoietin, Sasaki et al. (12) and Takeuchi et al. (23) noted that carbohydrate side chains containing multiple N-acetyllactosaminyl repeating units were more common in recombinant erythropoietin than in human urine erythropoietin. Molecules with this type of carbohydrate configuration may be more susceptible to uptake by the liver and, presumably, the bone marrow, even when fully sialated (87). On the other hand, Tsuda et al. argued that the presence of Gal(β1–3)GlcNAc sequence in native and recombinant erythropoietin preparations may impede hepatic uptake of the hormone (24). Takeuchi et al. also identified an unusual batch of recombinant erythropoietin con-

Table 10.4. Plasma Clearance Kinetics of G-CSF, GM-CSF, M-CSF, and Erythropoietin

Growth Factor (Ref.)	Distribution (α) Phase $T_{1/2}$, min	Elimination (β) Phase $T_{1/2}$, h
rG-CSF* (92)	30	3.8
(93)	8	1.8
rGM-CSF† (94)	5	2.5
‡(95)	7	1.5
mCSF-1§ (96)	10	N.D.
rErythropoietin¶ (31)	53	3.0

Abbreviations: r, recombinant; m, mouse; N.D., not determined.
*Hamsters.
†Humans.
‡Monkeys.
§Mice.
¶Rats.

taining more biantennary side chains than human urine or other batches of recombinant erythropoietin (91). The biantennary form of the hormone was more active in vitro than was conventional erythropoietin but had virtually no activity in vivo, suggesting that the type of branching pattern may influence in vivo survival. Recently, Steinberg and colleagues observed a rapid plasma distribution (α) phase for erythropoietin obtained from hypoxic rats (43). The plasma clearance of the homologous hormone seemed similar to that of asialoerythropoietin or erythropoietin that contains multiple lactosaminyl repeating units (87). It is thus tempting to speculate that, under hypoxic stress, the erythropoietin produced may be different with respect to its carbohydrate side chains than the erythropoietin produced under normal steady state conditions and, therefore, more easily transferred from the blood to the marrow.

A Comparison of Erythropoietin with Other Hematopoietic Growth Factors

As mentioned initially, erythropoietin is unique among the hematopoietic growth factors because it is the only one that behaves like a hormone. Therefore, it was of interest to compare the pharmacokinetics of erythropoietin with macrophage colony-stimulating factor (CSF-1), granulocyte colony-stimulating factor (G-CSF), and granulocyte-macrophage colony-stimulating factor (GM-CSF). As indicated in Table

Table 10.5. Organ Accumulation of Recombinant Erythropoietin or GM-CSF in the Rat

Growth Factor*	$T_{1/2}$, min†		
	Plasma	Liver	Kidney
r Erythropoietin	85	7	3
r Asialoerythropoietin	21	71	7
r GM-CSF	47	3	34
r Asialo-GM-CSF	28	52	12

*The r indicates recombinant.

†At 15 minutes after injection for GM-CSF and at 20 minutes for erythropoietin. r GM-CSF data are from Reference 96. Erythropoietin data are from Reference 31.

10.4, all of the colony-stimulating factors seem to conform to a two-compartment exponential model with respect to their plasma clearance, although this has been carefully evaluated only for G-CSF (92,93). For G-CSF, GM-CSF, and CSF-1, it seems that the bulk of the protein is cleared from the circulation during the α phase of plasma clearance, in contrast to erythropoietin. Differences in the extent and type of glycosylation and molecular weight are not reflected in the plasma clearance times (Table 10.4). CSF-1 is heavily glycosylated, whereas G-CSF is not. CSF-1 may be unique in that its plasma clearance seems to be mediated by the cells whose survival and proliferation it promotes (96,97). This is certainly not true for erythropoietin, and the extent to which G-CSF and GM-CSF are metabolized by their target cells is unknown.

The N-linked carbohydrates of GM-CSF seem to have an important role in maintaining this growth factor in the circulation; even the loss of one N-linked side chain accelerates its plasma clearance (98). GM-CSF, unlike erythropoietin (Table 10.5), has a substantial renal clearance. Like erythropoietin, however, asialo-GM-CSF is cleared rapidly by the liver (98). It is clear from the above data that determinants other than carbohydrates are involved in the plasma clearance of the hematopoietic growth factors, although, in contrast to erythropoietin, the other growth factors are not hormones and seem to be produced and to act locally.

Conclusion

Studies of erythropoietin production and pharmacokinetics suggest that the hormone normally is distributed between the plasma and the extravascular space. The distribution volume of erythropoietin seems to vary among individuals, as does its plasma concentration. The fact that the extravascular acceptor sites for the hormone are normally not saturated suggests that neither the available quantity of erythropoietin nor tissue demands for it influence erythropoietin production. This contention is supported by observations that the rate of erythropoietin production is independent of its plasma concentration and that, within limits, the plasma clearance of erythropoietin is not influenced by its plasma concentration. Erythropoietin is cleared from the plasma in an exponential fashion, and its clearance is slower than that of the other hematopoietic growth factors. The fate of eliminated erythropoietin is unknown. Only a small portion of the hormone is lost in the urine or catabolized by the kidneys, and catabolism by erythroid cells does not seem to constitute a significant source of hormone elimination. Although sialic acid residues protect the hormone from hepatic uptake and degradation, this protection is not complete with respect to erythropoietin molecules that contain multiple lactosaminyl repeating units. Nevertheless, recognition by hepatic galactosyl receptors cannot account for the observed elimination kinetics of erythropoietin because asialoagalactoerythropoietin, which is biologically inert, has the same elimination kinetics as has intact erythropoietin. Another unanswered question about the metabolism of erythropoietin concerns the mechanism by which it is transported across the sinus endothelium, which represents the blood-bone marrow barrier. Galactosyl receptors are displayed by sinus endothelial cells, but no mechanism for desialation of erythropoietin has been identified. The pharmacokinetics of recombinant human erythropoietin expressed in Chinese hamster ovary cells are identical to those of native human urine erythropoietin, and repeated administration of the recombinant protein has not been associated with a significant acceleration of its catabolism. The physiologic significance of the heterogeneity of glycosylation of native erythropoietin between individuals has yet to be explored. Experience with recombinant erythropoietin has thus far been based on the human hormone sequence expressed and glycosylated in a Chinese hamster ovary cell line. Expression of the human sequence in a human cell line may provide further insight into the significance of the heterogeneity of glycosylation patterns (99).

REFERENCES

1. Reissmann KR. Studies on the mechanism of erythropoietin stimulation in parabiotic rats during hypoxia. Blood 1956;5:372–80.

2. Spivak JL. The mechanism of action of erythropoietin. Int J Cell Cloning 1986;4:139–66.

3. Stohlman F Jr., Howard D. Humoral regulation of erythropoiesis IX. The rate of disappearance of erythropoietin from the plasma. In: Jacobson LO, Doyle M, eds. Erythropoiesis. New York: Grune and Stratton, 1962:120–4.

4. Reissmann KR, Diederich DA, Ito K, Schmaus JW. Influence of disappearance rate and distribution space on plasma concentration of erythropoietin in normal rats. J Lab Clin Med 1965;65:967–75.

5. Weintraub AH, Gordon AS, Becker EL, et al. Plasma and renal clearance of exogenous erythropoietin in the dog. Am J Physiol 1964;207:523–9.

6. Roh BL, Paula LG, Thompson J, Fisher JW. Plasma disappearance of ^{125}I-labeled erythropoietin in anesthetized rabbits. Proc Soc Exp Biol Med 1972;141:268–70.

7. Keighley G. The metabolic fate of plasma erythropoietin. In: Jacobson LO, Doyle M, eds. Erythropoiesis. New York: Grune and Stratton, 1962:106–10.

8. Naets JP, Wittek M. Erythropoietic activity of marrow and disappearance rate of erythropoietin in the rat. Am J Physiol 1969;217:297–301.

9. Sherwood JB, Goldwasser E. A radioimmunoassay for erythropoietin. Blood 1979;54:885–93.

10. Egrie JC, Cotes PM, Lane J, et al. Development of radioimmunoassays for human erythropoietin using recombinant erythropoietin as tracer and immunogen. J Immunol Methods 1987;99:235–41.

11. Davis JM, Strickland TW, Yphantis DA. Characterization of recombinant human erythropoietin produced in Chinese hamster ovary cells. Biochemistry 1987;26:2633–8.

12. Sasaki HB, Bothner B, Dell A, Fukuda M. Carbohydrate structure of erythropoietin expressed in Chinese hamster ovary cells by a human erythropoietin cDNA. J Biol Chem 1987;262:12059–76.

13. Dordal MS, Wang FF, Goldwasser E. The role of carbohydrate in erythropoietin action. Endocrinology 1985;116:2293–9.

14. Shoemaker CB, Mitsock LD. Murine erythropoietin gene: cloning, expression, and gene homology. Mol Cell Biol 1986;6:849–58.

15. McDonald JD, Lin F-K, Goldwasser E. Cloning, sequencing, and evolutionary analysis of the mouse erythropoietin gene. Mol Cell Biol 1986;6:842–8.

16. Jacobs K, Shoemaker C, Rudersdorf R, et al. Isolation and characterization of genomic and cDNA clones of human erythropoietin. Nature 1985;313:806–9.

17. Lin F-K, Suggs S, Lin C-H, Browne JK, et al. Cloning and expression of the human erythropoietin gene. Proc Natl Acad Sci USA 1985;82:7580–4.

18. Beru N, McDonald J, Lacombe C, Goldwasser E. Expression of the erythropoietin gene. Mol Cell Biol 1986;6:2571–5.

19. Bondurant MC, Koury MJ. Anemia induces accumulation of erythropoietin mRNA in the kidney and liver. Mol Cell Biol 1986;6:2731–3.

20. Spivak JL, Hogans BB. Clinical evaluation of a radioimmunoassay for serum erythropoietin using reagents derived from recombinant erythropoietin [Abstract]. Blood 1987;70:143a.

21. Moccia G, Miller ME, Garcia JF, Cronkite EP. The effect of plethora on erythropoietin levels. Proc Soc Exp Biol Med 1980;163:36–8.

22. Recny MA, Scoble HA, Kim Y. Structural characterization of natural

human urinary and recombinant DNA-derived erythropoietin. J Biol Chem 1987;262:17156–63.

23. Takeuchi M, Takasaki S, Miyazaki H, et al. Comparative study of the asparagine-linked sugar chains of human erythropoietins purified from urine and the culture medium of recombinant Chinese hamster ovary cells. J Biol Chem 1988;263:3657–63.

24. Tsuda E, Goto M, Murakami A, et al. Comparative structural study of N-linked oligosaccharides of urinary and recombinant erythropoietins. Biochemistry 1988;27:5646–54.

25. Sasaki H, Ochi N, Dell A, Fukuda M. Site-specific glycosylation of human recombinant erythropoietin: analysis of glycopeptides or peptides at each glycosylation site by fast atom bombardment mass spectrometry. Biochemistry 1988;27:8618–26.

26. Dube S, Fisher JW, Powell JS. Glycosylation at specific sites of erythropoietin is essential for biosynthesis, secretion, and biological function. J Biol Chem 1988;263:17516–21.

27. Nielsen OJ, Schuster SJ, Kaufman R, et al. Regulation of erythropoietin production in a human hepatoblastoma cell line. Blood 1987;70:1904–9.

28. Wojchowski DM, Orkin SH, Sytkowski AJ. Active human erythropoietin expressed in insect cells using a baculovirus vector: a role for N-linked oligosaccharide. Biochim Biophys Acta 1987;910:224–32.

29. Goldwasser E, Kung CK-H, Eliason J. On the mechanism of erythropoietin-induced differentiation. XII. The role of sialic acid in erythropoietin action. J Biol Chem 1974;249:4202–6.

30. Lukowsky WA, Painter RH. Studies on the role of sialic acid in the physical and biological properties of erythropoietin. Can J Biochem 1972;50:909–17.

31. Spivak JL, Hogans BB. The in vivo metabolism of recombinant human erythropoietin in the rat. Blood 1989;73:90–9.

32. Schuster SJ, Wilson JH, Erslev AJ, Caro J. Physiologic regulation and tissue localization of renal erythropoietin messenger RNA. Blood 1987;70:316–8.

33. Schuster SJ, Badiavas EV, Costa-Giomi P, et al. Stimulation of erythropoietin gene transcription during hypoxia and cobalt exposure. Blood 1989;73:13–6.

34. Goldberg MA, Dunning SP, Bunn HF. Regulation of the erythropoietin gene: evidence that the oxygen sensor is a heme protein. Science 1988;242:1412–4.

35. Koury ST, Bondurant MC, Koury MJ. Localization of erythropoietin synthesizing cells in murine kidneys by in situ hybridization. Blood 1988;71:524–7.

36. Lacombe C, DaSilva L, Bruneval P, et al. Peritubular cells are the site of erythropoietin synthesis in the murine hypoxic kidney. J Clin Invest 1988;81:620–3.

37. Koury ST, Koury MJ, Bondurant MC, et al. Quantitation of erythropoietin-producing cells in kidneys of mice by in situ hybridization: correlation with hematocrit, renal erythropoietin mRNA, and serum erythropoietin concentration. Blood 1989;74:645–51.

38. Schooley JC, Mahlmann LJ. Evidence for the de novo synthesis of erythropoietin in hypoxic rats. Blood 1972;40:662–70.

39. Goldberg MA, Gaut CC, Bunn HF. Erythropoietin mRNA levels are gov-

erned by both the rate of gene transcription and posttranscriptional events. Blood 1991;77:1–3.

40. Abbrecht PH, Littell JK. Plasma erythropoietin in men and mice during acclimatization to different altitudes. J Appl Physiol 1972;32:54–8.

41. Jelkmann W. Temporal pattern of erythropoietin titers in kidney tissue during hypoxic hypoxia. Pflugers Arch 1982;393:88–91.

42. Milledge JS, Cotes PM. Serum erythropoietin in humans at high altitude and relation to plasma renin. J Appl Physiol 1985;59:360–4.

43. Steinberg SE, Mladenovic J, Matzke GR, Garcia JF. Erythropoietin kinetics in rats: generation and clearance. Blood 1986;67:646–9.

44. Hughes RT, Cotes PM, Oliver DO, et al. Correction of the anaemia of chronic renal failure with erythropoietin: pharmacokinetic studies in patients on haemodialysis and CAPD. Contrib Nephrol 1989;76:122–30.

45. Emmanouel DS, Goldwasser E, Katz AI. Metabolism of pure human erythropoietin in the rat. Am J Physiol 1984;247:F168–76.

46. Fu J-S, Lertora JJL, Brookins J, et al. Pharmacokinetics of erythropoietin in intact and anephric dogs. J Lab Clin Med 1988;111:669–76.

47. Mladenovic J, Eschbach JW, Koup JR, et al. Erythropoietin kinetics in normal and uremic sheep. J Lab Clin Med 1985;105:659–63.

48. Waldman T. Discussion on the metabolic fate of erythropoietin. In: Jacobson LO, Doyle M, eds. Erythropoiesis. New York: Grune and Stratton, 1962:136–9.

49. Eckardt K-U, Boutellier U, Kurtz A, et al. Rate of erythropoietin formation in humans in response to acute hypobaric hypoxia. J Appl Physiol 1989;66:1785–8.

50. Urabe A, Takaku F, Mizoguchi H, et al. Effect of recombinant human erythropoietin on the anemia of chronic renal failure. Int J Cell Cloning 1988;6:179–91.

51. Flaharty KK, Caro J, Erslev A, et al. Pharmacokinetics and erythropoietic response to human recombinant erythropoietin in healthy men. Clin Pharmacol Ther 1990;47:557–64.

52. Kampf D, Kahl A, Passlick J, et al. Single-dose kinetics of recombinant human erythropoietin after intravenous, subcutaneous and intraperitoneal administration. Contrib Nephrol 1989;76:106–11.

53. Neumayer H-H, Brockmoller J, Fritschka E, et al. Pharmacokinetics of recombinant human erythropoietin after SC administration and in long-term IV treatment in patients on maintenance hemodialysis. Contrib Nephrol 1989;76:131–42.

54. Muirhead N, Keown PA, Slaughter D, et al. Recombinant human erythropoietin in the anaemia of chronic renal failure: a pharmacokinetic study [Abstract]. Nephrol Dial Transplant 1988;3:499.

55. Kindler J, Eckardt K-U, Ehmer B, et al. Single-dose pharmacokinetics of recombinant human erythropoietin in patients with various degrees of renal failure. Nephrol Dial Transplant 1989;4:345–9.

56. Egrie JC, Eschbach JW, McGuire T, Adamson JW. Pharmacokinetics of recombinant human erythropoietin (rHuEpo) administered to hemodialysis (HD) patients [Abstract]. Kidney Int 1988;33:262.

57. Wikstrom B, Salmonson T, Grahnen A, Danielson BG. Pharmacokinetics of recombinant human erythropoietin in haemodialysis patients [Abstract]. Nephrol Dial Transplant 1988;3:503.

58. Cotes PM, Pippard MJ, Reid CDL, et al. Characterization of the anaemia

of chronic renal failure and the mode of its correction by a preparation of human erythropoietin (r-HuEPO). An investigation of the pharmacokinetics of intravenous erythropoietin and its effects of erythrokinetics. Q J Med 1989;70:113–37.

59. MacDougall IC, Neubert P, Coles GA, et al. Pharmacokinetics of recombinant human erythropoietin in patients on continuous ambulatory peritoneal dialysis. Lancet 1989;1:425–7.

60. Lim VS, DeGowin RL, Zavala D, et al. Recombinant human erythropoietin treatment in pre-dialysis patients. Ann Intern Med 1989;110:108–14.

61. Maxwell AP, Douglas JF, Afrasiati M, et al. Erythropoietin pharmacokinetics and red cell metabolism in haemodialysis patients [Abstract]. Nephrol Dial Transplant 1989;4:476.

62. McMahon FG, Vargas R, Ryan M, et al. Pharmacokinetics and effects of recombinant human erythropoietin after intravenous and subcutaneous injections in healthy volunteers. Blood 1990;76:1718–22.

63. Embury SH, Garcia JF, Mohandas N, et al. Effects of oxygen inhalation on endogenous erythropoietin kinetics, erythropoiesis, and properties of blood cells in sickle-cell anemia. N Engl J Med 1984;311:291–5.

64. Chandra M, Clemons GC, McVicar M, et al. Serum erythropoietin levels and hematocrit in end-stage renal disease: influence of the mode of dialysis. Am J Kidney Dis 1988;12:208–13.

65. Bommer J, Samtleben W, Koch KM, et al. Variations of recombinant human erythropoietin application in hemodialysis patients. Contrib Nephrol 1989;76:149–58.

66. Eschbach JW, Kelly MR, Haley NR, et al. Treatment of the anemia of progressive renal failure with recombinant human erythropoietin. N Engl J Med 1989;321:158–63.

67. Lui SF, Chung WWM, Leung CB, et al. Pharmacokinetics and pharmacodynamics of subcutaneous and intraperitoneal administration of recombinant human erythropoietin in patients on continuous ambulatory peritoneal dialysis. Clin Nephrol 1990;33:47051.

68. Dukes PP, Goldwasser E. On the utilization of erythropoietin. In: Jacobson LO, Doyle M, eds. Erythropoiesis. New York: Grune and Stratton, 1962:125–7.

69. Koury MJ, Bondurant MC. Erythropoietin retards DNA breakdown and prevents programmed death in erythroid progenitor cells. Science 1990;248:378–81.

70. Spivak JL, Pham TH, Isaacs MA, Hankins WD. Erythropoietin is a mitogen for erythropoietin-dependent cells. Blood (in press).

71. Cotes PM, Brozovic B. Dirunal variation of serum immunoreactive erythropoietin in a normal subject. Clin Endocrinol 1982;17:419–22.

72. Wide L, Bengtsson C, Birgegard G. Circadian rhythm of erythropoietin in human serum. Br J Haematol 1989;72:85–90.

73. Burke WT, Morse BS. Studies on the production and metabolism of erythropoietin in rat liver and kidney. In: Jacobson LO, Doyle M, eds. Erythropoiesis. New York: Grune and Stratton, 1962:111–9.

74. Roh BL, Paulo LG, Fisher JW. Metabolism of erythropoietin by isolated perfused livers of dogs treated with SKF 525-A. Am J Physiol 1972;223:1345–8.

75. Kukral JC, Carney AL, Ebroon E, et al. The role of the liver and surgical stress in erythropoietin metabolism. Surg Forum 1968;19:348–9.

76. Nielsen OJ, Egfjord M, Hirth P. Erythropoietin metabolism in the isolated perfused rat liver. Contrib Nephrol 1989;76:90–7.

77. Dinkelaar RB, Engels EY, Hart AAM, et al. Metabolic studies on erythropoietin (Ep): II. The role of liver and kidney in the metabolism of Ep. Exp Hematol 1981;9:796–803.

78. Fried W. The liver as a source of extrarenal erythropoietin production. Blood 1972;40:671–7.

79. Naughton BA, Kaplan SM, Roy M, et al. Hepatic regeneration and erythropoietin production in the rat. Science 1977;196:301–2.

80. Naets JP, Wittek M. A role of the kidney in the catabolism of erythropoietin in the rat. J Lab Clin Med 1974;84:99–106.

81. Alexanian R. Correlations between erythropoietin production and excretion. J Lab Clin Med 1969;74:614–22.

82. Sawyer ST, Krantz SB, Goldwasser E. Binding and receptor-mediated endocytosis of erythropoietin in Friend virus-infected erythroid cells. J Biol Chem 1987;262:5554–62.

83. Alexanian R. Erythropoietin excretion in bone marrow failure and hemolytic anemia. J Lab Clin Med 1973;82:438–45.

84. Miller ME, Cronkite EP, Okula R, Shiue G. Plasma clearance of erythropoietin (Ep) in mice with perturbed erythropoiesis [Abstract]. Blood 1982;60:22a.

85. Piroso E, Flaharty K, Caro J, Erslev A. Erythropoietin half-life in rats with hypoplastic and hyperplastic bone marrows [Abstract]. Blood 1989; 74:270a.

86. Goldwasser E, Kung CK-H. Progress in the purification of erythropoietin. Ann NY Acad Sci 1968;149:49.

87. Fukuda MN, Sasaki H, Lopez L, Fukuda M. Survival of recombinant erythropoietin in the circulation: the role of carbohydrates. Blood 1989;73:84–9.

88. Kataoka M, Tavassoli M. Identification of lectin-like substances recognizing galactosyl residues of glycoconjugates on the plasma membrane of marrow sinus endothelium. Blood 1985;65:1163–71.

89. Tavassoli M, Kishimoto T, Kataoka M. Liver endothelium mediates the hepatocyte's uptake of ceruloplasmin. J Cell Biol 1986;102:1298–1303.

90. Regoeczi E, Chindemi PA, Hatton MWC, Berry LR. Galactose specific elimination of human asialotransferrin by the bone marrow in the rabbit. Arch Biochem Biophys 1980;205:76–84.

91. Takeuchi M, Inoue N, Strickland TW, et al. Relationship between sugar chain structure and biological activity of recombinant human erythropoietin produced in Chinese hamster ovary cells. Proc Natl Acad Sci USA 1989; 86:7819–22.

92. Cohen AM, Zsebo KM, Inoue H, et al. In vivo stimulation of granulopoiesis by recombinant human granulocyte colony-stimulating factor. Proc Natl Acad Sci USA 1987;84:2484–8.

93. Morstyn G, Souza LM, Keech J, et al. Effect of granulocyte colony stimulating factor on neutropenia induced by cytotoxic chemotherapy. Lancet 1988; 1:667–72.

94. Cebon J, Dempsey P, Fox R, et al. Pharmacokinetics of human granulocyte-macrophage colony-stimulating factor using a sensitive immunoassay. Blood 1988;72:1340–7.

95. Donahue RE, Wang EA, Stone DK, et al. Stimulation of haematopoiesis

in primates by continuous infusion of recombinant human GM-CSF. Nature 1986;321:872–5.

96. Bartocci A, Mastrogiannis DS, Migliorati G, et al. Macrophages specifically regulate the concentration of their own growth factor in the circulation. Proc Natl Acad Sci USA 1987;84:6179–83.

97. Tushinski RJ, Oliver IT, Guilbert LJ, et al. Survival of mononuclear phagocytes depends on a lineage-specific growth factor that the differentiated cells selectively destroy. Cell 1982;28:71–81.

98. Donahue RE, Wang EA, Kaufman RJ, et al. Effects of N-linked carbohydrate on the in vivo properties of human GM-CSF. Cold Spring Harbor Symp Quant Biol 1986;51:685–92.

99. Yanagi H, Yoshima T, Ogawa I, Okamoto M. Recombinant human erythropoietin produced by Namalwa cells. DNA 1989;8:419–27.

Chapter 11

Erythropoietin in Health and Disease

P. Mary Cotes and Jerry L. Spivak

Initial recognition of erythropoietin in body fluids and of its increase during anemia or in response to any hypoxic stimulus depended upon observations made in a range of species, including humans (1,2). It is now apparent that the hormone is a major factor in the control of red cell formation and that estimates of its concentration in body fluids provide information about the physiologic regulation of red cell formation and its disorders. This chapter reviews recent information about erythropoietin in plasma in humans and indicates the place of estimates in diagnosis and as a guide to possible benefit from therapy. For the most part we draw upon data based on immunoassay estimates of erythropoietin, for other assays are less satisfactory for tests on large numbers of plasma samples. In vivo bioassays require larger amounts of erythropoietin than may be available from physiologic samples, and in vitro bioassays are liable to interference from matrix constituents of serum and plasma. Such effects are particularly likely to give invalid estimates of potency when erythropoietin is present in plasma in a low or normal concentration. The significance of changes in the concentration of erythropoietin in plasma needs first to be considered in relation to the formation of the hormone and its entry into and removal from the plasma. For this reason these topics are considered here although discussed in greater detail elsewhere.

The Origin of Plasma Erythropoietin and Its Removal from the Circulation

The main site of formation of erythropoietin is probably interstitial cells (3,4) or tubular cells (5) of the renal cortex, with some erythropoietin, perhaps 5 to 15 percent, formed extrarenally, mainly in the liver (6,7). The results of hybridization studies indicate that some formation may possibly occur in normal bone marrow, probably in macrophages (8). There is no evidence that erythropoietin is stored in any organ so changes in the concentration of erythropoietin in plasma reflect changes in the rates of synthesis or removal of the hormone. Synthesis is increased after any hypoxic stimulus, and the oxygen sensor may well be a heme protein (9) located in or near the cells that synthesize the hormone (10).

Anemia is associated with an increase in renal erythropoietin mRNA, demonstrable 2 hours after blood loss in mice (6). With an increase in the severity of anemia, the number of renal cortical cells that express erythropoietin mRNA increases exponentially; in mice, an increase in serum erythropoietin is directly related to the number of erythropoietin-producing cells in the kidney (4). Thus, we expect and indeed find exponential rather than arithmetic modulation of the concentration of erythropoietin in plasma. Results of other studies in mice indicate that erythropoietin mRNA has a relatively short half-life, with the disappearance of some 50 percent of renal erythropoietin mRNA within 1 hour of the termination of a short period of hypoxia (10). There is a single copy of the erythropoietin gene located on chromosome 7 (11,12). This encodes for a 193-residue peptide from which a 27-residue leader peptide is cleaved. There is also further specific modification involving loss of the arginyl residue from the COOH terminus, leaving a 165-residue peptide (13) that, after glycosylation, gives the complete erythropoietin molecule, with a molecular mass of some 30.4 kd (14).

Removal of erythropoietin from the circulation involves at least three pathways. These are: (a) renal excretion, which probably accounts for no more than 1 to 5 percent of the erythropoietin entering the circulation; (b) removal by binding to specific (and probably mainly high-affinity) erythropoietin effector receptors on red cell progenitors (15); and (c) removal by binding to noneffector receptors that may not be specific for erythropoietin but which include receptors for specific carbohydrate units likely to be important in the removal of partly degraded erythropoietin (16). Estimates of the half-life of native erythropoietin in the circulation in humans vary from a range of 1.5 to 2.9 hours in patients with sickle cell disease (17) to 5.2 hours in normal subjects (18). These estimates may be compared with estimates ranging from 2.3 to 7.3 hours for the half-life of exogenous human erythropoietin derived from recombinant DNA (recombinant human erythropoietin—

rHuEpo) in patients with end-stage renal disease (19). It is still uncertain whether the binding of erythropoietin to specific effector receptors contributes significantly to the removal of the hormone from the circulation. Patients with end-stage renal disease before and after treatment with rHuEpo provide a model for human subjects in whom the erythron (and numbers of erythropoietin effector receptors) is reduced before treatment and increased to nearly normal by treatment. In such subjects the $T_{1/2}$ of exogenous rHuEpo was not influenced by increase in the size of the erythron ($T_{1/2}$ pretreatment mean $\pm$ SD, 4.9 ± 1.7 hours; after approximate doubling of the erythron, 4.2 ± 0.5 hours) (19). In contrast, other studies in patients with renal disease showed shortening of the $T_{1/2}$ of rHuEpo between the first and later doses (20,21).

In the case of macrophage growth factor (CSF-1), removal from the circulation is by binding to specific receptors on macrophages, which are its mature target cells, and this is the main mechanism by which the concentration of CSF-1 in the circulation is controlled (22,23). For most polypeptide hormones, however, there is no evidence that binding to effector receptors is a controlling factor in the removal of hormone from the circulation. Nor is it clear how important are receptors for specific carbohydrate structures in the normal removal of erythropoietin from the circulation. Sialylated tetra-antennary saccharides are major carbohydrate units of erythropoietin and a portion contain N-acetyllactosamine repeats. When galactose residues of rHuEpo are exposed (for example, by treatment with sialidase), the resulting asialo rHuEpo is more rapidly cleared from the circulation than is untreated rHuEpo (16,24,25). However, it is not known whether cleavage of carbohydrate is normally a first step in erythropoietin degradation. Thus, there is no clear evidence for variation or control of the removal of erythropoietin from the circulation by its binding to specific or nonspecific receptors or by changing its excretion in the urine. There is undoubtedly some heterogeneity in the glycosylation of both native human erythropoietin (26,27) and rHuEpo (25). In the latter, molecules containing three N-acetyllactosamine repeats were rapidly removed from the circulation by receptors in liver (25). It is to be anticipated that different patterns of glycosylation in native erythropoietin, as in other glycoprotein hormones (28,29), will be associated with different rates for its removal from the circulation. There is the possibility that this may contribute to regulation of its biologic activity or to variation in the erythropoietin response elicited by different stimuli to production of the hormone. For the most part, however, changes in the concentration of erythropoietin in the plasma seem to reflect changes in the production of the hormone.

The Control of Erythropoietin Production

An increase in erythropoietin production requires a hypoxic stimulus of adequate severity and duration (30). Examples studied include the effects of acute blood loss (31–33) and hypobaric exposure (18, 34,35). After a hypoxic stimulus but before an increase in red cell mass or other mechanisms provide complete correction or compensation for the hypoxia, there is downregulation of erythropoietin production if the marrow is capable of responding to the erythropoietic stimulus of the hormone. Thus, in mice and humans, prolonged hypobaric exposure is accompanied by an initial increase in plasma erythropoietin which returns to a nearly normal concentration long before complete acclimatization (34,35). In contrast, there is no apparent downregulation of erythropoietin production in patients with a persistent anemia. In these, the concentration of erythropoietin in plasma can remain increased indefinitely. In other circumstances the erythropoietin response is enhanced, as in mice in which the marrow erythroid response is reduced by irradiation or the injection of 5-fluorouracil. Here, the erythropoietin response to a hypoxic challenge is greater than in controls (36). This is one of a number of observations which are most easily explained if the size or the potential of the erythron to expand in response to erythropoietin influences the concentration of erythropoietin in plasma. Thus, an increase in serum immunoreactive erythropoietin may occur after treatment with cytostatic drugs, even in the absence of any fall in hemoglobin concentration (37–39). Another phenomenon that may be explained by a similar mechanism is the fall in serum erythropoietin that occurs immediately after the administration of iron to patients with an iron deficiency anemia and before any improvement in oxygen delivery or increase in reticulocyte count (40). This immediate fall in serum erythropoietin is not limited to the correction of iron deficiency; it has also been seen immediately after the administration of B_{12} in pernicious anemia and at the beginning of spontaneous recovery from aplastic anemia (41–43).

There is also a negative feedback by which erythropoietin production is reduced after increased provision of oxygen. This is demonstrable after blood transfusion (44,45) or oxygen breathing (17,18,46) and in patients with severe congestive cardiac failure, in whom clinical improvement after treatment with enalapril was associated with a reduction in serum erythropoietin (47).

The Estimation of Erythropoietin in Plasma

Earliest estimates of erythropoietin were based upon the induction of an increase in circulating red cell mass in intact animals, usually rats (for example, see References 1 and 48). Smaller doses of erythropoietin became detectable when endogenous erythropoietin production and baseline erythropoiesis in intact animals were suppressed by starvation (49) or polycythemia (50,51) and when stimulation of the incorporation of iron 59 into new red cells replaced the increase in total red cell mass as the response parameter (49). The stimulation of incorporation of iron 59 into new red cells of mice made polycythemic by exposure to hypoxia (51) has served as a definitive bioassay for erythropoietin (National Committee for Clinical Laboratory Standards USA, TS6, 1980) and is still widely used for the calibration of rHuEpo for therapeutic use. However, bioassays for erythropoietin using mice in vivo are expensive in time and resources and require larger amounts of erythropoietin (a minimum of 25 to 50 mIU/animal) than are practicable for many clinical studies unless samples are concentrated before assay with appropriate correction for loss of erythropoietin (52). Radioimmunoassays for erythropoietin based on reagents derived from rHuEpo are now widely available and can give estimates of erythropoietin which are similar to estimates by bioassay in vivo (53). Both tracer antigen and erythropoietin antibody contribute to the specificity of each individual radioimmunoassay, and it cannot be assumed that all will show identical specificity. A further generation of sandwich-type immunoassays is now being developed, and some use monoclonal antibodies to erythropoietin (54,55). These offer the possibility of tailoring assays to selected specificities and can use an enzyme indicator in place of a radioactive label. The immunoradiometric assays offer potentially greater sensitivity than do radioimmunoassays. Erythropoietin is relatively stable in serum so that samples frozen at or below $-20°C$ can be stored for many months before assay (56–58).

Several reports draw attention to the occasional invalidity of estimates of erythropoietin from the heterogeneity of serum constituents showing erythropoietin immunoreactivity and the associated nonparallelism of dose-response lines given by such samples compared with a standard preparation of erythropoietin (59–61). It is not yet possible to predict which serum samples will show nonparallelism and, to exclude invalid estimates, sera should be assayed at more than one dose level so that the consistency of potency estimates can be assessed using different regions of the assay dose-response curve.

Erythropoietin in Normal Subjects

Diurnal Changes

In many normal subjects the concentration of erythropoietin in plasma is stable throughout the 24-hour day (62). However, in some (two of eight studied [32]) diurnal changes are seen with highest values toward midnight (63). Similar diurnal changes occurred in 81 percent of patients with chronic hypoxic lung disease (62) and 44 percent of hospitalized patients in whom serum erythropoietin sampled between 8 AM and noon was within the range for normal subjects (64). The reason for the diurnal changes is not understood. All are certainly not attributable to nocturnal hypoxia. In magnitude, the mean deviation of serum erythropoietin may be some 20 percent above the 24-hour mean value.

Adults, Children, Pregnancy, the Fetus, and the Premature Infant

In normal adults the concentration of erythropoietin in plasma is essentially independent of gender. In two studies the mean concentration was higher in women than in men, but there was almost total overlap of the ranges of individual values (65,66). The concentration of erythropoietin in plasma is independent of age in adults (62,67); in healthy children aged 3 months to 16 years, estimates are identical with those in adults (68) (Fig 11.1). For normal infants, data on changes during the first 3 months of life are scanty (68). In the normal human fetus, plasma erythropoietin increases with gestation (69) and is independent of the concentration of erythropoietin in maternal plasma (70). At delivery, cord blood serum erythropoietin is influenced by factors that affect fetal oxygen supply before delivery. After normal gestation and delivery the concentration of erythropoietin in cord serum is very variable. Then, during the first days of life, the concentration of erythropoietin in serum continues to vary widely and is not significantly related to hemoglobin, hematocrit, PaO_2, SaO_2, or arterial oxygen (71). In preterm infants with the anemia of prematurity, concentrations of erythropoietin in serum are inversely related to hemoglobin but lower than in adults, despite lower "available oxygen" (72), and estimates of serum erythropoietin are of no value in determination of the need for transfusion (73). During pregnancy, maternal erythropoietin increases with gestation, although the magnitude of the increase varies greatly among individuals and the stimulus to increased production is not clearly understood (70).

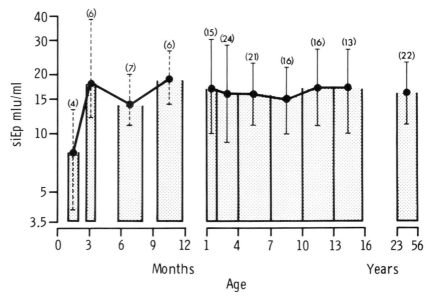

Figure 11.1. Estimates of erythropoietin in serum (siEp) and their relation to age in healthy children and adults. The estimates are shown as the arithmetic mean with ranges (dashed brackets) or the geometric mean with the calculated 95 percent range for the observations (solid brackets). The numbers of subjects are shown in parentheses. Stippled areas indicate the age range of the subjects included in the derivation of each data point. The figure does not include anomalous data for two children whose serum samples were subsequently found to contain a cross-reactant of erythropoietin (60). *Source: Adapted from Reference 68*

Erythropoietin in Umbilical Cord Plasma and Amniotic Fluid as an Indicator of Fetal Risk

Because hypoxia is the main stimulus to increased production of erythropoietin, estimates of erythropoietin in umbilical cord serum and plasma have been studied extensively as possible indicators of fetal hypoxia. The concentration of erythropoietin in amniotic fluid is related to that in umbilical cord plasma (74) so that estimates of amniotic fluid erythropoietin can provide an accessible indicator of fetal erythropoietin production and fetal well-being (75). In Rh-immunized pregnancies, anemia in the fetus induces an increase in cord serum erythropoietin which falls if the anemia is corrected (69); however, an increasing concentration of erythropoietin in amniotic fluid is a useful indicator of fetal distress (76). Abnormal fetal heart rate records are associated with an increase in cord plasma erythropoietin (77) and in amniotic fluid erythropoietin (78). In acute fetal hypoxia cord plasma erythropoietin is not increased (79), although products of adenosine triphosphate (ATP) accumulate rapidly. In contrast, in maternal pre-eclampsia when fetal oxygen supply is likely to be chronically compromised, umbilical plasma erythropoietin is increased (79). With reduction in the time for assay completion, it becomes practicable to assess whether estimates of erythropoietin will contribute to the management of pregnancy.

Anemia

Although the erythropoietin system responds to anemia with an exponential increase in the production of erythropoietin, studies of the relation between hemoglobin concentration and the concentration of erythropoietin in plasma led to the conclusion that, even in the absence of renal disease, the plasma erythropoietin response is not necessarily identical in all anemias of seemingly comparable severity. In renal disease, damage to sites of production of erythropoietin is associated with an inappropriately low concentration of erythropoietin in plasma if assessed in relation to the severity of renal anemia (Fig 11.2). Treatment with acetazolamide also impairs production of erythropoietin, probably because blocking of sodium reabsorption, preferentially in the proximal renal tubule, leads to a decrease in tubular oxygen consumption and change in the signal at the renal oxygen sensor (80,81).

Acute Blood Loss

Acute loss of 450 ml of blood, which reduces hemoglobin to a nadir at about 3 days, is associated with a progressive increase in plasma erythropoietin, which is still raised at 6 days. Among individuals there is great variation in response. At 6 days, however, with a mean increase of some 50 percent above baseline, the mean concentration of plasma erythropoietin is still within the normal range (31). From this fact and data in rats (82), it seems that very small changes in the concentration of erythropoietin in plasma may exert a significant regulatory function. Thus, under normal circumstances, control of erythropoiesis by erythropoietin is exerted on relatively mature red cell progenitors that are responsive to changes in the concentration of erythropoietin in the range of 5 to 50 mIU/ml (83). When blood is taken for autologous transfusion, even after a series of three or four 450-ml bleeds repeated at 3-

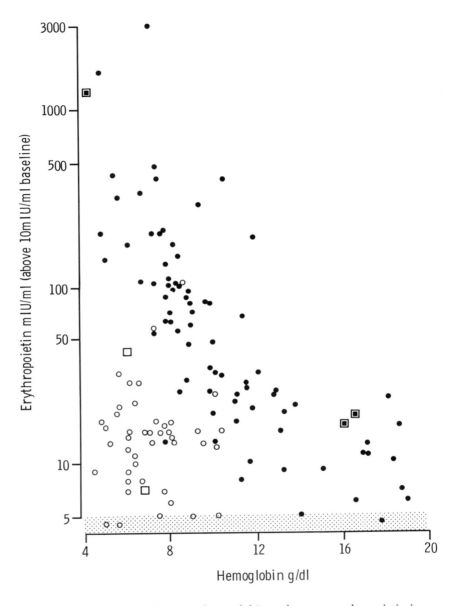

Figure 11.2. The relation between hemoglobin and serum erythropoietin in patients without renal disease (closed circles), patients with a functioning renal transplant (closed squares), and patients with anemia associated with renal failure managed by dialysis (nephric [open circles] and anephric [open squares] subjects). *Source: Reference 32*

Table 11.1. The Effect of Repeated Phlebotomy on Hematocrits and Serum Erythropoietin Levels in Autologous Blood Donors

Number of Phlebotomies	Men		Women	
	Hematocrit, %	Erythropoietin, units/litre	Hematocrit, %	Erythropoietin, units/litre
Normal range	0.41–0.53	4–26	0.36–0.46	4–26
1	0.42 ± 0.01* (18)†	12.6 ± 1.3 (18)	0.40 ± 0.04 (24)	14.0 ± 1.5 (24)
2	0.40 ± 0.01 (18)	15.5 ± 1.4 (18)	0.37 ± 0.04‡ (24)	21.6 ± 2.2§ (24)
3	0.39 ± 0.01 (12)	21.7 ± 4.9§ (12)	0.36 ± 0.06‡ (7)	27.0 ± 3.5§ (8)
4	0.36 ± 0.01‡ (7)	23.4 ± 4.5§ (5)	0.36 ± 0.08‡ (5)	22.0 ± 5.4 (5)

Source: Reference 33. Copyright 1988 by the American Medical Association.
*Values are means ± SEM.
†Numbers in parentheses, numbers of subjects.
‡Value is significantly different from value for first sample ($P < 0.01$).
§Value is significantly different from value for first sample ($P < 0.05$).

to 7-day intervals, the mean increase in serum erythropoietin is about 80 percent and in some subjects the concentration still remains within the normal range for the population (33) (Table 11.1). Acute reduction in total red cell mass by 20 percent by erythraphoresis increased serum erythropoietin by 10 mIU/ml from 16 to 26 mIU/ml (still within the normal range). We infer that this change induced an increase in red cell production to restore red cell mass (84). These observations emphasize that, without extensive baseline data, the erythropoietin response to phlebotomy may be difficult to discern, is of little use as a test to assess normal function of the erythropoietin secretory mechanism, and is of doubtful value in the elucidation of polycythemia. In uncomplicated iron deficiency, serum erythropoietin may not increase above the upper limit of the normal range until hemoglobin falls below 10.5 g/dl (85). The much greater erythropoietin responses in patients with more severe anemia or during acute hypobaric exposure may represent emergency responses. Thus, in mice, reduction in hematocrit from 0.50 to 0.35 by a single bleed (4) is a much more severe challenge than that from a similar reduction in hematocrit brought about gradually by repeated venesection in humans; the former induced a sevenfold increase in serum erythropoietin from 26 to 180 mIU/ml. This and higher concentrations of erythropoietin, which can range up to 10 or 20 IU/ml, influence the maturation and division of progressively earlier red cell progenitors, as well as of more mature ones, and thus have the potential to induce greater increases in red cell mass than can result from effects on late progenitors only.

Renal Disease

Progressive renal disease is usually associated with impaired production of erythropoietin, and this is the main cause of the anemia of renal failure. During the development of renal failure, severity of anemia is related to plasma creatinine, which tends to reflect the extent of renal damage (86). In end-stage renal disease, there is loss of the normal direct relation between the severity of anemia and the log-concentration of erythropoietin in plasma (19,86,87) and most but not all of the erythropoietin in plasma is extrarenal, probably hepatic in origin. In anephric patients serum erythropoietin and hemoglobin tend to be lower than in uremic nephric patients (88), although serum erythropoietin may remain in the range for normal subjects and can increase if hepatitis occurs (89,90). As anemia develops, however, the available erythropoietin seems to be insufficient to induce the expansion of the erythron which would correct the anemia (19). The retention of the erythropoietin hematocrit feedback circuit is demonstrable by a reduction in plasma erythropoietin after transfusion (91) or an increase in erythropoietin production with hypoxia (92).

In patients with polycystic kidney disease, the hemoglobin level may be higher than in other patients with end-stage renal failure (93,94) as a result of autonomous oxygen-independent production of erythropoietin by certain interstitial cells closely associated with proximal tubular cysts (95).

Chronic Disorders and Infection

Gross impairment of erythropoietin formation is uniquely a feature of renal disease. There is also evidence that inappropriately low increases in the concentration of erythropoietin in serum may contribute to the anemia of chronic disorders. In the anemia associated with rheumatoid arthritis, serum erythropoietin is lower than in patients with iron deficiency matched for the severity of anemia (96,97). An inappropriately low concentration of erythropoietin in plasma is also a feature of the anemia associated with the acquired immunodeficiency syndrome (98) (Fig 11.3) and of the anemias associated with malignancy (99) (Fig 11.4), with the exception of hepatocellular carcinoma, in which there may be increased hepatic production of erythropoietin (100). Likewise, in patients with severe hepatic failure, serum erythropoietin may be higher than in patients with iron deficiency matched for the severity of anemia (101). In ulcerative colitis, taken as a model for chronic inflammatory bowel disease, serum erythropoietin tended

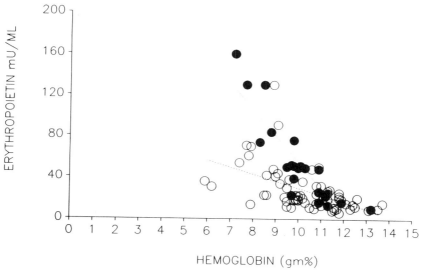

Figure 11.3. The relationship between hemoglobin and serum immunoreactive erythropoietin in 55 anemic, untreated patients with AIDS (open circles) and 23 patients with iron-deficiency anemia (closed circles). For the AIDS patients, the equation for the regression line was $y = -6.6x + 96.1$ ($r = 0.5$, $P < 0.01$). For the patients with iron deficiency, the equation for the regression line was $y = -25.8x + 316$ ($r = 0.9$, $P < 0.01$). The difference between the slopes was significant ($P < 0.01$). *Source: Reference 98. Copyright 1989 by the American Medical Association.*

to be lower than in patients with anemia of comparable severity associated with leukemia (102).

Malnutrition

There is evidence that, in protein-deprived animals, the erythropoietin secretory response to hypoxia is impaired (103,104). In patients with renal disease, increased dietary protein increased serum erythropoietin (105). In Nigerian children, however, protein energy malnutrition did not prevent the typical direct relation between the severity of anemia and the logarithm of the concentration of erythropoietin in serum (106). Serum erythropoietin in control Nigerian children (107) was higher and more variable than that in healthy Norwegian children (68); thus, it is difficult to assess the adequacy of the erythropoietin response to malnutrition in the Nigerian study.

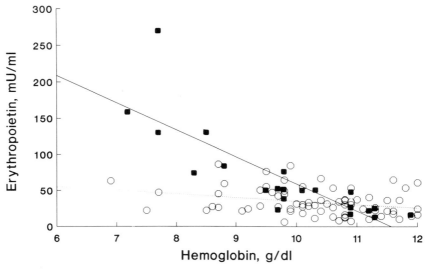

Figure 11.4. Hemoglobin concentrations in relation to serum immunoreactive erythropoietin concentrations in 74 nonhypoxemic anemic patients with cancer (open circles) and 24 patients with iron-deficiency anemia (closed squares). For the cancer patients, the equation for the regression line was $y = -4.9x + 85$ ($r = -0.30$, $P = 0.48$). For the patients with iron deficiency (the controls), the equation for the regression line was $y = -45.0x + 518$ ($r = -0.71$, $P = 0.001$). *Source: Reference 99. Reprinted by permission of the New England Journal of Medicine.*

Miscellaneous

In the anemia of thermal injury, urinary erythropoietin increases with increasing severity of anemia (107). Thus, impaired production of erythropoietin is not consistently a major factor in this anemia, which is almost certainly multifactorial in etiology (108).

Erythrocytosis and Apropriate and Inappropriate Production of Erythropoietin

An increased hematocrit without significant increase in total red cell volume, variously called stress polycythemia or Gaisbock's syndrome, is not associated with any abnormality of erythropoietin production, and estimates of erythropoietin in serum are normal and make no contribution to diagnosis (109) (Fig 11.5, column 4). In contrast, in patients with erythrocytosis, an estimate of erythropoietin in plasma or serum may be a useful diagnostic indicator.

We consider erythrocytosis under three categories: (a) secondary erythrocytosis associated with hypoxia, (b) secondary erythrocytosis from inappropriate overproduction of erythropoietin (which is sometimes familial), and (c) polycythemia rubra vera.

Erythrocytosis Secondary to Hypoxia

Secondary erythrocytosis associated with hypoxia is a heterogeneous grouping, and information is available about the concentration of erythropoietin in plasma in several more homogeneous groups of subjects. In patients with erythrocytosis secondary to hypoxic lung disease, serum erythropoietin is increased above normal in about 50 percent (84). Serum erythropoietin is consistently normal in patients with severe hypoxic lung disease who do not develop erythrocytosis. These patients do not show the same severity of nocturnal hemoglobin oxygen desaturation which occurs in patients in whom red cell mass is increased. In this study neither the duration or severity of nocturnal desaturation nor smoking history (despite the fact that smoking alone may induce polycythemia [110]) indicated the polycythemic patients in whom serum erythropoietin was above normal. We infer that the normal concentrations of serum erythropoietin occur from the same down-regulatory phenomenon that gives a fall in erythropoietin production after the initial increase in response to chronic exposure to hypobaric hypoxia from high-altitude exposure or during simulated altitude exposure. In these circumstances, the initial hypoxic stimulus induces an almost immediate increase in serum erythropoietin within about 2 hours (18,30,32); the increase continues until about 48 hours (34). There is then downregulation of production with a decrease in serum erythropoietin to nearly normal values. This occurs well before acclimatization is complete and while hemoglobin is still increasing (34,35). Despite downregulation of production, the oxygen sensor is still able to respond to an increase in the severity of hypoxia (from ascent to a higher altitude) with a further increase in erythropoietin production (35).

Congenital cyanotic cardiac disease, which usually induces erythrocytosis, provides a further model for study of the control of erythropoietin production. As in climbers after the initial phase of exposure to a high altitude, serum erythropoietin is usually in the range for normal subjects (111). In a small proportion of cases, an atypically small in-

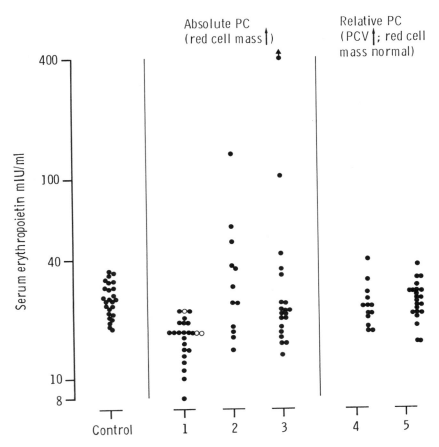

Figure 11.5. Estimates of serum immunoreactive erythropoietin in the investigation of patients with a raised hematocrit, with or without erythrocytosis, compared with normal controls. Column 1 indicates patients with polycythemia (PC) rubra vera (closed and open circles; open circles indicate those treated with radioactive phosphorus); Column 2, patients with secondary erythrocytosis; Column 3, patients with erythrocytosis of unknown cause after a full investigation except for erythropoietin estimation; Column 4, patients without erythrocytosis but with a raised packed red cell volume (PCV) and reduced plasma volume (stress polycythemia or Gaisbock's syndrome); Column 5, patients with raised hematocrit at first test but normal total red cell volume and normal plasma volume. *Source: Reference 109. Reprinted by permission of the New England Journal of Medicine.*

crease in hemoglobin, an exceptionally low Pao_2, or a low mixed venous oxygen saturation and tension are associated with an increase in serum erythropoietin (111–113). Thus, as in other hypoxic conditions, down-regulation of erythropoietin production occurs only if there is an "adequate" hemoglobin response. Findings in these three studies contrast with an earlier report (114) that mean serum erythropoietin is increased in patients with cyanotic congenital heart disease.

Overall, there is now a considerable amount of data indicating that the conventional textbook wisdom that patients with secondary hypoxic erythrocytosis usually have plasma erythropoietin values above the normal range is misleading. In about 50 percent of patients with secondary erythrocytosis associated with hypoxia, plasma erythropoietin is in the range found in normal subjects. In some patients values are above normal. It is essentially true that, in these patients, despite erythrocytosis, there is never suppression of plasma erythropoietin below normal values. In this respect, these patients are different from those with polycythemia rubra vera and from animal models with polycythemia from hypertransfusion (115).

Erythrocytosis from Inappropriate Overproduction of Erythropoietin

This is an uncommon but well-recognized occurrence. It may be associated with a localized erythropoietin-producing lesion; in these instances abolition of the erythrocytosis by correction or excision of the lesion provides proof of the diagnosis. In addition to localized renal lesions (116), including renal artery stenosis (117), a number of ectopic sites of erythropoietin production have been described (116).

In all of these instances an estimate of erythropoietin in serum is only sometimes increased above normal. Typical of such cases is a nephroblastoma with erythrocytosis corrected by nephrectomy despite a normal concentration of erythropoietin in venous blood draining from the tumor (118). In erythrocytosis associated with cerebellar hemangioblastoma, erythropoietin may be detected in cerebrospinal fluid (119). Regenerating hepatocytes have increased capacity for production of erythropoietin, and this probably accounts for increases in hemoglobin in hemodialysis patients during viral hepatitis (120,123) and during a period of transient liver enzyme abnormalities (89).

However, it is in cases of inappropriate overproduction of erythropoietin without any localized site for its production and in the absence of abnormal blood oxygen affinity that diagnosis depends upon an abnormally high concentration of erythropoietin in body fluids (Fig 5, column 3). Overproduction may occur intermittently and is not excluded by a single normal estimate (109). This condition is sometimes familial (121,122).

Polycythemia Rubra Vera

In this clonal disorder of which erythrocytosis is one manifestation, the increased red cell mass exerts the normal negative feedback control on erythropoietin production. Serum or plasma erythropoietin is reduced, although in many patients values remain in the normal range (109). Differences in reports of the discriminatory value of estimates of erythropoietin in differentiating between polycythemia rubra vera and secondary hypoxic polycythemia may be accounted for by differences in assay specificity or in patient selection (65,109,114). An estimate of serum or plasma erythropoietin that is below or near the lower limit of normal is a useful indicator of polycythemia rubra vera. An increased value excludes it.

Conclusion

Immunoassays now permit direct estimation of erythropoietin in serum and plasma. Such determinations provide insight into the regulation of erythropoietin production and are of use in the investigation of anemia and erythrocytosis and in the identification of patients who might benefit from therapy with recombinant human erythropoietin.

REFERENCES

1. Gordon AS. Hemopoietine. Physiol Rev 1959;39:1–40.
2. Erslev A. Humoral regulation of erythropoiesis. Blood 1953;8:349–57.
3. Lacombe C, De Silva JL, Bruneval P, et al. Peritubular capillary cells are the site of erythropoietin synthesis in the murine hypoxic kidney. J Clin Invest 1988;81:620–3.
4. Koury ST, Koury MJ, Bondurant MC, Caro J, Grabar SE. Quantitation of erythropoietin-producing cells in kidneys of mice by in situ hybridization: correlation with hematocrit, renal erythropoietin mRNA, and serum erythropoietin concentration. Blood 1989;74:645–51.
5. Maxwell AP, Lappin TR, Johnston CF, Bridges JM, McGeown MG. Erythropoietin production in kidney tubular cells. Br J Haematol 1990;74:535–9.
6. Bondurant MC, Koury MJ. Anemia induces accumulation of erythropoietin mRNA in the kidney and liver. Mol Cell Biol 1986;6:2731–3.

7. Beru N, McDonald J, Lacombe C, Goldwasser E. Expression of the erythropoietin gene. Mol Cell Biol 1986;6:2571–5.

8. Vogt C, Pentz S, Rich IN. A role for the macrophage in normal hemopoiesis: III. In vitro and in vivo erythropoietin gene expression in macrophages detected by in situ hybridization. Exp Hematol 1989;17:391–7.

9. Goldberg MA, Dunning SP, Bunn HF. Regulation of the erythropoietin gene: evidence that the oxygen sensor is a heme protein. Science 1988;242: 1412–4.

10. Schuster SJ, Wilson JH, Erslev AJ, Caro J. Physiologic regulation and tissue localization of renal erythropoietin messenger RNA. Blood 1987;70: 316–8.

11. Powell JS, Berkner KL, Lebo RV, Adamson JW. Human erythropoietin gene: high level expression in stably transvected mammalian cells and chromosome expression. Proc Natl Acad Sci USA 1986;83:6465–9.

12. Law ML, Cai G-Y, Lin F-K, et al. Chromosomal assignment of the human erythropoietin gene and its DNA polymorphism. Proc Natl Acad Sci USA 1986;83:6920–4.

13. Recny MA, Scoble HA, Kim Y. Structural characterization of natural human urinary and recombinant DNA-derived erythropoietin. J Biol Chem 1987;262:17156–65.

14. Davis JM, Strickland TW, Yphantis DA. Characterization of recombinant human erythropoietin produced in Chinese hamster ovary cells. Biochemistry 1987;26:2633–8.

15. Sawyer ST, Krantz SB, Goldwasser E. Binding and receptor-mediated endocytosis of erythropoietin in Friend-virus infected erythroid cells. J Biol Chem 1987;262:5554–62.

16. Spivak JL, Hogans BB. The in vivo metabolism of recombinant human erythropoietin in the rat. Blood 1989;73:90–9.

17. Embury SH, Garcia JF, Mohandas N, Pennathur-Das R, Clark MR. Effects of oxygen inhalation on endogenous erythropoietin kinetics, erythropoiesis and properties of blood cells in sickle-cell anemia. N Engl J Med 1984;311:291–5.

18. Eckardt K, Boutellier U, Kurtz A, Schopen M, Koller EA, Bauer C. Rate of erythropoietin formation in humans in response to acute hypobaric hypoxia. J Appl Physiol 1989;66:1785–8.

19. Cotes PM, Pippard MJ, Reid CDL, Winearls CG, Oliver DO, Royston JP. Characterization of the anaemia of chronic renal failure and the mode of its correction by a preparation of human erythropoietin (r-HuEPO). An investigation of the pharmacokinetics of intravenous erythropoietin and its effects on erythrokinetics. Q J Med New Ser 1989;70:113–37.

20. Egrie JC, Eschbach JW, McGuire T, Adamson JW. Pharmacokinetics of recombinant human erythropoietin (r-HuEPO) administered to hemodialysis (HD) patients. Kidney Int 1988;33:Abstract 152.

21. Lim VS, DeGowin RL, Zavala D, et al. Recombinant human erythropoietin treatment in pre-dialysis patients. Ann Intern Med 1989;110:108–14.

22. Tushinski RJ, Oliver IT, Guilbert LJ, Tynan PW, Warner JR, Stanley ER. Survival of mononuclear phagocytes depends on a lineage-specific growth factor that the differentiated cells selectively destroy. Cell 1982;28:71–81.

23. Bartocci A, Mastrogiannis DS, Migliorati G, Stockert RJ, Wolkoff AW. Macrophages specifically regulate the concentration of their own growth factor in the circulation. Proc Natl Acad Sci USA 1987;84:6179–83.

24. Lukowsky WA, Painter RH. Studies on the role of sialic acid in the physical and biological properties of erythropoietin. Biochemistry 1972;50:909–17.

25. Fukada MN, Sasaki H, Lopez L, Fukuda M. Survival of recombinant erythropoietin in the circulation: the role of carbohydrates. Blood 1989;73: 84–9.

26. Miyaki T, Kung CK-H, Goldwasser E. Purification of human erythropoietin. J Biol Chem 1977;252:5558–64.

27. Yanagawa S, Hirade K, Ohnota H, et al. Isolation of erythropoietin with monoclonal antibodies. J Biol Chem 1984;259:2707–10.

28. Robertson DM, VanDamme M-P, Dixzfalusy E. Biological and immunological characterization of human luteinizing hormone: I. Biological profile in pituitary and plasma samples after electrofocusing. Mol Cell Endocrinol 1977;9:45–56.

29. Wide L. The regulation of metabolic clearance rate of human FSH in mice by variation of the molecular structure of the hormone. Acta Endocrinol (Copenh) 1986;112:336–44.

30. Schooley JC, Mahlmann LJ. Evidence for the de novo synthesis of erythropoietin in hypoxic rats. Blood 1972;40:662–70.

31. Miller ME, Cronkite EP, Garcia JF. Plasma levels of immunoreactive erythropoietin after acute blood loss in man. Br J Haematol 1982;52:545–9.

32. Cotes PM. Physiological studies of erythropoietin in plasma. In: Jelkman W, Gross AJ, eds. Erythropoietin. Berlin: Springer-Verlag, 1989;57–79.

33. Kickler TS, Spivak JL. Effect of repeated whole blood donations on serum immunoreactive erythropoietin levels in autologous donors. JAMA 1988;260:65–7.

34. Abbrecht PH, Littell JK. Plasma erythropoietin in men and mice during acclimatization to different altitudes. J Appl Physiol 1972;32:54–8.

35. Milledge JS, Cotes PM. Serum erythropoietin in humans at high altitude and its relation to plasma renin. J Appl Physiol 1985;59:360–4.

36. Barceló AC, Bozzini CE. Erythropoietin formation during hypoxia in mice with impaired responsiveness to erythropoietin induced by irradiation or 5-fluorouracil injection. Experientia 1982;38:504–5.

37. Birgegard G, Wide L, Simonsson B. Marked erythropoietin increase before fall in Hb after treatment with cytostatic drugs suggests mechanism other than anaemia for stimulation. Br J Haematol 1989;72:462–6.

38. Piroso E, Erslev AJ, Caro J. Inappropriate increase in erythropoietin titres during chemotherapy. Am J Hematol 1989;32:248–54.

39. Hellebostad M, Marstrander J, Slordahl S, Cotes PM, Refsum HE. Serum immunoreactive erythropoietin in children with acute leukaemia at various stages of disease and the response to treatment. Eur J Haematol 1990;44: 159–64.

40. Bjarnason I, Cotes PM, Knowles S, Reid C, Wilkins R, Peters TJ. Giant lymph node hyperplasia (Castleman's disease) of the mesentry. Observations on the associated anemia. Gastroenterology 1984;87:216–23.

41. Ortega JA, Shore NA, Hammond D. Erythropoiesis and erythropoietin during recovery from severe anemia [Abstract]. Blood 1969;34:838.

42. Zalusky R. Erythropoietin (ESF) "utilisation" in nutritional anemias [Abstract]. Clin Res 1967;15:291.

43. Finne PH, Skoglund R, Wetterhus S. Urinary erythropoietin during initial treatment of pernicious anaemia. Scand J Haematol 1973;10:62–8.

44. Cotes PM. Immunoreactive erythropoietin in serum. I. Evidence for the

validity of the assay method and the physiological relevance of estimates. Br J Haematol 1982;50:427–38.

45. Berglund B, Hemmingsson P, Birgegard G. Detection of autologous blood transfusions in cross-country skiers. Int J Sports Med 1987;8:66–70.

46. Cotes PM, Lowe RD. The influence of renal ischaemia on red cell formation. Memoirs Soc Endocrinol 1963;13:187–94.

47. Fyhrquist F, Karppinen K, Honkanen T, Saijomaa O, Rosenlof K. High serum levels are normalized during treatment of congestive heart failure with enalapril. J Int Med 1989;226:257–60.

48. Garcia JF, Van Dyke DC. Dose-response relationships of human urinary erythropoietin. J Appl Physiol 1959;14:233–6.

49. Plzak LF, Fried W, Jacobson LD, Bethard WF. Demonstration of stimulation of erythropoiesis by plasma from anemic rats using Fe⁵⁹. J Lab Clin Med 1955;46:671–8.

50. Jacobson LO, Goldwasser E, Gurney CW. Transfusion-induced polycythaemia as a model for studying factors influencing erythropoiesis. In: Wolstenholme GEW, O'Connor M, eds. Haemopoiesis. Ciba Foundation Symposium. London: Churchill, 1960:423–52.

51. Cotes PM, Bangham DR. Bioassay of erythropoietin in mice made polycythaemic by exposure to air at a reduced pressure. Nature 1961;191:1065–7.

52. Erslev AJ, Caro J, Kansu E, Miller O, Cobbs E. Plasma erythropoietin in polycythemia. Am J Med 1979;66:243–7.

53. Egrie JC, Cotes PM, Lane J, Gaines Das RE, Tam RC. Development of radioimmunoassays for human erythropoietin using recombinant erythropoietin as tracer and immunogen. J Immunol Methods 1987;99:235–41.

54. Goto M, Murakami A, Akai K, et al. Characterization and use of monoclonal antibodies directed against human erythropoietin that recognize different antigenic determinants. Blood 1989;74:1415–23.

55. Wogum AW, Lansdorp PM, Eaves AC, Krystal G. An enzyme linked immunosorbent assay for erythropoietin using monoclonal antibodies, tetrameric immune complexes, and substrate amplification. Blood 1989;74:622–8.

56. Cotes PM, Canning CE. Stability of immunoreactive erythropoietin in blood, plasma and serum. Blood 1982;60(Suppl 1):85a.

57. Mizoguchi H, Ohta K, Suzuki T, et al. Basic conditions for radioimmunoassy of erythropoietin and plasma levels of erythropoietin in normal subjects and anemic patients. Acta Haematol Jpn 1987;50:15–24.

58. Eckardt K-U, Kurtz A, Hirth P, Scigalla P, Wieczorek L, Bauer C. Evaluation of the stability of human erythropoietin in samples for radioimmunoassay. Klin Wochenschr 1988;66:241–5.

59. Cotes PM, Canning CE, Gaines Das RE. Modification of a radioimmunoassay for human serum erythropoietin to provide increased sensitivity and investigate nonspecific serum responses. In: Hunter WM, Corrie JET, eds. Immunoassays for clinical chemistry. Edinburgh: Churchill Livingstone, 1983:106–12, 124–7.

60. Cotes PM, Tam RC, Reed PJ, Hellebostad M. An immunological cross-reactant of erythropoietin in serum which may invalidate erythropoietin radioimmunoassay. Br J Haematol 1989;73:265–8.

61. Sherwood JB, Carmichael LD, Goldwasser E. The heterogeneity of circulating human serum erythropoietin. Endocrinology 1988;122:1472–7.

62. Miller ME, Garcia JF, Cohen RA, Cronkite EP, Moccia G, Acevedo J.

Diurnal levels of immunoreactive erythropoietin in normal subjects and subjects with chronic lung disease. Br J Haematol 1981;49:189–200.

63. Cotes PM, Brozovic B. Diurnal variation of serum immunoreactive erythropoietin in a normal subject. Clin Endocrinol (Oxf) 1982;17:419–22.

64. Wide L, Bengtsson C, Birgegard G. Circadian rhythm of erythropoietin in human serum. Br J Haematol 1989;72:85–90.

65. Garcia JF, Ebbe SN, Hollander L, Cutting HO, Miller ME, Cronkite EP. Radioimmunoassay of erythropoietin: circulating levels in normal and polycythemic human beings. J Lab Clin Med 1982;99:624–35.

66. Rhyner K, Egli F, Niemöller M, Wieczorek A, Greminger P, Vetter W. Serum erythropoietin werte bei verschiedenen Krankheitszuständen. Nephron 1989;51(Suppl 1):39–46.

67. Mori M, Murai Y, Hirai M, et al. Serum erythropoietin titres in the aged. Mech Ageing Dev 1988;46:105–9.

68. Hellebostad M, Hågå P, Cotes PM. Serum immunoreactive erythropoietin in healthy normal children. Br J Haematol 1988;70:247–50.

69. Thomas RM, Canning CE, Cotes PM, et al. Erythropoietin and cord blood haemoglobin in the regulation of human fetal erythropoiesis. Br J Obstet Gynaecol 1983;90:795–800.

70. Cotes PM, Canning CE, Lind T. Changes in serum immunoreactive erythropoietin during the menstrual cycle and normal pregnancy. Br J Obstet Gynaecol 1983;90:304–11.

71. Hågå P, Cotes PM, Till JA, Shinebourne EA, Halvorsen S. Is oxygen supply the only regulator of erythropoietin levels? Serum immunoreactive erythropoietin during the first 4 months of life in term infants with different levels of arterial oxygenation. Acta Paediatr Scand 1987;76:907–13.

72. Brown MS, Garcia JF, Phibbs RH, Dallman PR. Decreased response of plasma immunoreactive erythropoietin to "available oxygen" in anemia of prematurity. J Pediatr 1984;105:793–8.

73. Keyes WG, Donohue PK, Spivak JL, Jones D, Oski FA. Assessing the need for transfusion of premature infants and role of hematocrit, clinical signs and erythropoietin level. Pediatrics 1989;84:412–7.

74. Teramo KA, Widness JA, Clemons GK, Voutilainen P, McKinlay S, Schwartz R. Amniotic fluid erythropoietin in normal and abnormal pregnancy. Obstet Gynecol 1987;69:710–6.

75. Harkness RA, Cotes PM, Gordon H, McWhinney N. Prolonged pregnancy and fetal energy supply: amniotic fluid concentrations of erythropoietin, hypoxanthine, xanthine and uridine in uncomplicated prolonged pregnancy. J Obstet Gynaecol 1988;8:235–42.

76. Voutilainen PEJ, Widness JA, Clemons GK, Schwartz R, Teramo KA. Amniotic fluid erythropoietin predicts fetal distress in Rh-immunized pregnancies. Am J Obstet Gynecol 1989;160:429–34.

77. Widness JA, Teramo KA, Clemons GK, et al. Correlation of the interpretation of fetal heart rate records with cord plasma erythropoietin levels. Br J Obstet Gynaecol 1985;92:326–32.

78. Smith JH, Anand KJS, Cotes PM, et al. Antenatal fetal heart rate variation in relation to the respiratory and metabolic status of the compromised human fetus. Br J Obstet Gynaecol 1988;95:980–9.

79. Ruth V, Fyhrquist F, Clemons G, Raivio KO. Cord plasma vasopressin, erythropoietin and hypoxanthine as indices of asphyxia at birth. Pediatr Res 1988;24:490–4.

80. Miller ME, Rorth M, Parving HH, et al. pH effect on erythropoietin response to hypoxia. N Engl J Med 1973;288:706–10.

81. Eckardt K-U, Kurtz A, Bauer C. Regulation of erythropoietin production is related to proximal tubular function. Am J Physiol 1989;256:F942–7.

82. Miller ME, Garcia JF, Shiue GG, Okula RM, Clemons GK. Humoral regulation of erythropoiesis. In: Killmann SVA, Cronkite EP, Mullerberat CN, eds. Haemopoietic stem cells. Copenhagen: Munksgaard, 1983:217–33. (Alfred Benzon Symposium Series; vol 18.)

83. Monette FC. Cell amplification in erythropoiesis: in vitro perspectives. In: Dunn CDR, ed. Current concepts in erythropoiesis. New York: Wiley, 1983:21–57.

84. Wedzicha JA, Cotes PM, Empey DW, Newland AC, Royston JP, Tam RC. Serum immunoreactive erythropoietin in hypoxic lung disease with and without polycythaemia. Clin Sci 1985;69:413–22.

85. Spivak JL, Hogans BB. Clinical evaluation of a radioimmunoassay for serum erythropoietin using reagents derived from recombinant erythropoietin [Abstract]. Blood 1987;70(Suppl 1):143a.

86. McGonigle RJS, Wallin JD, Shadduck RK, Fisher JW. Erythropoietin deficiency and inhibition of erythropoiesis in renal insufficiency. Kidney Int 1984;25:437–44.

87. Gimenez LF, Watson AF, Spivak JL. Serum immunoreactive erythropoietin in patients with end stage renal disease. In: The biology of hematopoiesis (in press).

88. Caro J, Brown S, Miller O, Murray T, Erslev AJ. Erythropoietin levels in uremic nephric and anephric patients. J Lab Clin Med 1979;93:449–58.

89. Brown S, Caro J, Erslev AJ, Murray TA. Spontaneous increase in erythropoietin and hematocrit value associated with transient liver enzyme abnormalities in an anephric patient undergoing hemodialysis. Am J Med 1980; 68:280–4.

90. Simon P, Boffa G, Ang KS, Menault M. Polyglobulie chez une hémodialysée anéphrique ayant une hépatite. Mise en évidence d'une sécrétion d'érythropoiétine. Nouv Presse Med 1982;11:1401–3.

91. Walle AJ, Wong GY, Clemons GK, Garcia JF, Niedermayer W. Erythropoietin-hematocrit feedback circuit in the anemia of end-stage renal failure. Kidney Int 1987;31:1205–9.

92. Chandra M, Clemons GK, McVicar MI. Relation of serum erythropoietin levels to renal excretory function: evidence for lowered set point for erythropoietin production in chronic renal failure. J Pediatr 1988;113:1015–21.

93. Chandra M, Miller ME, Garcia JF, Mossey RT, McVicar M. Serum immunoreactive erythropoietin levels in patients with polycystic kidney disease as compared with other hemodialysis patients. Nephron 1985;39:26–9.

94. Shalhoub RJ, Rajan U, Kim VV, Goldwasser E, Kark JA, Antoniou LD. Erythrocytosis in patients on long term hemodialysis. Ann Intern Med 1982; 97:686–90.

95. Eckardt K-U, Mollmann M, Neumann R, et al. Erythropoietin in polycystic kidneys. J Clin Invest 1989;84:1160–6.

96. Baer A, Dessypris EN, Goldwasser E, Krantz SB. Blunted erythropoietin response to anaemia in rheumatoid arthritis. Br J Haematol 1987;66:559–64.

97. Hochberg MC, Arnold CM, Hogans BB, Spivak JL. Serum immunoreactive erythropoietin in rheumatoid arthritis: impaired response to anaemia. Arthritis Rheum 1988;31:1318–21.

98. Spivak JL, Barnes DC, Fuchs E, Quinn TC. Serum immunoreactive erythropoietin in HIV-infected patients. JAMA 1989;261:3104–7.

99. Miller CB, Jones RJ, Piantadosi S, Abeloff MD, Spivak JL. Decreased erythropoietin response in patients with anemia of malignancy. N Engl J Med 1990;322:1689–92.

100. Kew MC, Fisher JW. Serum erythropoietin concentrations in patients with hepatocellular carcinoma. Cancer 1986;58:2485–8.

101. Harris ML, Spivak JL. Serum immunoreactive erythropoietin levels in patients with liver disease or inflammatory bowel disease [Abstract]. Gastroenterology 1988;94:172a.

102. Johannsen H, Jelkmann W, Wiedemann G, Otte M, Wagner T. Erythropoietin/haemoglobin relationship in leukaemia and ulcerative colitis. Eur J Haematol 1989;43:201–6.

103. Reissmann KR. Protein metabolism and erythropoiesis. I. The anemia of protein deprivation. Blood 1964;23:137–45.

104. Anagnastou A, Schade S, Ashkinaz M, Barone J, Fried W. Effect of protein deprivation on erythropoiesis. Blood 1977;50:1093–7.

105. Rosenberg ME, Howe RB, Zanjani ED, Hostelter TH. The response of erythropoietin to dietary protein in renal disease. J Lab Clin Med 1989; 113:735–42.

106. Wickramasinghe S, Cotes PM, Gill DS, Tam RC, Grange A, Akinyanju OO. Serum immunoreactive erythropoietin in protein-energy malnutrition. Br J Haematol 1985;60:515–24.

107. Andes WA, Rogers PW, Beason JW, Pruitt BA. The erythropoietin response to the anemia of thermal injury. J Lab Clin Med 1976;88:584–92.

108. Wallner SF, Vautrin R. The anemia of thermal injury: mechanism of inhibition of erythropoiesis. Proc Soc Exp Biol Med 1986;181:144–50.

109. Cotes PM, Dore CJ, Yin JAL, et al. Determination of serum immunoreactive erythropoietin in the investigation of erythrocytosis. N Engl J Med 1986;315:283–7.

110. Smith JR, Landaw SA. Smokers' polycythemia. N Engl J Med 1978; 298:6–10.

111. Hågå P, Cotes PM, Till JA, Minty BD, Shinebourne EA. Serum immunoreactive erythropoietin in children with cyanotic and acyanotic congenital heart disease. Blood 1987;70:822–6.

112. Giddings SS, Stockman JA. Erythropoietin in cyanotic heart disease. Am Heart J 1988;116:128–32.

113. Tyndall MR, Teital DF, Lutin WA, Clemons GK, Dallman PR. Serum erythropoietin levels in patients with congenital heart disease. J Pediatr 1987; 110:538–44.

114. Koeffler HP, Goldwasser E. Erythropoietin radioimmunoassay in evaluating patients with polycythemia. Ann Intern Med 1981;94:44–7.

115. Moccia G, Miller ME, Garcia JF, Cronkite EP. The effect of plethora on erythropoietin levels. Proc Soc Exp Biol Med 1980;163:36–8.

116. Thorling EB. Paraneoplastic erythrocytosis and inappropriate erythropoietin production. Scand J Haematol 1976; Suppl 17:1–16.

117. Bacon BR, Rothman SA, Ricanati ES, Rashad FA. Renal artery stenosis with erythrocytosis after renal transplantation. Arch Intern Med 1980;140: 1206–11.

118. Reman O, Troussard X, Boutard P, Lacombe C, Mandard JC, Leporrier

M. Nèphroblastome de l'adulte révèlé par une polyglobulie. Presse Med 1988; 17:78–9.

119. Jankovic GM, Ristić MS, Pavlovic-Kentera V. Cerebellar haemangioblastoma with erythropoietin in cerebrospinal fluid. Scand J Haematol 1986; 36:511–4.

120. Kolk-Vegter AJ, Bosch E, Van Leeuwen AM. Influence of serum hepatitis on haemoglobin level in patients on regular haemodialysis. Lancet 1971; 1:526–8.

121. Adamson JW. Familial polycythemia. Semin Hematol 1975;12:383–96.

122. Hellmann A, Rotoli B, Cotes PM, Luzzatto L. Familial erythrocytosis with over production of erythropoietin. Clin Lab Haematol 1983;5:335–42.

123. Klassen DK, Spivak JL. Hepatitis-related hepatic erythropoietin production. Am J Med 1990;89:684–6.

II. Clinical Trials

Recombinant Human Erythropoietin (Epoetin Alfa) in Patients on Hemodialysis: United States

Joseph W. Eschbach

Anemia, an almost universal complication of progressive renal failure, is a major factor causing the increased morbidity that limits rehabilitation with dialysis therapy, despite adequate biochemical control of uremia. The anemia is primarily due to the inability of the diseased kidney to produce adequate amounts of erythropoietin, although mild hemolysis and blood loss secondary to uremic platelet dysfunction may contribute (1). Therapy for the anemia traditionally has been limited to red cell transfusions and androgens. However, such therapy is incomplete and associated with potential complications (2). Definitive therapy with erythropoietin replacement was not possible until the erythropoietin gene was cloned and expressed and was shown to be effective in animals (3,4).

Recombinant human erythropoietin (epoetin alfa) became available for Phase I–II clinical trials in late 1985 (5), and reports of its use in anemic hemodialysis patients (6–14), including a Phase III clinical trial in the United States (15), indicated that almost all responded with an effective increase in erythropoiesis, cessation of transfusions, and improved well-being. This chapter summarizes the results of intravenous epoetin alfa (epoetin) therapy in the largest number of hemodialysis patients studied in the United States.

Patients, Materials, and Methods

Four hundred ninety-eight hemodialysis patients from 13 dialysis centers entered the study.* Patient entry began on December 3, 1985,

*University of Alabama (E. Rutsky, K. Zuckerman), University of Arizona (D. Ogden,

and concluded on November 17, 1988. Many have been followed for more than 4 years. Criteria for entry included hematocrit of <30 percent, adequate iron stores, no disease that might impair a response to epoetin, controlled hypertension, no history of seizures, and a history of being on hemodialysis for at least 3 months. Of the 498 patients, 56 percent were women, and the mean age was 50 years (range, 18–81).

Recombinant human erythropoietin (epoetin alfa, Epogen; Amgen Inc., Thousand Oaks, California) was given three times per week, at the end of each hemodialysis, into the venous return tubing. The treatment protocols were devised, monitored, and funded by Amgen, Inc. Initial doses varied between 1.5 and 1500 units/kg; most patients received either 150 or 300 units/kg. Subsequent doses were adjusted to maintain the hematocrit at 35 ± 3 percent (SEM). Further adjustments in the epoetin dose were made by increments of ±12.5–25 units/kg every 2 weeks if necessary.

In the Phase I–II clinical trial in Seattle, 35 patients were treated (5). The initial 15 patients did not respond to epoetin doses of 1.5, 5.0, and 15 units/kg except for one anephric, iron-overloaded patient. With 15 units/kg, this patient had a rise in hematocrit from 15 to 27.5 which then plateaued at 23.5 until the dose was increased. Some of the other patients were retreated at higher doses so that a total of 23 patients responded to initial doses of 50 to 1500 units/kg.

The Phase III clinical trial involved 333 patients at nine centers (University of Alabama; University of Arizona; Cleveland Clinic; Downstate Medical Center, New York; University of Missouri; Rush-Presbyterian-St. Luke's Medical Center, Chicago; UCLA; Vanderbilt University; and the University of Washington/Northwest Kidney Center) (15). Patients initially received epoetin, either 300 or 150 units/kg, three times per week. These doses were reduced to 75 units/kg when the target hematocrit was reached and were readjusted thereafter to maintain a hematocrit of 35 ± 3 percent.

A double-blind, placebo-controlled clinical study involved three centers (Harvard University, Henry Ford Medical Center, and Johns Hopkins University) and 101 patients (data on file; Amgen, Inc., Thousand

J. Stivelman, J. Van Wyck), Cleveland Clinic (M. Abdulhadi, E. Paganini), Downstate Medical Center, New York (B. Delano, A. Lundin, E. Friedman), Harvard University (J. M. Lazarus), Henry Ford Medical Center (N. Levine, R. Michaels, R. Mohini), Johns Hopkins University (A. Watson), Mayo Clinic (W. Johnson, J. McCarthy, T. Yanagihara), University of Missouri (J. Van Stone), Rush-Presbyterian-St. Luke's Medical Center, Chicago (S. Korbet), U.C.L.A. (A. Nissenson), Vanderbilt University (S. Krantz, W. Stone, P. Teschan), and University of Washington/Northwest Kidney Center (J. Adamson, J. Eschbach, N. Haley).

Oaks, California). Fifty patients were initially treated with placebo (0.25 percent human albumin in sterile, buffered saline) intravenously three times per week for 12 weeks. Forty-nine completed placebo therapy and subsequently were treated with epoetin.

A serial study of hemodynamics was begun in 20 and carried out in 18 Seattle patients at either 50 or 150 units/kg intravenously thrice weekly to determine whether the dose of epoetin or the rate of rise in hematocrit contributed to the rise in blood pressure, if it occurred (16).

Because seizures occurred in several patients in the first clinical trials, a study was initiated to determine if epoetin or a rising hematocrit adversely affected cerebral or cutaneous blood flow. Ten anemic, hemodialysis patients were given intravenous epoetin, 150 units/kg thrice weekly. In five patients, frequent phlebotomy maintained the baseline hematocrit (25 $\pm$ 2); the other five patients were not phlebotomized and their hematocrits increased to 33 $\pm$ 2 (17).

The effectiveness of therapy was determined by serial blood counts with measurement of corrected reticulocytes, serum iron, total iron binding capacity, and serum ferritin. A quality of life questionnaire was completed by a large proportion of the patients at baseline and after approximately 6 and 10 months of epoetin therapy. These results were previously reported (18).

The safety of therapy was evaluated in all patients by serial histories and physical examinations, blood chemistries, other hematologic values, chest x-ray films, electrocardiograms, and determinations of epoetin antibodies. Cerebral blood flow, whole blood viscosity, and transcutaneous oxygen tension were measured serially in one subgroup of patients, and serial, noninvasive hemodynamic measurements of cardiac output and peripheral vascular resistance were measured in another subgroup.

Laboratory results are expressed as means $\pm$ standard error.

Results

The Efficacy of Epoetin

Erythropoiesis. Four hundred forty-nine anemic hemodialysis patients completed 12 weeks of therapy with epoetin alfa in five clinical trials. The mean baseline hematocrit of 22.3 $\pm$ 0.2 percent increased to 32 to 38 percent or increased 6 percent over baseline. This was considered an effective response. The mean corrected reticulocyte count at baseline was 1.1 $\pm$ 0.4 percent; it increased to 2.5 $\pm$ 0.1 percent by the onset of the maintenance phase. The epoetin dosage needed to maintain a

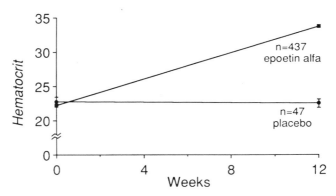

Figure 12.1. Change in the hematocrit after 12 weeks of therapy with epoetin alfa in 437 hemodialysis patients, compared to placebo therapy in 47 hemodialysis patients.

hematocrit of 35 ± 3.0 percent ranged from 12.5 to 525 units/kg, with a median dose of 75 units/kg intravenously thrice weekly. None of the placebo-treated patients (47 completed 12 weeks of "therapy") had a significant rise in hematocrit (22.8 ± 0.9 percent to 22.5 ± 1.2 percent) (Fig 12.1) or corrected reticulocytes (1.1 ± 0.2 percent to 0.9 ± 0.1 percent).

The epoetin-induced increased erythropoiesis subsequently decreased the need for red cell transfusions, decreased iron overload, and improved quality of life.

Transfusions. In 473 patients, 1173 red cell transfusions were required during the 6 months before the initiation of epoetin therapy—an average of 0.41 transfusion per month per patient. All patients ceased requiring transfusions within 2 months of epoetin therapy. Occasional transfusions have been required since then, following blood losses related to surgery or hemorrhage, or when epoetin therapy was interrupted.

Reduction of Iron Overload. Eighty-three of 443 patients (19 percent) had iron overload as defined by a serum ferritin level greater than 1000 ng/ml. In these patients, after 6 months of epoetin therapy, the mean serum ferritin level decreased 38 percent, from 3387 ± 73 to 2116 ± 62 ng/ml.

Quality of Life. Over 300 patients completed questionnaires at baseline and after approximately 6 and 10 months of epoetin therapy. There was almost a twofold increase in the number of patients who stated that they had no complaints and/or were able to carry on normal activity after 6 and 10 months of therapy (37 at baseline vs. 50 and 48 percent at 6 and 10 months, respectively), by Karnofsky scoring, while the number that were mildly to moderately impaired at baseline decreased after therapy (69 vs. 46 vs. 48 percent at baseline, 6, and 10 months, respectively) (18). According to the Nottingham Health Profile, energy level improved from a baseline score of 50 to 24 after 6 months and to 23 after 10 months of therapy ($P = 0.001$) (100 = complete limitation, 0 = absence of limitation) (18).

Follow-up. Of the 449 patients who completed 12 weeks of therapy, 96 percent responded to epoetin. Of the 16 patients who initially failed to respond to epoetin, 3 eventually responded at the initial doses and 1 with the α-thalassemia trait responded after the dose was increased to 1200 units/kg, thrice weekly. Myelofibrosis, osteomyelitis, and acute and/or chronic blood loss were present in the remaining patients. Of the 49 patients not completing 12 weeks of epoetin therapy, 12 patients received inadequate doses (1.5–15 units/kg) and the remaining patients withdrew for personal or medical reasons or received a kidney transplant.

Of 424 patients beginning epoetin therapy, 335 received 1 year of therapy, 241 remained on epoetin as of March 1, 1989, and 195 were on therapy as of March 1, 1990. These latter patients have had epoetin treatment for 2¼ to 4 years. The reasons for withdrawal from the study were renal transplantation (10 percent), death (9 percent), possible toxicity (4 percent), voluntary withdrawal (4 percent), and miscellaneous reasons (2 percent).

The Safety of Epoetin

The adverse effects of epoetin treatment can be divided into those directly related to the administration of epoetin and those indirectly related to the increase in red cell mass.

Direct Effects. Sixteen patients (4 percent) had myalgias and a flulike syndrome within 60 to 90 minutes after receiving epoetin. These cleared with repeated injections, except for two patients, who discontinued epoetin therapy because of these symptoms (15). Ten patients developed injected conjunctivae. Some others experienced headaches or flank pain. These effects eventually cleared and did not prevent continued therapy.

No antibodies to epoetin have developed in >3 years of intravenous administration (J. C. Egrie, Ph.D., personal communication). Increasing the red cell mass by epoetin therapy has resulted in most of the perceived adverse effects: iron deficiency, hypertension, seizures, increased dialyzer clotting, and hyperkalemia and hyperphosphatemia.

Iron Deficiency. Two hundred nineteen of 437 patients (50 percent) developed evidence of absolute or relative iron deficiency as defined by a serum ferritin of <30 ng/ml and a percentage of transferrin saturation of <20 or by a percentage of transferrin saturation of <20 associated with a normal serum ferritin, respectively (5). This occurred at any time during the course of epoetin therapy and depended on the quantity of iron stores at the beginning of therapy (19). Most patients required and received either oral or intravenous iron during the acute phase of epoetin therapy. Despite this, the serum ferritin levels decreased from a mean baseline of 987 ± 24 to 638 ± 20 ng/ml in 354 patients by the onset of the maintenance phase. In 17 patients treated for at least 3 years, the mean serum ferritin level decreased from 1330 ± 339 to 192 ± 63 ng/ml (20) (Fig 12.2). Iron stores were unchanged in the placebo-treated patients.

Hypertension. In 103 of 330 (31 percent) evaluable patients, a rise in diastolic blood pressure of ≥10 mm Hg occurred or an increase in antihypertensive medication was needed. Of the 330 patients, 225 (68 percent) had baseline hypertension. However, an equal percentage of normotensive and hypertensive patients had clinically significant increases in their blood pressure after responding to epoetin therapy. Four of 50 (8 percent) placebo-treated patients had a ≥10-mm Hg rise in diastolic blood pressure (double-blind, placebo-controlled clinical study—data on file; Amgen, Inc., Thousand Oaks, California).

One concern has been whether a more rapid rise in hematocrit from higher doses of epoetin would accentuate this pressor response. The results of the Phase III clinical trial indicated that there was no difference between the incidence of hypertension in those treated with 300 or 150 units/kg (15). For further evaluation of this issue, 18 patients underwent monthly noninvasive hemodynamic studies for up to 5 months and at 1 year. The pressor response in 10 patients receiving 150 units/kg intravenously, thrice weekly, was compared to that in 8 patients receiving 50 units/kg. Because an earlier study indicated that severe anemia (hematocrit <20) was a risk factor for patients to become more hypertensive after epoetin therapy (21), we purposely included more

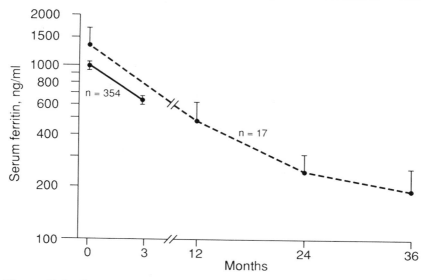

Figure 12.2. Change in serum ferritin levels during epoetin alfa therapy: during acute therapy in 354 hemodialysis patients (solid line) and over 3 years in 17 hemodialysis patients (dashed line).

severely anemic patients in the lower dose group; their baseline hematocrit was 20.4 ± 0.6. The baseline hematocrit in the higher dose group was 24.5 ± 0.9.

The peripheral vascular resistance increased in both groups along with normalization of the elevated cardiac output; mean arterial blood pressure increased equally in both groups. In the group receiving 50 units/kg, new or additional antihypertensive medication was required in four of the eight patients after 2 months of epoetin therapy and was usually associated with a hematocrit that was rising to above 29 (22). Subsequent hemodynamic measurements were difficult to interpret in light of the extra antihypertensive medications. The blood pressure response in the higher (150 units/kg) dose group was similar, with one exception; the response occurred earlier because the red cell mass increased at a more rapid rate.

Seizures. Eighteen of 424 patients (4 percent) experienced seizures. In 10 patients, the seizures occurred within the first 3 months of epoetin therapy when the hematocrit was increasing, and these seizures were often related to a sudden increase in blood pressure.

For assessment of the role of epoetin and an increasing red cell mass on central nervous system function, cerebral blood flow, whole blood viscosity, and transcutaneous oxygen tension were measured in two groups of anemic patients treated with epoetin (17). All received 150 units/kg intravenously thrice weekly for 4 months. Five patients responded with hematocrits increased to 33 ± 0.9, while the other five patients had periodic phlebotomy and supplemental iron therapy to keep their hematocrits at baseline of 26 ± 0.9. In those whose hematocrits increased to 33 ± 0.9, whole blood viscosity increased to normal, cerebral blood flow decreased from above normal to normal, and transcutaneous oxygen tension increased. There was no increase in blood pressure or development of seizures. In the patients who also received epoetin but whose hematocrits did not change because of periodic phlebotomies, there was no change in whole blood viscosity, blood pressure, or transcutaneous oxygen tension, and cerebral blood flow remained elevated (17).

Effects on Vascular Access Clotting. Forty-seven of 386 patients experienced 72 episodes of access clotting during the initial 6 to 12 months of epoetin therapy. This represents an incidence of access clotting of 0.26 episode per patient year, an incidence no greater than that observed in 1111 hemodialysis patients not receiving epoetin (15).

The mean platelet count increased from 224 ± 4 to 252 ± 5 × 10^9/litre ($P < 0.0005$) in 356 patients during the acute phase but did not change thereafter. The platelet count also increased slightly but without significance in 47 patients treated with placebo for 12 weeks (210 ± 3 to 222 ± 4 × 10^9/litre). Prothrombin and partial thromboplastin times and fibrinogen levels did not change with epoetin therapy.

Adequacy of Hemodialysis. This was determined by serial measurements of predialysis serum creatinine, urea nitrogen, potassium, and phosphorous concentrations. There were no significant increases in urea nitrogen levels. In 400 patients, the serum creatinine levels increased from 13.3 ± 0.3 to 13.9 ± 0.4 mg/dl ($P < 0.0005$), the serum potassium (n = 325) increased from 5.1 ± 0.04 to 5.2 ± 0.06 meq/litre, and serum phosphorus levels (n = 320) increased from 5.5 ± 0.1 to 6.3 ± 0.2 mg/dl ($P < 0.0005$) after the hematocrit had increased from 22.3 ± 0.2 percent to 34.0 ± 0.2 percent during the first 12 to 24 weeks of epoetin therapy. Although serum potassium levels rose only slightly, they are the most critical, and hyperkalemia has resulted in the deaths of 2 epoetin-treated patients in the clinical trials due to dietary noncompliance. In 17 patients treated for more than 3 years, there was an increase in predialysis serum creatinine and phosphorus levels within 1 year of therapy, which remained stable thereafter (20).

Other Effects. In over 4 years of epoetin therapy, there have been no consistent changes in liver function tests; serum uric acid, lipids, calcium, or alkaline phosphatase; white blood count; or electrocardiograms. Serial chest x-ray films have demonstrated no changes in pulmonary status, but the transverse diameter of the heart has decreased in most patients who had baseline cardiomegaly (21).

Discussion

The results of these United States trials with epoetin alfa extend the observations of smaller initial trials with epoetin (5–15). More than 96 percent of 449 anemic hemodialysis patients responded and achieved the target hematocrit (32–38 percent) within 12 weeks of the initiation of epoetin therapy. Regular red cell transfusions were eliminated. Maintaining a stable hematocrit has not been difficult, and no patient has become refractory to treatment after initially responding unless iron deficiency or inflammation has supervened. Patients who dialyzed at home had no difficulty injecting the epoetin alfa into the dialysis circuit, and nurses easily made the injections part of the routine dialysis protocol. The symptoms of anemia (easy fatigability, coldness, poor appetite, insomnia and/or sleepiness, and depression) often improved as the result of increasing the hematocrit to approximately 32–38 percent.

The health of dialysis patients has been positively affected by epoetin in three major ways: elimination of routine transfusions and their associated complications, improved quality of life, and improved tissue/organ function as a result of better tissue perfusion.

Elimination of routine transfusions will greatly decrease the incidence of transfusion-related complications. Transmission of blood-borne infections such as hepatitis C, which has an incidence of 1 in 25 transfusions (23), should be markedly reduced, resulting in less mortality and hospitalization for this complication. Elimination of transfusions has also resulted in a serial reduction in HLA antibody formation as expressed by T and B cell panel reactive activity (24). This has resulted in an increased number of previously transfused patients now able to benefit from renal transplantation. Elimination of transfusions has also reduced iron stores and will eventually eliminate the risks from iron overload. These risks include cardiac, liver, pancreatic, and pituitary dysfunction (25), proximal myopathy (26), infection (27), and cancer (28). The need for the iron chelate, deferrioxamine, will also be decreased, reducing the risk of mucormycosis (29). Serum ferritin levels decrease spontaneously as a result of decreased iron intake (no more transfused hemoglobin iron), a shift of reticuloendothelial iron into more new red cells (erythropoiesis is increased by two- to threefold [30]), and continued losses of hemoglobin-iron remaining in the dialyzer after use. Of patients, 19 percent had iron overload as defined by a serum ferritin of greater than 1000 ng/ml. In these patients, after 6 months of epoetin therapy the mean serum ferritin level decreased 38 percent. In 17 patients treated for at least 3 years, the mean serum ferritin level decreased from 1139 to 186 ng/ml. Iron overload can be reduced more rapidly if regular phlebotomy is combined with higher epoetin doses, as shown by Lazarus et al. (31). (This Amgen-sponsored study was not included in the present analysis of epoetin-treated patients.) This indicates that iron overload, with its potential for associated side effects, will not be a medical problem for dialysis patients in the future.

Quality of life, as determined by subjective and objective responses to serial questionnaires, has increased in a significant number of patients. Over 300 of the 424 patients treated with epoetin were evaluated serially and disclosed improvement in energy and activity level, functional ability, sleep and eating behavior, satisfaction with health, sex life, and happiness (18).

Improved tissue oxygenation has resulted in a reduction in "feeling cold" and elimination of a Raynaud's syndrome (7), improved central nervous system function (32–35), improved exercise tolerance (36,37), and a decrease in the anemia-induced elevated cardiac output with an associated reduction in cardiac enlargement (38,39). Retinal circulation improved in one patient, leading to improved vision.

There were three major adverse consequences from correcting the anemia with epoetin: iron deficiency, hypertension, and seizures. Increased vascular access clotting and underdialysis were not clinically significant problems.

Elemental iron is a requirement for adequate hemoglobin formation. Epoetin therapy at the usual doses increases erythropoiesis by two to threefold (30). This results in the mobilization of reticuloendothelial iron for hemoglobin synthesis and leads to a decrease in serum iron, percentage of transferrin saturation, and serum ferritin. In addition, because red cell transfusions are eliminated, less exogenous iron enters the body and, because hemodialyzers always retain some blood after use, red cell or iron loss continues. As a result of these three mechanisms, iron deficiency is now much more common in the hemodialysis patient than before epoetin therapy.

Iron deficiency, either absolute or relative, developed in 50 percent of the patients. In these patients, iron replacement therapy, either as daily oral iron compounds (100–150 mg elemental iron) or periodic intravenous iron dextran (100–500 mg), was necessary to maintain the percentage of transferrin saturation at >20 for optimal epoetin response. Iron deficiency is technically a preventable complication unless the patient is both allergic to intravenous iron dextran and unable to tolerate oral iron.

Hypertension is a common manifestation in patients with chronic renal failure. In dialysis patients blood pressure often may be controlled without antihypertensive medications by maintaining euvolemia. The anemia may also contribute to the improvement in blood pressure control as a result of peripheral vasodilatation. However, 31 percent of the patients in this study (vs. 8 percent of placebo-treated hemodialysis patients) had a significant increase in blood pressure associated with near correction of their anemia. This complication has also been noted by others (6–9). Reversal of the vasodilatation may explain this phenomenon, as hypertension has also occurred in very anemic subjects with normal renal function whose anemia was corrected by other hematopoietic agents (40–42). Whole blood viscosity increases as the hematocrit increases, but it is not solely responsible for the increase in blood pressure; many patients do not become hypertensive with correction of anemia. In a subgroup of patients, two risk factors were identified that increased the likelihood that blood pressure would increase after an erythropoietic response to epoetin: a baseline hematocrit of ≤20 and the baseline blood pressure (21). A baseline pressure of 85 to 90 mm Hg could predispose to significant hypertension because the diastolic blood pressure often increased by 10 mm Hg when the hematocrit reached approximately 30. These hemodynamic changes are similar to those observed when the anemia is corrected with red cell transfusions (43). Factors that are not associated with a rising diastolic pressure include the rate of rise in hematocrit and the dose of epoetin.

It, therefore, seems that the pressor response is more a function of an increasing red cell mass than of its rate of rise but that, if the rate of rise is too rapid, there is less time to intervene successfully with appropriate antihypertensive therapy. Why every dialysis patient does not have a pressor response is not clear; perhaps only some have an increased vascular sensitivity to changes in adrenergic tone (44).

Although epoetin has recently been shown to stimulate endothelial cell proliferation in vitro (45), the pressor response is probably not due to the direct effects of epoetin in vivo. A pressor response does not occur with the infusion of epoetin into isolated arterioles (46), hypertension has not occurred in patients with normal renal function treated short-term or long-term with epoetin (47–50), and hypertension is not aggravated in anemic hemodialysis patients treated with recombinant human erythropoietin when baseline hematocrit levels are maintained by periodic phlebotomy (17).

Grand mal seizures occurred in 4 percent of the patients and were associated with a sudden increase in blood pressure in about one half of these patients. To determine if epoetin has a direct adverse effect on cerebral circulation, one study carried out at the Mayo Clinic prevented the rise in red cell mass that would have occurred if periodic phlebotomy had not been used. This study reaffirmed that epoetin does not have a direct effect on cerebral blood flow, does not result in microvascular thrombi that could decrease cutaneous circulation and presumably that of other vascular beds, and does not directly affect viscosity. Rather, the epoetin-induced improvement in anemia actually has beneficial effects on cerebral circulation and does not decrease it to below normal levels.

Careful monitoring and medicinal control of blood pressure in epoetin-treated patients are necessary, particularly when the hematocrit is rising. Inasmuch as hypertension and seizures are relatively common in patients with chronic renal failure and these complications have not been observed in other patient populations treated with epoetin (47–50), it is likely that the hemodynamic effects due to the correction of the anemia in a patient population at higher risk for seizures (51) lead to the increased incidence of seizures.

Although platelet function is known to improve with correction of the anemia of dialysis patients (8), this was not deleterious for the patients in these studies. Specifically, arteriovenous fistula clotting, while occasionally accentuated, did not increase in frequency even after 4 years of epoetin therapy. However, increased fibrin formation and clotting in the extracorporeal circuit may occur in approximately one third of epoetin-treated patients when the hematocrit increases to 30 or above. A small increase in heparin is usually sufficient to maintain good dialyzer blood flows and reuse techniques (2). Epoetin-treated patients, including those with diabetes mellitus, have shown no increased incidence of small or large vessel thromboses, such as strokes, myocardial infarctions, or peripheral vascular disease.

Underdialysis, a potential concern because dialyzer clearances decrease as the plasma volume contracts, was not a clinical problem, even though predialysis serum creatinine levels increased by 4.5 percent. Mean serum potassium levels increased minimally, but the potential for serious hyperkalemia is increased because appetite increases in many epoetin-treated patients. Three noncompliant patients had a hyperkalemic cardiac arrest, and two of these died. Therefore, serum potassium should be carefully monitored. Dialyzer potassium must be adjusted downward, and dietary counseling may be required more frequently in some epoetin-treated patients, especially during the first 6 to 9 months of epoetin therapy. Serum phosphorus levels increased, partly because of a decrease in dialyzer clearance but probably more because of an increase in food intake.

The influence of epoetin on the health of dialysis patients is impressive. Red cell transfusions are eliminated. Iron overload will eventually cease to be a complication. More patients will be eligible for renal transplantation because they will have fewer HLA antibodies or, better yet, will not develop HLA antibodies because the need for transfusions will be eliminated or reduced. Because the prolonged bleeding time of uremia shortens toward normal with partial correction of the anemia by epoetin (52), chronic blood loss accentuated by uremia should decrease. Exercise performance improves, sexual function may improve (53), depression decreases, and appetite increases. Longer-term studies will determine whether hospitalization rates decrease and longevity increases through correction of the anemia with epoetin. None of the many prior studies of quality-of-life assessments in dialysis patients has documented such an improvement as that achieved by epoetin.

Epoetin is effective, well tolerated, and safe if blood pressure and serum potassium levels are carefully monitored during the initial correction of the anemia. Epoetin should become standard therapy in the management of patients with the anemia of chronic renal failure whose hematocrit levels are less than 30 percent and should result in higher energy levels, decreased morbidity, and better patient rehabilitation.

REFERENCES

1. Eschbach J, Adamson J. Modern aspects of the pathophysiology of renal anemia. Contrib Nephrol 1988;66:63–70.

2. Eschbach JW. The anemia of chronic renal failure: pathophysiology and the effects of recombinant erythropoietin. Kidney Int 1989;35:134–48.

3. Lin F-K, Suggs S, Lin CH, et al. Cloning and expression of the human erythropoietin gene. Proc Natl Acad Sci USA 1985;82:7580–4.

4. Egrie JC, Strickland TW, Lane J, et al. Characterization and biological effects of recombinant human erythropoietin. Immunobiology 1986;72: 213–24.

5. Eschbach J, Egrie J, Downing M, Browne J, Adamson J. Correction of the anemia of end-stage renal disease with recombinant human erythropoietin. N Engl J Med 1987;316:73–8.

6. Winearls G, Oliver D, Pippard M, Reid C, Downing M, Cotes P. Effect of human erythropoietin derived from recombinant DNA on the anaemia of patients maintained by chronic haemodialysis. Lancet 1986;2:1175–8.

7. Bommer J, Alexiou C, Muller-Buhl E, Eifer J, Ritz E. Recombinant human erythropoietin therapy in haemodialysis patients: dose determination and clinical experience. Nephrol Dial Transplant 1987;2:238–42.

8. Casati S, Passerini P, Campise M, et al. Benefits and risks of protracted treatment with human recombinant erythropoietin in patients having haemodialysis. Br Med J 1987;295:1017–20.

9. Bommer J, Kugel M, Schoeppe W, et al. Dose-related effects of recombinant human erythropoietin on erythropoiesis: results of a multicenter trial in patients with end-stage renal disease. Contrib Nephrol 1988;66:85–93.

10. Schaefer R, Buerner B, Zech M, Denninger G, Borneff C, Heidland A. Treatment of the anemia of hemodialysis patients with recombinant human erythropoietin. Int J Artif Organs 1988;11:249–54.

11. Akizawa T, Koshikawa S, Takaku F, et al. Clinical effect of recombinant human erythropoietin on anemia associated with chronic renal failure: a multi-institutional study in Japan. Int J Artif Organs 1988;11:343–50.

12. Sobota JT. Recombinant human erythropoietin in patients with anemia due to end-stage renal disease. Contrib Nephrol 1989;76:166–78.

13. Suzuki M, Hirasawa Y, Hirashima K, et al. Dose-finding, double blind, clinical trial of recombinant human erythropoietin (Chugai) in Japanese patients with end-stage renal disease. Contrib Nephrol 1989;76:179–92.

14. Kreis H, Zins B, Naret C, et al. Recombinant erythropoietin: personal experience with a new treatment for the anemia of chronic renal failure. Transplant Proc 1989;21:55–61.

15. Eschbach JW, Abdulhadi MH, Browne JK, et al. Recombinant human erythropoietin in anemic patients with end-stage renal disease. Ann Intern Med 1989;111:992–1000.

16. Davidson RC, Haley NR, Easterling TR, Ahmad S, Adamson JW, Eschbach JW. Serial hemodynamic changes following recombinant erythropoietin (rHuEPO) therapy [Abstract]. Kidney Int 1990;37:237.

17. Johnson WJ, McCarthy JT, Yanagihara T, et al. Effects of recombinant human erythropoietin (EPO) on blood flow and blood coagulability. Kidney Int 1990;38:919–24.

18. Evans RW, Rader R, Manninen OL, et al. The quality of life of hemodialysis patients treated with recombinant human erythropoietin. JAMA 1990; 263:85–30.

19. Van Wyck DB, Stivelman JC, Ruiz J, Kirlin LF, Katz MA, Ogden DA. Iron status in patients receiving erythropoietin for dialysis-associated anemia. Kidney Int 1989;35:712–16.

20. Eschbach JW, Haley NR, Aquilling T, et al. Three years of erythropoietin (rHuEPO) therapy [Abstract]. Kidney Int 1990;37:237.

21. Buckner FS, Eschbach JW, Haley NR, Davidson RC, Adamson JW. Hypertension following erythropoietin therapy in anemic hemodialysis patients. Am J Hypertension 1990;3:947–55.

22. Haley NR, Davidson RC, Eschbach JW, Easterling TR, Adamson JW. Patterns of development of hypertension with recombinant human erythropoietin (rHuEpo) therapy: a prospective study [Abstract]. Am J Hypertension 1989; 2:56.

23. Huggins C. Hazards of transfusions and ways to reduce their risk: blood conservation. Transplant Proc 1989;21:43–4.

24. Paganini EP, Braun WE, Latham D, Abdulahadi MH. Renal transplantation: results in hemodialysis patients previously treated with recombinant human erythropoietin. Trans Am Soc Artif Intern Organs 1989;35:535–8.

25. Schafer AI, Cheron RG, Dluhy R, et al. Clinical consequences of acquired transfusional iron overload in adults. N Engl J Med 1981;304:319–24.

26. Bregman H, Winchester JF, Knepshield JH, Gelfand MC, Manz HJ, Schreiner GE. Iron-overload-associated myopathy in patients on maintenance haemodialysis: a histocompatibility-linked disorder. Lancet 1980;2:882–5.

27. Seifert A, Von Herrath D, Schaefer K. Iron overload, but not treatment with desferrioxamine favours the development of septicemia in patients on maintenance hemodialysis. Q J Med 1987;65:1015–24.

28. Stevens RG, Jones DY, Micozzi MS, Taylor PR. Body iron stores and the risk of cancer. N Engl J Med 1988;319:1047–52.

29. Coburn JW, St Jan AZ. Mucormycosis in dialysis patients: update from International Registry [Abstract]. In: Proceedings of the XIth International Congress of Nephrology, Tokyo, Japan, 1990:240.

30. Eschbach JW, Haley NR, Adamson JW. The use of recombinant erythropoietin in the treatment of the anemia of chronic renal failure. In: Orlic D, ed. Molecular and cellular controls of hematopoiesis. New York: New York Academy of Sciences, 1989;554:225–30.

31. Lazarus JM, Hakim RM, Newell J. Recombinant human erythropoietin and phlebotomy in the treatment of iron overload in chronic hemodialysis patients. Am J Kidney Dis 1990;16:101–8.

32. Nissenson AR. Recombinant human erythropoietin; impact on brain and cognitive function, exercise tolerance, sexual potency, and quality of life. Semin Nephrol 1989;9:25–31.

33. Wolcott DL, Marsh JT, LaRue A, et al. Recombinant human erythropoietin treatment may improve quality of life and cognitive function in chronic hemodialysis patients. Am J Kidney Dis 1989;14:478–85.

34. Di Paolo B, Vocino V, Amoroso L, et al. Electrophysiological variations following recombinant human erythropoietin (r-HuEPO) treatment in standard hemodialysis patient (RDT) [Abstract]. Kidney Int 1990;37:392.

35. Nissenson AR, Marsh JT, Brown WS, et al. Anemia is a reversible cause of brain dysfunction in uremic patients [Abstract]. Kidney Int 1990;37:313.

36. Mayer G, Thum J, Cada EM, et al. Working capacity is increased following recombinant human erythropoietin treatment. Kidney Int 1988;34: 525–8.

37. Robertson HT, Haley NR, Guthrie M, Cardenas D, Eschbach JW, Adamson JW. Increase in maximal exercise capacity in hemodialysis (HD) patients following correction of the anemia with recombinant human erythropoietin (rHuEpo). Am J Kidney Dis 1990;20:325–32.

38. Löw I, Grützmacher P, Bergman M, Schoeppe W. Echocardiographic

findings in patients on maintenance hemodialysis substituted with recombinant human erythropoietin. Clin Nephrol 1989;31:26–30.

39. London GM, Zins B, Pannier B, et al. Vascular changes in hemodialysis patients in response to recombinant human erythropoietin. Kidney Int 1989; 36:878–82.

40. Ellis LB, Faulkner JM. The heart in anemia. N Engl J Med 1939; 220:943–52.

41. Porter WB. Heart changes and physiologic adjustment in hookworm anemia. Am Heart J 1937;13:550–79.

42. Cropp GJA. Cardiovascular function in children with severe anemia. Circulation 1969;39:775–84.

43. Neff M, Kim K, Persoff M, Onesti G, Swartz C. Hemodynamics of uremic anemia. Circulation 1971;43:876–83.

44. Baldamus CA, Pollock M, Steffen HM, et al. Adrenergic system in renal anemia, corrected with recombinant human erythropoietin (rHuEPO) [Abstract]. Kidney Int 1990;37:208.

45. Anagnostou A, Lee ES, Kessinian N, Levinson R, Steiner M. Erythropoietin has a mitogenic and positive chemotactic effect on endothelial cells. Proc Natl Acad Sci USA 1990;87:5978–82.

46. Pagel H, Jelkmann W, Wiess C. Erythropoietin and blood pressure. Horm Metab Res 1989;21:224.

47. Goodnough LT, Rudnick S, Price TH, et al. Increased preoperative collection of autologous blood with recombinant human erythropoietin therapy. N Engl J Med 1989;321:1163–8.

48. Means RT, Olsen NF, Krantz SB, et al. Treatment of the anemia of rheumatoid arthritis with recombinant human erythropoietin: clinical and in vitro studies. Arthritis Rheum 1989;32:638–42.

49. Fischl M, Galpin JE, Levine JD, et al. Recombinant human erythropoietin for patients with AIDS treated with Zidovudine. N Engl J Med 1990; 322:1488–93.

50. Ludwig H, Fritz E, Kotzmann H, Hocker P, Gissling H, Barnas U. Erythropoietin treatment of anemia associated with multiple myeloma. N Engl J Med 1990;322(24):1693–99.

51. Raskin NH, Fishman RA. Neurologic disorders in renal failure. N Engl J Med 1976;294:143–8.

52. Moia M, Vizzotto L, Cattaneo M, et al. Improvement in the haemostatic defect of uraemia after treatment with recombinant human erythropoietin. Lancet 1987;2:1227–9.

53. Delano BG. Improvements in quality of life following treatment with rHuEpo in anemic hemodialysis patients. Kidney Dis 1989;14:14–8.

Chapter 13

Recombinant Human Erythropoietin (Epoetin Alfa) in Patients with Renal Anemia: Japan

Tadao Akizawa, Nobuhide Mimura,
Teiryo Maeda, and Fumimaro Takaku

Clinical studies of recombinant human erythropoietin (rHuEpo) (epoetin alfa) in patients with renal insufficiency began in July 1986 in Japan. By November 1988, many studies had been made in 830 patients with renal anemia under the leadership of the Recombinant Human Erythropoietin Investigating Committee. This chapter reviews the results of these studies.

The Efficacy of rHuEpo Therapy for Renal Anemia

In early Phase II studies in which the dose of recombinant human erythropoietin was increased stepwise at 4-week intervals from 50 units/kg to 100 and 200 units/kg, improvement of anemia was noted in 65 of 66 patients with stable renal insufficiency undergoing hemodialysis whose hematocrit levels were less than 20 percent (1). The dose levels upon completion of the treatment were 50 units/kg or less, 50 to 100 units/kg, 100 units/kg, and 200 units/kg in 30 percent, 12 percent, 25 percent, and 20 percent of the patients, respectively. The cumulative dose per kg needed to increase the hematocrit by 1 percent varied widely, as illustrated in Figure 13.1. In high responders, however, the iron saturation index was significantly higher and the unsaturated iron-binding capacity was significantly lower than in other patients, suggesting that the iron reserve is a rate-limiting factor for the improvement of anemia. No correlation was observed between the responses to the

227

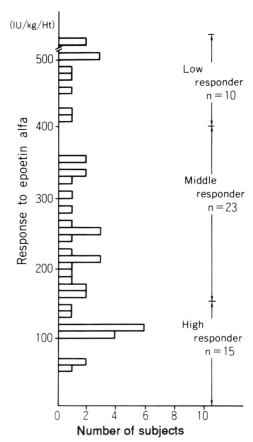

Figure 13.1. Responses to epoetin alfa. IU/kg/Ht indicates the cumulative dose per kg needed to increase the hematocrit by 1 percent.

rHuEpo and ΔAl determined after desferrioxamine loading (a parameter that reflects the accumulated amount of aluminum in the body), carboxy terminal of parathyroid hormone (C-PTH), β_2-microglobulin, or levels of endogenous erythropoietin (Table 13.1).

Because the effective initial dose of rHuEpo was found to be 100 units/kg in about 80 percent of patients with renal anemia, an 8-week randomized, double-blind trial was conducted in 89 hemodialysis patients weighing 40 to 60 kg with hematocrit values of 23 percent or less using 1500, 3000, and 6000 units/kg hemodialysis to determine the optimal initial dose (2). The rate of increase of the hematocrit (Fig 13.2) and increases in the reticulocyte index and platelet counts were dose-dependent. Serum iron and ferritin levels decreased as the treatment was continued but increased again after the treatment was discontinued. Although the improvement of anemia was achieved most rapidly in the group receiving 6000 units/kg, the incidence of side effects, mainly hypertension, was significantly higher in this group than in any other group (Table 13.2). Therefore, the safest initial dose was determined to be 3000 units/kg hemodialysis three times per week.

In Japan, mepitiostane, an anabolic steroid, is approved for the treatment of renal anemia (3). A 14-week, double-blind clinical trial was conducted using the double-dummy method in 71 hemodialysis patients with hematocrit values of 23 percent or less. Patients were randomly assigned to receive either mepitiostane, 20 mg/day (34 cases) or rHuEpo, 3000 units (37 cases). Both the hematocrit elevation rate (Fig 13.3) and the increases in reticulocytes were significantly greater in the rHuEpo group than in the mepitiostane group after the 1st week of treatment. Anemia was improved in 94.6 percent of the patients in the rHuEpo group, compared to only 55.9 percent in the mepitiostane group. The incidence of side effects, such as voice change, hirsutism, and other skin symptoms, was significantly higher in the mepitiostane group. Thus, rHuEpo proved to be superior to mepitiostane in the treatment of renal anemia.

Table 13.1. The Effects of Biochemical Parameters on the Response of Anemia to Epoetin Alfa

	Group*	Mean $\pm$ SD	P
ΔAl (μg/litre)	H	133.0 $\pm$ 57.3	
	M	114.4 $\pm$ 69.6	NS[†]
	L	75.4 $\pm$ 55.6	
c-PTH (ng/ml)	H	4.9 $\pm$ 3.9	
	M	4.6 $\pm$ 5.1	NS
	L	2.8 $\pm$ 1.7	
β_2-microglobulin (mg/l)	H	43.2 $\pm$ 10.2	
	M	44.6 $\pm$ 7.5	NS
	L	45.6 $\pm$ 3.9	
Erythropoietin (mU/ml)	H	13.0 $\pm$ 8.4	
	M	10.4 $\pm$ 3.9	NS
	L	14.9 $\pm$ 6.8	

*H, high responder; M, middle responder; L, low responder.
†NS, not significant.

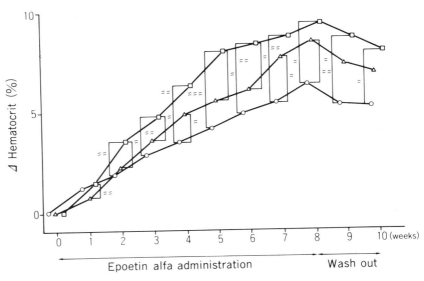

Figure 13.2. The increase in the hematocrit value after the administration of epoetin alfa during a randomized, double-blind, dose-response study. Hematocrit values in all three groups increased significantly ($P < 0.001$) after the 1 week. Open circles indicate 1500 units hemodialysis; open triangles, 3000 units hemodialysis; open squares, 6000 units hemodialysis; #, $P < 0.05$; ##, $P < 0.01$; ###, $P < 0.001$, intergroup comparison.

Table 13.2. The Incidence of Side Effects Related to the Dosage Level of rHuEpo (Epoetin Alfa)

Side Effect	Number of Cases at Dose of:		
	1500 units	3000 units	6000 units
Headache	2	1	3
Hypertension	1	0*	7*
Malaise	0	1	1
Total	3/28	2/31	11/30

*Comparing the incidence of hypertension in patients receiving 3000 vs. 6000 units gave a P value of <0.05.

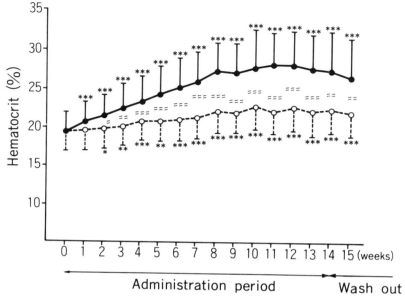

Figure 13.3. Changes in the hematocrit value after the administration of epoetin alfa (closed circles) or mepitiostane (open circles) during a randomized, double-blind study. *, $P < 0.05$; **, $P < 0.01$; ***, $P < 0.001$ vs. 0 week; #, $P < 0.05$; ##, $P < 0.01$; ###, $P < 0.001$, intergroup comparison.

Up to 6000 units of rHuEpo was administered at each hemodialysis for 48 weeks to 109 patients with hematocrit values of 23 percent or less (4). The improvement of the anemia was maintained throughout the treatment period. The analysis of doses conducted at 12-week intervals showed continuous increase in patients on low dosages (4500 units/week or less); these patients accounted for about 70 percent of the total upon completion of the study (Fig 13.4). The number of patients on large dosages (9000 units/week) remained virtually unchanged throughout the study period, suggesting that some patients need large dosages for maintenance therapy, although the maintenance dosage can be gradually tapered in the majority of patients (Fig 13.4). Various factors, such as the patient's background, serum iron, ferritin, percentage of transferrin saturation, serum aluminum, c-PTH, and β_2-microglobulin levels, were determined, but none was closely related to the differences in responsiveness.

In another long-term study (5), rHuEpo was administered one to

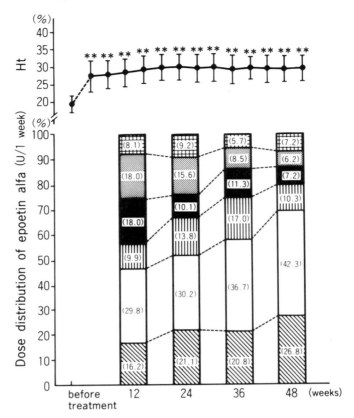

Figure 13.4. Changes in the hematocrit (Ht) and dose distribution (D) of epoetin alfa during 48 weeks of treatment. **, *P* < 0.01 vs. before treatment; ⬚ = D ≤ 3000 units per week, ☐ = 3000 < D ≤ 4500 units per week, ⧈ = 4500 < D ≤ 6000 units per week, ■ = 6000 < D ≤ 7500 units per week, ▨ = 7500 < D ≤ 9000 units per week, ⊞ = 9000 units per week < D.

three times per week for 24 weeks to 251 patients on hemodialysis, including 9 patients on continuous ambulatory peritoneal dialysis, with hematocrit values of 25 percent or less. Anemia was also markedly improved in this study, and the maintenance dose could be tapered. The optimal maintenance dosage regimen was 1500 units three times per week for the greatest number of patients (27.6 percent), followed by 1500 units twice a week and 3000 units twice a week. Once-weekly treatment produced optimal efficacy in 10.6 percent of patients (Table 13.3).

The number of blood transfusions decreased markedly, reflecting the improvement of anemia by rHuEpo in all of the above-mentioned studies. The reduction rate was 80 to 87.5 percent in the early studies (1,2) and 92 to 96 percent in the long-term studies (4,5). Blood transfusion was required only in occasional situations, such as the recurrence of hemorrhagic complications.

rHuEpo was administered intravenously at least once a week to 13 patients on continuous ambulatory peritoneal dialysis (6). The anemia improved to the same extent in the patients on continuous ambulatory peritoneal dialysis as in the patients on hemodialysis, although the dosage level was lower in the former (6000 $\pm$ 5000 units per week) than in the latter (9000 $\pm$ 5000 units per week). The drug improved the anemia even when administered only once every other week if large doses (12,000 to 24,000 units) were used (7).

rHuEpo was administered at 1500 to 21,000 units per week for 20.2 $\pm$ 8.4 weeks to nine predialysis patients (baseline hematocrit, 21.1 $\pm$ 2.6 percent) with serum creatinine levels of 7.2 $\pm$ 1.6 mg/dl. The anemia improved in all cases, and the responsiveness to the drug was similar to that observed in patients on hemodialysis. The renal function exacerbation rate, as determined by the slope of 1/creatinine − time plots, did not accelerate after treatment with rHuEpo and improvement of the anemia (8).

Table 13.3. The Maintenance Administration Interval of rHuEpo (Epoetin Alfa)

rHuEpo Dosage	Number of Patients	%
1500 units/wk		
1500 units × 1/wk	13	5.1
3000 units/wk		
1500 units × 2/wk	60	23.6
3000 units × 1/wk	14	5.5
4500 units/wk		
1500 units × 3/wk	70	27.6
6000 units/wk		
3000 units × 2/wk	56	22.0
9000 units/wk		
3000 units × 3/wk	36	14.2
Other	5	2.0
Total	254	100.0

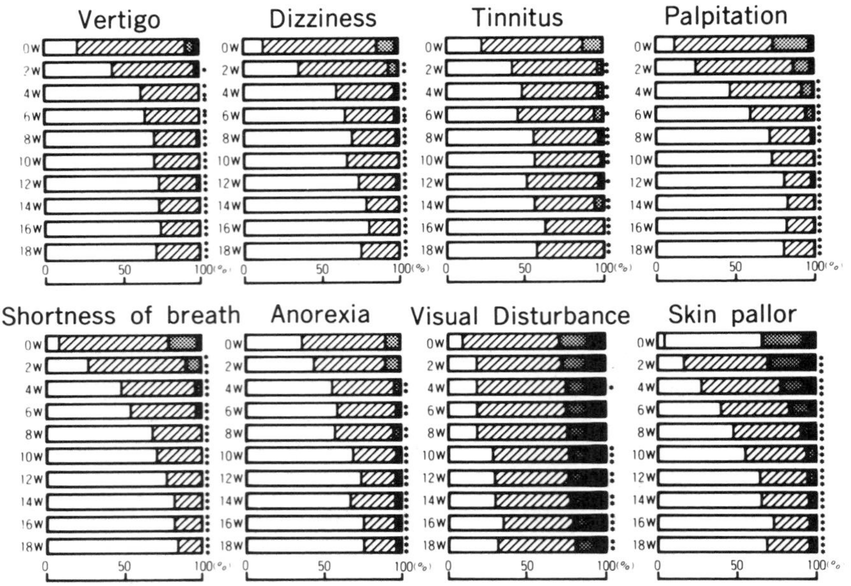

Figure 13.5. Subjective and objective symptoms during treatment with epoetin alfa. □ = none, ▨ = mild, ▦ = moderate, ■ = severe. *, $P < 0.05$, **, $P < 0.01$, ***, $P < 0.001$ vs. 0 week. *Source: Data from Reference 6*

Treatment with rHuEpo did not result in the improvement of anemia in 24 of 417 cases (5.8 percent) in the early studies (1,2,6). The failure of the treatment was attributable to iron deficiency in 6 cases and to insufficient dosage levels in 7 cases because of side effects at higher doses. Other reasons for the failure included the presence of hemorrhagic lesions (2 cases), splenic hyperfunction (chronic infection) (1 case), and severe aluminum bone disease (1 case). The reasons for the failure remained unclear in 7 cases. Transient decreases in efficacy during long-term treatment were seen in patients with infections, bone fracture, surgery, and hemorrhagic complications (4).

Accessory Effects of rHuEpo Therapy and the Improvement of Anemia

The improvement of anemia had favorable effects on subjective and objective symptoms in an analysis of 267 treated patients (Fig 13.5) (6). A patient questionnaire survey showed that the improvement of these symptoms resulted in greater activities of daily life and helped patients to resume a more active social life.

rHuEpo was administered to 21 hemodialysis patients with hematocrit values of 19.6 ± 2.2 percent. Cardiac hemodynamics were determined at baseline and after increases in hematocrit values to at least 30 percent or to at least 10 percent above baseline (Table 13.4) (9). The circulating plasma volume remained unchanged, while the total peripheral resistance index showed significant increases associated with compensatory decreases in the cardiac index. The thickness of the left ventricular posterior wall increased, reflecting decreases in the cardiac index. Decreases in the cardiac load were supported by decreases in the cardiothoracic ratio and in levels of human atrial natriuretic peptide.

After treatment with rHuEpo, 7 patients had an increase in blood pressure to at least 160/90 mm Hg (hypertensive group) and 14 had unchanged blood pressure (normotensive group) (10). While the total peripheral resistance index increased in both groups, the cardiac index decreased in the normotensive group and remained unchanged in the hypertensive group, suggesting that the increase in blood pressure was due to insufficient decreases in the cardiac index in response to increases in the total peripheral resistance index.

An exercise tolerance test of the same strength was carried out before rHuEpo treatment in 25 hemodialysis patients with hematocrit values

Table 13.4. Changes in Hemodynamic Parameters by Treatment with rHuEpo (Epoetin Alfa)

	Observation Period	Treatment Period	P Value*
Systolic BP‡ (mm Hg)	128.43 ± 25.35†	138.05 ± 29.66	NS
Diastolic BP (mm Hg)	67.52 ± 18.65	77.24 ± 13.91	0.05
Mean BP (mm Hg)	87.81 ± 19.01	97.57 ± 18.03	0.01
Stroke volume (ml/m²)	57.35 ± 16.32	53.42 ± 12.36	NS
Heart rate (/min)	73.24 ± 11.97	67.86 ± 9.06	0.05
Cardiac index (litres/min/m²)	4.13 ± 1.15	3.59 ± 0.77	0.01
TPRI (mm Hg/litre/min/m²)	22.65 ± 5.42	28.25 ± 7.88	0.001
CTR (%)	50.32 ± 4.66	49.04 ± 4.44	0.05
LVPWth (mm)	10.22 ± 2.20	11.29 ± 2.03	0.01
α-hANP (pg/ml)	143 ± 62	113 ± 77	0.05
Plasma volume (ml/kg)	65.26 ± 11.39	64.16 ± 11.25	NS

*Wilcoxon test; NS, not significant.
†Mean ± SD.
‡BP, blood pressure; TPRI, total peripheral resistance index; CTR, cardiothoracic rate; LVPWth, left ventricular posterior wall thickness; hANP, human atrial natriuretic peptide.

of 22.7 ± 1.5 percent. The test was repeated when hematocrit values increased to 29.0 ± 2.2 percent. The heart rate, perceived exertion, postloading lactic acid levels, and preloading creatine phosphokinase levels decreased significantly and the number of patients who were able to complete the test increased after treatment. The improvement of anemia increases exercise tolerance, presumably through an improvement in anaerobic muscle metabolism, muscle ischemia, and cardiac function (11).

Bone marrow puncture was carried out before rHuEpo treatment in 20 patients with hematocrit values of 19.3 ± 2.1 percent. Marrow puncture was repeated when hematocrit values increased to 30.0 ± 3.2 percent. Medullary findings showed no significant differences in nuclear cell and megakaryocyte counts before and after treatment. However, the medullary erythroblast ratio, as well as the number of colony-forming units-erythroid (CFU-E) and burst-forming units-erythroid (BFU-E) (cultured by the methylcellulose method), increased significantly after treatment (12).

rHuEpo was administered at 3000 units per hemodialysis for 12 weeks to 18 hemodialysis patients with baseline hematocrit values of 22.9 ± 3.1 percent. Ivy bleeding time, platelet function, and coagulation factors were determined before treatment, during treatment (hematocrit, 31.0 ± 3.0 percent), and 6 to 8 weeks after discontinuation of rHuEpo (hematocrit, 26.2 ± 4.2 percent). The Ivy bleeding time, which was markedly prolonged before treatment, decreased significantly during treatment but increased after treatment was discontinued. The median platelet volume, median value of platelet distribution, platelet retention, and von Willebrand factor antigen also increased during treatment. However, other coagulation factors, as well as thromboxane B_2 and 6-keto-prostaglandin $F_{1\alpha}$, remained unchanged. Thus, the improvement of anemia by treatment with rHuEpo in hemodialysis patients resulted in improved hemostatic function, probably due to rheologic effects and increases in juvenile platelets and von Willebrand factor antigen (13).

rHuEpo was administered to 18 hemodialysis patients with hematocrit values of 20.8 ± 2.4 percent in the same way as described in the previous section, and immunologic parameters were compared before treatment, during treatment (hematocrit, 29.7 ± 4.4 percent), and after treatment was discontinued (hematocrit, 23.7 ± 4.2 percent). No significant differences were seen at the three time points with respect to white blood count, lymphocytes, lymphocyte subpopulation, subset (OKT4, OKT8, OKT4/OKT8, and OKI_{a1}), natural killer cell activity, or lymphoblast formation. The lymphocytes' ability to produce interleukin 2, which was low before treatment, increased significantly during treatment, suggesting that the improvement of anemia may have favorable effects on the immunodeficiency of hemodialysis patients (14).

rHuEpo was administered at 3000 units per hemodialysis to 10 female (hematocrit, 21.8 ± 3.2 percent) and 6 male (hematocrit, 23.0 ± 2.3 percent) patients on hemodialysis. Changes in pituitary and sex hormones before and after the luteinizing hormone/thyrotropin-releasing hormone loading test were evaluated before treatment, during treatment, and 6 to 8 weeks after treatment was discontinued. In the female patients, basal hormone levels and percentage changes in luteinizing hormone, follicle-stimulating hormone, prolactin, growth hormone, and thyroid-stimulating hormone determined before and after 30 minutes loading with luteinizing hormone and thyrotropin-releasing hormone showed no significant differences during rHuEpo treatment (hematocrit, 30.7 ± 3.3 percent) and after treatment was discontinued (hematocrit, 26.5 ± 3.1 percent), as compared to those observed before treatment. Pituitary hormone levels determined before and after loading with luteinizing hormone and thyrotropin-releasing hormone also remained unchanged in male patients during the 3-month rHuEpo treatment period (hematocrit, 30.3 ± 6.2 percent) and after treatment (hematocrit, 24.2 ± 3.8 percent), as compared to before treatment. E_1, E_2, progesterone, free testosterone, and sex hormone-binding globulin levels remained unchanged in both men and women before, during, and after treatment. In men, changes in these hormones were compared between patients who reported improvement of impotence in the questionnaire survey after treatment with rHuEpo and those who did not. However, no differences in hormonal changes were noted between the two groups. From these findings, one can say that it is unlikely that rHuEpo treatment and improvement in anemia have any significant effect on the production of pituitary and sex hormones in male hemodialysis patients or in women who have regular menstruation and biphasic basal body temperature patterns (15).

Adverse Effects of rHuEpo (1–6)

Side effects (124 events) occurred in 96 of 830 patients (11.6 percent) treated with rHuEpo (Table 13.5). The side effect with the highest incidence was an increase in blood pressure (6.9 percent), followed by headache (2.9 percent). A number of side effects were noted, each in a small number of patients. Treatment was discontinued in 6 patients be-

Table 13.5. The Incidence of Side Effects and Abnormal Laboratory Findings during Treatment with rHuEpo (Epoetin Alfa)

Finding	Number of Events*
Side effect	
Hypertension	57 (6.9%)
Headache	24 (2.9)
Fever	7 (0.9)
Itching	6 (0.7)
Nausea	4 (0.5)
Malaise	4 (0.5)
Clotting of A-V fistula[†]	3 (0.3)
Arthralgia or myalgia	3 (0.3)
Skeletal pain	1 (0.1)
Other	15 (1.8)
Total number/total patients	124/830 (14.9)
Abnormal laboratory test	
Increase in LDH[†]	4 (0.5)
Increase in potassium	8 (1.0)
Eosinophilia	4 (0.5)
Increase in GOT, GPT, γ-GPT	5 (0.6)
Increase in Alp	2 (0.2)
Other	4 (0.5)
Total number/total patients	27/830 (3.3)

*Numbers of patients who showed side effects and abnormal laboratory findings were 96 (11.6%) and 22 (2.7%), respectively.
†A-V fistula, arteriovenous fistula; LDH, lactate dehydrogenase; GOT, glutamic oxaloacetic transaminase; GPT, glutamic pyruvic transaminase; γ-GTP, γ-guanosine-5'-triphosphate; Alp, alkaline phosphatase.

cause of difficulties in controlling hypertension with antihypertensive drugs.

The incidence of a flulike syndrome was low, with fever occurring in seven cases, arthralgia in two, general ostealgia in one, and myalgia in one.

Clotting of an arteriovenous fistula occurred in three patients. Retinal vein thrombosis occurred in four patients, although the relationship to rHuEpo is unknown. Patients treated with rHuEpo whose anemia improves may develop thrombotic complications due to the improved platelet function and fibrinogen levels observed with long-term rHuEpo treatment (4).

Abnormal laboratory tests were noted in 27 patients. About half of these abnormalities were related to changes in the efficiency of the dialysis and dietary intake, such as increases in potassium and uric acid levels. The incidence of hepatic disorders, other than increases in lactate dehydrogenase and bilirubin associated with increases in hemolysis, was only 0.6 percent. A similar incidence of eosinophilia was observed.

Regarding the efficiency of the dialysis, decreases in creatinine and uric acid clearance associated with an increase in the hematocrit were reported in many studies. In one study, the dialysis efficiency, residual blood in the extracorporeal circuit, and heparin requirement were evaluated in 65 patients before and after a 10 percent increase in the hematocrit. In this study, creatinine and uric acid reduction rate decreased, showing an inverse correlation with increases in the hematocrit (16). However, these decreases did not significantly increase the predialysis maintenance values of serum creatinine and uric acid. Both maintenance serum levels and clearance remained unchanged for blood urea nitrogen, while maintenance serum levels increased for both potassium and phosphate, probably because of decreases in clearance and increases in dietary intake. The amount of residual blood in the extracorporeal circuit did not increase despite the increase in blood viscosity. No major modification in conventional hemodialysis techniques was required when rHuEpo treatment resulted in improvement in the anemia. Neither antierythropoietin antibody nor anti-Chinese hamster ovary antibody formation has been reported in any patient treated with rHuEpo for more than three years.

Conclusion

Treatment with rHuEpo markedly improved not only the anemia but also various associated complications in hemodialysis patients, resulting in significant improvement in the patients' quality of life. Adverse effects, such as an increase in blood pressure, can be minimized by using appropriate dosage levels and antihypertensive treatment. No major modification is required for conventional techniques of hemodialysis. Although thrombotic complications may increase, rHuEpo therapy is expected to significantly improve the quality of life and prognosis of patients on hemodialysis.

REFERENCES

1. Akizawa T, Koshikawa S, Takaku F, et al. Clinical effect of recombinant human erythropoietin on anemia associated with chronic renal failure: a multidimensional study in Japan. Int J Artif Organs 1988;11:343–50.

2. Takaku F, Mimura N, Maeda T, et al. Clinical effect of recombinant human erythropoietin (KRN5702) on anemia associated with chronic renal failure: double blind clinical trial for dose finding. Kidney Dial 1989;26:279–305.

3. Fujimi S, Hori K, Takaku F, et al. Clinical evaluation of recombinant human erythropoietin (KRN5702) on renal anemia: double blind comparative study with Mepitiostane. Igaku No Ayumi 1989;11:759–73.

4. Kawaguti Y, Takaku F, Maeda T, et al. Results of recombinant human erythropoietin (KRN5702) in long-term treatment on anemia associated with chronic renal failure. J Clin Ther Med 1988;4:2075–100.

5. Kubo K, Ota K, Takaku F, et al. Maintenance dosage of recombinant human erythropoietin on anemic patients with chronic renal failure. Jpn J Clin Dial 1989;135:603–19.

6. Maeda T, Sezai Y, Takaku F, et al. Clinical evaluation of recombinant human erythropoietin (KRN5702) on anemic patients with renal failure on regular treated hemodialysis. Kidney Dial 1989;26:1115–36.

7. Kawaguti Y, Aizawa S, Suzuki M, et al. A trial of pulse administration of high dose of recombinant erythropoietin (r-HuEPO) in CAPD patients [Abstract]. Kidney Int 1990;37:330.

8. Akizawa T, Koshikawa S, Maeda T, et al. Clinical effects of recombinant human erythropoietin on renal anemia of predialysis patients. Jpn J Clin Dial 1989;5:109–20.

9. Kamata K, Masuda S, Satou K, et al. Effects of KRN5702 (recombinant human erythropoietin) on hemodynamics of hemodialysis patients with anemia. Kidney Dial 1988;25:1083–91.

10. Kori k, Marumo F, Onoyama K, et al. Clinical effects of recombinant human erythropoietin (r-HuEPO) on hemodynamics on anemic patients with chronic renal failure. Biomedica 1989;4:372–6.

11. Nakamura T, Watanabe Y, Sakamoto N, et al. Effects of recombinant human erythropoietin on exercise tolerance in patients on chronic hemodialysis treatment. J Jpn Soc Dial Ther 1989;22:1211–18.

12. Hino M, Miyazono K, Takaku F, et al. Effects of recombinant human erythropoietin on hematopoietic progenitors of chronic hemodialysis patients in vitro and in vivo. Int J Cell Cloning 1988;6:179–91.

13. Akizawa T, Kinugawa E, Kosikawa S, et al. Effects of rHuEPO and correction of anemia on platelet function in hemodialysis patients. Nephron (in press).

14. Kinugasa E, Akizawa T, Koshikawa S. Immunological effects of corrections of anemia with r-HuEPO in hemodialysis patients. J Jpn Soc Dial Ther (in press).

15. Akizawa T, Kinugawa E, Kosikawa S, et al. Changes in endocrinological functions in hemodialysis patients associated with improvements in anemia after recombinant human erythropoietin therapy. Contrib Nephrol (in press).

16. Kinugasa E, Nakayama F, Akizawa T, et al. Changes in dialysis procedure by the correction of anemia with r-HuEPO [Abstract]. Artif Organs 1989; 13:323.

Chapter 14

Recombinant Human Erythropoietin (Epoetin Alfa) in Anemic Patients on Hemodialysis: Canada

Norman Muirhead

Until recently, anemia was an inseparable part of the uremic syndrome, especially in patients on hemodialysis (1). The isolation of the gene for human erythropoietin and subsequent production of recombinant human erythropoietin (rHuEpo) in clinically useful amounts (2,3) revolutionized the approach to the management of anemia related to end-stage renal disease.

Although of major importance, anemia is not the sole cause of ill health among patients with end-stage renal disease. This fact coupled with early reports of significant adverse events related to rHuEpo therapy, particularly hypertension and seizures (4,5) led the Canadian Erythropoietin Study Group to focus on issues of quality of life and to rely principally on placebo-controlled trials in its studies of rHuEpo.

Canadian studies of rHuEpo are listed in Table 14.1. Clinical trials of rHuEpo began in Canada in early 1987 with a small placebo-controlled pilot study of 24 maintenance hemodialysis patients from a single center in London, Ontario. The main objectives of this study were to evaluate the safety and efficacy of rHuEpo and to examine the pharmacokinetics of erythropoietin after intravenous administration. The quality of life instruments used during the Canadian Multicentre Erythropoietin Study were developed and validated in the London Pilot Study.

Subsequent studies in Canada were concerned mainly with the short- and long-term effects of rHuEpo on quality of life in hemodialysis patients and the efficacy, dose requirements, and morbidity associated with long-term rHuEpo therapy. Currently under way in Canada is a

Table 14.1. Canadian Studies of rHuEpo

Study Number	Name	Purpose
EP86-001/003	London Pilot Study	Efficacy/pharmacokinetics
EP86-005/005X	London Maintenance Study	Efficacy/dose frequency
EP86-004	Canadian Multicentre Study	Quality of life/exercise capacity
EP88-101	Canadian Maintenance Study	Quality of life/long-term morbidity/efficacy
EP88-102	Erythropoietin High Risk Study	Efficacy/adverse events

study of rHuEpo in patients considered to be at high risk for adverse events. This study is concerned mainly with safety, efficacy, morbid event rates, and, to a limited extent, quality of life. As this study is incomplete, it will not be discussed further.

The Canadian studies of rHuEpo all have as their theme some aspect of quality of life. Each study is reviewed in some detail in this chapter, and these discussions necessarily include data that have already been published.

The London Pilot Study

Study Outline

The purpose of this study (EP86-001/003) was to evaluate the safety, efficacy and pharmacokinetics of rHuEpo in a population of stable hemodialysis patients. The study lasted 9 weeks in total: an initial 3-week period addressing safety issues and 24-hour pharmacokinetic profiles and a subsequent 6-week period directed primarily toward an evaluation of efficacy.

This was a randomized, double-blind, placebo-controlled study with 24 patients allocated to four treatment groups: placebo; rHuEpo, 50 units/kg intravenously three times per week; rHuEpo, 100 units/kg intravenously three times per week; or rHuEpo, 200 units/kg intravenously three times per week. All of the patients studied were aged 18 to 75 years, had been stable on hemodialysis for a minimum of 3 months, and were not transfusion dependent. This latter criterion was included to reduce the chance of unblinding of the patients during the course of this short study by their continued requirement for blood transfusion during treatment with rHuEpo.

All of the patients received, when indicated, intravenous iron dextran in a dosage of 100 to 450 mg/week to maintain serum ferritin at >500 ng/ml. Patients were cared for by two teams. A blinded team consisting of a nephrologist, a study nurse, and dialysis personnel was responsible for the day-to-day care of the patient and the administration of outcome measures. A second, unblinded team consisting of a second nephrologist and a pharmacist was responsible for recording hemoglobin measurements and for prescribing rHuEpo, iron, and blood transfusions as indicated.

Hematologic parameters measured during the 65 days of the study included hemoglobin, hematocrit, platelet count, radioisotopic blood volume, and ferritin. Pharmacokinetic profiles were obtained after the initial rHuEpo administration and after 3 weeks of rHuEpo therapy. Nonhematologic parameters measured included blood pressure, serum chemistry, and adverse events.

The results are expressed as means ± standard deviation (SD). Between-group comparisons were made by a two-tailed t-test with $P < 0.05$ taken to indicate statistical significance.

Results

The main hematologic outcomes are summarized in Table 14.2. Hemoglobin, hematocrit, and reticulocyte count all increased after rHuEpo therapy, with no appreciable differences at the different dose

Table 14.2. The Effect of Treatment on Hematologic Measures of Outcome, London Pilot Study

Measure of Outcome	Treatment Group*				P
	Placebo	50 units/kg	100 units/kg	200 units/kg	
Reticulocytes ($\times$ 10⁹/litre)	-20 ± 31	25 ± 6	44 ± 31	96 ± 68	0.004
Hemoglobin (g/litre)	-5 ± 16	19 ± 20	31 ± 10	29 ± 23	0.024
Hematocrit (%)	-1 ± 4	6 ± 6	10 ± 4	9 ± 6	0.015
Total blood volume (ml/kg)	-2 ± 6	-3 ± 6	1 ± 3	-2 ± 15	NS
Red cell volume (ml/kg)	-2 ± 4	4 ± 5	7 ± 6	7 ± 6	0.072
Plasma volume (ml/kg)	0 ± 7	-7 ± 4	-7 ± 5	-9 ± 11	NS
Red cell volume/ platelet volume index (%)	-2 ± 7	11 ± 8	21 ± 17	21 ± 13	0.025
Platelets ($\times$ 10⁹/litre)	-42 ± 74	19 ± 8	26 ± 26	24 ± 67	NS
Ferritin (g/litre)	318 ± 414	139 ± 189	-8 ± 139	-40 ± 435	NS

*Results are given as means ± standard deviation absolute change from baseline. Statistical analysis was by the two-tailed t-test. NS, not significant.

levels. Total blood volume did not change during rHuEpo therapy, but red blood cell volume rose and plasma volume fell, resulting in a significant increase in the ratio of red blood cell count to plasma volume (RBC/PV) index at 9 weeks. No discernible effect on mean systolic or diastolic blood pressure or predialysis serum urea, creatinine, potassium, or phosphate values was apparent in this study. Although patients on rHuEpo reported more adverse events, the numbers of patients and adverse events reported were too small to allow meaningful group comparisons. The only serious adverse event occurred in a patient receiving 200 units/kg three times per week. This patient suffered an episode of transient right facial weakness that was thought to be a small completed stroke after 34 days of rHuEpo therapy. The hemoglobin value at the time of this event was 92 g/litre (starting hemoglobin, 76 g/litre), and blood pressure was 170/70 (initial blood pressure, 150/70). Therapy with rHuEpo was discontinued, and the patient made a full recovery from the facial hemiparesis.

A dose-response relationship was evident for the three dose levels (Fig 14.1). At the highest dose level, the hematocrit had diminished by day 65 because of dose reduction in two patients whose hematocrit had exceeded 35 percent. The increase in hematocrit in the placebo patients between days 40 and 50 reflects blood transfusion in four of the six patients.

The serum half-life of rHuEpo after intravenous injection ranged from 5.9 to 12 hours (mean, 8.6 ± 1.6 hour) after the first administration of rHuEpo and from 6.4 to 9.7 hours (mean, 7.4 ± 0.8 hours) after 3 weeks of rHuEpo therapy ($P < 0.05$). The volume of distribution of rHuEpo rose from 3.8 ± 0.91 to 4.3 ± 1.01 after 3 weeks. A representative pharmacokinetic profile for a patient receiving 200 units/kg is shown in Figure 14.2. It is likely that the reduction in pharmacologic $T_{1/2}$ seen with regular rHuEpo administration represents a change in the number or affinity of erythropoietin receptors in target tissues such as bone marrow. It is possible that the more rapid elimination represents more rapid metabolism, but the timing of the enhanced plasma disappearance is coincident with the onset of the erythropoietic response, making this less likely. No patient had any detectable antibodies to rHuEpo at any time during this study or during the subsequent long-term follow-up.

Conclusions

This study confirmed the efficacy of rHuEpo as reported by Eschbach et al. (5) and Winearls et al. (4). The pharmacokinetic data are consis-

r - HuEPO - HEMATOCRIT

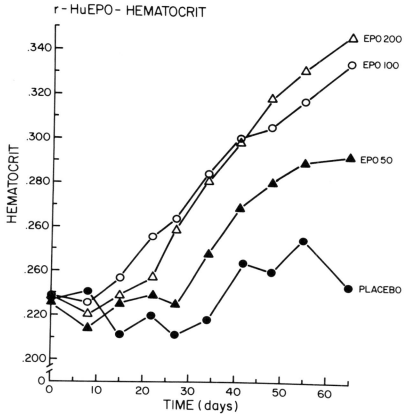

Figure 14.1. EP86-001/003. Summary of mean hematocrit response with time in the four treatment groups. The rise in the hematocrit between day 40 and day 55 in the placebo group reflects the need for blood transfusion in four of six patients. EPO, erythropoietin.

tent with those reported by others for rHuEpo (6,7). The incidence of adverse events, especially serious problems such as hypertension or seizures, was too low to permit any useful comment. Many adverse events, such as seizures, hypertension, and hyperkalemia, are common in hemodialysis patients. As further reports of serious adverse effects of rHuEpo therapy continued to appear (8,9), it became apparent that the only effective means of establishing the relationship of reported adverse events to rHuEpo therapy was to perform a large scale, randomized, placebo-controlled clinical trial.

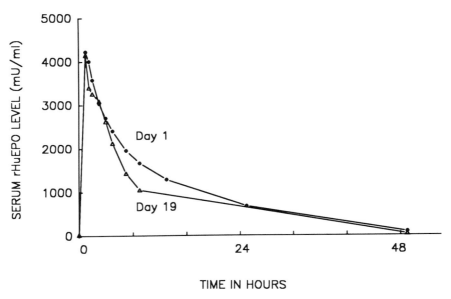

Figure 14.2. Representative pharmacokinetic profiles of days 1 and 19 for a patient receiving 200 units/kg of rHuEpo. The pharmacologic $T_{1/2}$ of rHuEpo was 9.1 hours on day 1 and 7.1 hours on day 19. mU, milliunits.

The London Maintenance Study

The 20 patients who completed the London Pilot Study entered a maintenance protocol (EP86-005/005X) designed to keep hemoglobin between 105 and 125 g/litre. Patients previously on placebo were begun on rHuEpo in a dose of 100 units/kg intravenously three times per week after dialysis. Once patients had been at their target hemoglobin for 4 consecutive weeks, they were randomized into a double-blind crossover protocol of once vs. thrice weekly rHuEpo administration. The intent of this study was to determine whether the frequency of rHuEpo dosing could be reduced. This was thought to be an important piece of information, particularly for home dialysis or limited care patients who would have less regular physician contact than would patients in center hemodialysis.

Results

The results of this study are displayed in Figure 14.3. Patients randomized to rHuEpo treatment one time followed by three times per

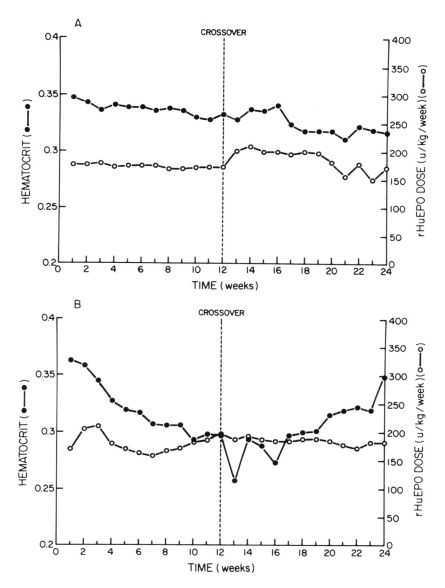

Figure 14.3. Results of EP86-005/005X. A, The hematocrit (closed circles) and rHuEpo dose (open circles) for patients initially on rHuEpo three times per week (left panel) followed by once a week. B, The hematocrit and rHuEpo dose for patients initially randomized to rHuEpo once a week (left panel) followed by three times per week. u, units.

week experienced a significant fall in mean hematocrit during once weekly administration (Fig 14.3), whereas those patients continued on rHuEpo treatment three times per week maintained their hematocrits during the first 12 weeks (Fig 14.3). After the crossover, hematocrit fell in patients switched to once weekly administration and rose in those on thrice weekly administration.

Conclusions

The main conclusion of this study was that, to maintain hematocrit, rHuEpo must be given more than once weekly, at least when the drug is given intravenously. There was a tendency for the total weekly dose to rise in patients on once weekly rHuEpo treatment so that, quite apart from any considerations of efficacy, once weekly intravenous rHuEpo is likely to be more expensive than thrice weekly administration.

The Canadian Multicentre Study

This study (EP86-004) is the main study performed to date in Canada and involved 118 patients from eight Canadian University centers. The selection criteria for this study were similar to those for the London pilot studies with the exception that anephric subjects were included so that there was a higher number of transfusion-dependent patients in the study.

The primary outcome measures assessed in this study were quality of life and exercise capacity. The opportunity was also taken to evaluate safety, efficacy, dose requirements, and the effect of increased hematocrit on predialysis blood chemistry. Particular attention was paid to a careful evaluation of changes in blood pressure and in echocardiographic parameters after 6 months of rHuEpo therapy. The study was double-blind and placebo controlled. Because quality of life was the principal outcome measure and the outcome on which sample size was determined, patients with conditions other than renal failure thought likely to have an independent effect on quality of life (e.g., diabetes, severe ischemic heart disease) were excluded.

The study design is summarized in Figure 14.4. Patients who met the eligibility criteria were randomly assigned to one of three groups—placebo, a medium target group where rHuEpo dose was adjusted to keep hemoglobin in the range 95–110 g/litre, and a high target group in whom rHuEpo dose was adjusted to maintain hemoglobin at 115–130 g/litre. The initial rHuEpo dose was 100 units/kg three times per week in all patients.

Canadian Multicentre rHuEpo Study

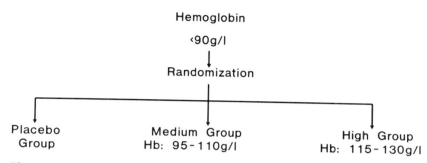

Figure 14.4. A schematic outline of the study design for EP86-004. Hb, hemoglobin.

Quality of life is a complex construct that is difficult to assess with any single instrument. Accordingly, three different quality-of-life measurements were used during the study: a disease-specific Kidney Disease Questionnaire (KDQ); the Sickness Impact Profile (SIP), a general health questionnaire used previously in chronic renal failure (10); and a measurement of utility using a time trade-off technique, again previously used in chronic renal failure (11). Exercise capacity was measured using a modified Naughton stress test and with a 6-minute walk test. Outcome measures for these tests were minutes and distance walked, respectively.

The KDQ is a disease-specific quality-of-life instrument targeted specifically at hemodialysis patients and developed at the Robarts Research Institute in London, Ontario. It was developed and validated in the London pilot studies of rHuEpo before being used in the Canadian Multicentre Study. The KDQ consists of 26 questions in five dimensions (fatigue, physical symptoms, relationships with others, frustration, and depression). The physical-symptoms dimension was patient specific (i.e., patients were asked at the initial encounter to identify their six most important physical symptoms, and these were then followed throughout the study). Questions were scored on a seven-point Likert scale with 7 indicating no problem at all and 0 indicating a severe problem. It is thought that a change in mean score of 0.5 on such a scale indicates a minimal clinically important difference and that a change of 1.0 represents a large clinical change (12).

Table 14.3. Reasons for Withdrawal in EP86-004

Reason	Number Who Withdrew		
	Placebo	Medium	High
Transplantation	5	2	3
Hypertension	0	1	2
Hypertension/seizure	0	1	0
Subarachnoid hemorrhage/seizure	0	1	0
Seizure/death	1	0	0
Noncompliance	1	0	0
Transfusion reaction	1	0	0
Pregnancy	0	1	0
Total	8	6	5

The Sickness Impact Profile (SIP) is a behaviorally based measure of overall health status consisting of 136 questions in 12 categories. Summary scores relating to physical and psychosocial dimensions and a global or overall score are obtained. The SIP was used previously in end-stage renal disease as part of the National Kidney Disease and Kidney Transplant Study (10). The best possible SIP score, indicating full health, is zero.

The time trade-off technique was used to derive a utility for each patient ranging from 1.0 (full health) to 0.0 (indifference between life and death). This measure has been used previously in end-stage renal disease and was able to distinguish readily among patients on center hemodialysis, on continuous ambulatory peritoneal dialysis, or with successful renal transplants in terms of their quality of life (11).

Results

Withdrawals. A total of 99 patients completed the study: 32 in the placebo group, 34 in the medium target group, and 33 in the high target group. The reasons for withdrawal of the 19 patients are given in Table 14.3. Six of the patients withdrew before the 2-month assessment, and the remaining 13 withdrew before the 4-month assessment. The patient who became pregnant while on rHuEpo was withdrawn from the study but continued to receive rHuEpo. She had a spontaneous abortion at 12 weeks gestation.

Hematologic Effects. The effect of rHuEpo on hemoglobin in the three treatment groups is displayed graphically in Figure 14.5. Mean hemo-

globin in the placebo group did not change during the 6 months of follow-up. Mean hemoglobin in the medium group reached the lower end
of the target range (95–110 g/litre) at 6 weeks. Mean hemoglobin in
the high target group reached the lower part of the target range (115–
130 g/litre) at 11 weeks. Mean hemoglobin remained within the specified target ranges throughout the study.

Total white blood cell count was unchanged during the 6 months of
follow-up, although there was a significant trend toward an increase in
white blood cell count in patients in the medium target range compared
to the placebo group. The changes in total white blood cell count were,
however, small and within the normal range (Table 14.4). Mean platelet
count rose in both treatment groups (Table 14.4), with the overall trend
being statistically significant (P = 0.032). The clinical relevance of a
mean increase of 23 to 35 × 10⁹/litre in platelet count is uncertain.

Biochemistry. There were no significant changes in predialysis serum
urea, creatinine, potassium, or phosphate values in any of the groups
throughout the 6 months of the study. A formal analysis of dialysis prescription was not undertaken. However, urea kinetic data were available
for 20 patients, 14 on rHuEpo and 6 on placebo, and the results are
summarized in Table 14.5. There were no significant changes in mean

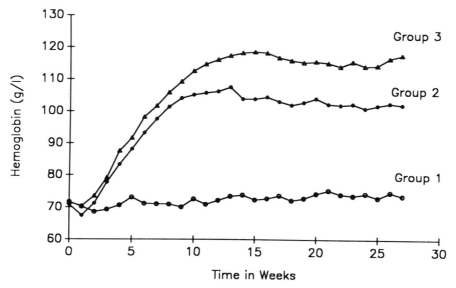

Figure 14.5. The mean hemoglobin throughout EP86-004 for the three treatment groups. Group 1 = placebo; group 2 = low target; group 3 = high target.

Table 14.4. Platelet and Total White Cell Counts for Patients in
EP86-004

Month	Placebo (n = 32)	Medium (n = 34)	High (n = 33)
	Mean Platelet Count ($\times$ 10⁹/litre)		
0	204.1 ± 57.4*	192 ± 62.6	205.8 ± 72.3
2	195.4 ± 55.5	217.7 ± 59.6	227.3 ± 78.8
4	197.7 ± 56.5	212.8 ± 62.4	215.5 ± 70.9
6	199.2 ± 60.1	217.4 ± 95.7	228.6 ± 72.1
	Mean Total White Blood Cell Count ($\times$ 10⁹/litre)		
0	6.3 ± 1.8	5.3 ± 1.7	6.2 ± 1.6
2	6.3 ± 1.8	6.0 ± 1.8	6.3 ± 1.7
4	6.3 ± 2.0	6.1 ± 2.1	6.3 ± 1.9
6	6.5 ± 2.3	5.9 ± 1.8	6.6 ± 1.6

*Results are expressed as means ± standard deviation.

dialyzer blood flow, Kt/V or protein catabolic rate between placebo and
rHuEpo patients at 0 and 6 months.

Quality of Life and Exercise Capacity. The scores for quality of life and
exercise capacity were comparable in the three groups before therapy,
with the exception that the duration of time walked in the exercise
stress test was significantly longer in the high target group ($P = 0.02$).
When the data analysis was repeated using each factor as an independent covariate, no effect of the differences in prestudy values on outcome was found.

As shown in Table 14.6, patients receiving rHuEpo showed statistically and clinically significant improvements in the fatigue and physical-symptoms dimensions of the KDQ, which were apparent after 2
months of rHuEpo therapy and were stable throughout the 6-month
follow-up period. Smaller, although still statistically significant, improvements were noted in the relationships and depression dimensions
of the KDQ. There was no significant change in the frustration dimension of the KDQ during rHuEpo therapy. Among specific physical
symptoms, significant improvemens occurred in fatigue and decreased
strength ($P < 0.01$). No improvement in sexual function was noted, but
only 18 of 118 patients had identified this as a major problem before
the study.

The global and physical-symptom summary scores in the SIP showed statistically and clinically significant improvements during rHuEpo therapy (Table 14.6). Again, this benefit was maximal after 2 months of therapy. Within the SIP, significant ($P < 0.05$) improvements occurred in body care and movement, home maintenance, ambulation, communication, and work. There was no improvement in the overall psychosocial summary score within the SIP. No overall improvement in quality of life was shown by the time trade-off utility score, although there was a trend toward improvement in the high target group.

There was a significant increase in time walked on the exercise stress test during rHuEpo therapy (Table 14.6; $P = 0.018$). There was no significant increase in distance walked in the 6-minute walk test, although there was a favorable trend in the high target group.

Although mean prerandomization hemoglobins were very similar in the three groups, individual hemoglobin levels varied widely. In addition, some patients did not achieve or maintain their target hemoglobin for the duration of the study. For these reasons, an assessment was made of the correlation between change in hemoglobin and change in quality of life and exercise capacity at 6 months. Significant correlations were found between change in hemoglobin and change in global, physical, and psychosocial scores on the SIP, all dimensions of the KDQ except frustration, and the duration of time walked on the exercise stress test.

Hypertension. Mean systolic and diastolic blood pressure throughout the study is shown in Table 14.7. There were no significant changes in systolic blood pressure during the study. Diastolic blood pressure rose significantly in rHuEpo patients compared to the placebo group ($P < 0.001$), with the most striking increase being in patients in the high target group. Among patients who completed the trial, antihypertensive

Table 14.5. Urea Kinetic Data for Patients in EP86-004

	Placebo			rHuEpo		
	Before	After	P	Before	After	P
Hemoglobin (g/litre)	73.7 ± 15.1*	69.3 ± 14.6	0.21	72.8 ± 8.8	109.6 ± 13.3	<0.01
Q_B (ml/min)	229.2 ± 36.6	244.2 ± 30.3	0.9	251.8 ± 62.1	261.8 ± 63.3	0.09
Kt/V	1.3 ± 0.3	1.2 ± 0.1	0.19	1.3 ± 0.3	1.4 ± 0.3	0.11
Protein catabolic rate	1.1 ± 0.2	0.9 ± 0.1	0.17	1.1 ± 0.3	1.0 ± 0.3	0.36

*Results are expressed as means ± standard deviation. Statistical analysis was by paired *t*-test.

Table 14.6. Scores for Quality of Life and Exercise Capacity in Placebo and Low and High Erythropoietin Patients in EP86-004

	Placebo (n = 32)			"Low" rHuEpo (n = 34)			"High" rHuEpo (n = 33)		
	0 mo	2 mo	6 mo	0 mo	2 mo	6 mo	0 mo	2 mo	6 mo
Kidney Disease Questionnaire									
Physical	4.2	4.7	4.6	3.6	4.7	5.2	3.9	5.0	5.3
Fatigue	4.4	4.7	4.5	4.1	4.7	5.0	4.2	5.2	5.3
Relationships	4.9	5.1	5.0	4.9	4.9	5.5	4.9	5.4	5.5
Depression	5.0	5.2	5.1	4.7	5.3	5.1	4.8	5.3	5.5
Frustration	4.9	4.9	4.9	4.9	5.0	4.9	4.5	4.8	4.9
Sickness Impact Profile									
Global	10.3	8.1	7.4	12.0	8.5	6.7	12.2	6.0	4.4
Physical	4.9	3.2	4.2	6.4	4.0	2.6	6.5	3.3	2.4
Psychosocial	9.1	5.9	4.8	10.9	8.1	6.0	11.8	5.2	3.4
Time Trade Off	0.42	0.46	0.42	0.49	0.51	0.51	0.52	0.58	0.58
Stress Test (minutes walked)	11.4	13.0	13.2	11.2	14.2	14.8	16.1	19.8	19.7
Six-Minute Walk (distance walked in metres)	421	437	440	418	456	451	470	509	521

Source: Adapted from Reference 13
Note: Results given are mean scores in each group. Statistical analysis was based on the change in mean scores from baseline (see text for details).

Table 14.7. EP86-004: Mean Blood Pressure in the Three Treatment Groups at 0 and 6 Months

	Mean Blood Pressure, mm Hg						Significance*	
	Placebo		"Low" Erythropoietin		"High" Erythropoeitin		Among Groups	Erythropoietin vs. Placebo
	0 mo	6 mo	0 mo	6 mo	0 mo	6 mo		
Systolic	147	143	137	137	144	144	NS	NS
Diastolic	80	79	76	78	78	83	0.023	<0.001

*Statistical analysis was by analysis of variance for repeated measures. NS, not significant.

Table 14.8. The Number of Patients Reporting Adverse Events Other than Hypertension in EP86-004

Adverse Event	Number of Patients		
	Placebo	"Low" Erythropoietin	"High" Erythropoietin
Seizure	1	2	0
Access clotting*	1	4	7
Dialyzer clotting	4	4	4
Chest pain	6	7	6
Hemorrhage/epistaxis	7	5	5
Headache	19	13	13
Red eyes†	0	2	3
Flulike symptoms	12	9	9
Bone/muscle aches	9	8	12

*$P = 0.01$, erythropoietin vs. placebo.
†$P = 0.04$, erythropoietin vs. placebo.

medications were increased or initiated in 3 of 32 placebo patients compared to 18 of 67 patients on rHuEpo therapy ($P = 0.06$). Four patients (2 in the low and 2 in the high target group) were withdrawn because of hypertension at 1, 2, 12, and 13 weeks after randomization. None had been on antihypertensive medication before the study, and none had obvious sequelae from their hypertension.

Other Side Effects. The incidence of side effects other than hypertension is given in Table 14.8. There were positive associations between rHuEpo therapy and vascular access clotting ($P = 0.01$) and eye redness. The relationship of rHuEpo therapy and vascular access clotting is discussed in more detail below.

Conclusions

This study confirmed the efficacy of rHuEpo in increasing the hemoglobin concentration of over 90 percent of patients receiving it (13). In addition, the reduction in anemia was accompanied by a clinically significant improvement in quality of life and exercise capacity, especially in those areas related to fatigue and energy level. The incidence of adverse events was low, with only access failure and red eyes occurring more commonly in rHuEpo-treated patients. A significant increase in diastolic, but not systolic, blood pressure occurred in rHuEpo-treated patients and persisted throughout follow-up despite an overall increase

in antihypertensive prescription. Because neither the clinical significance of the change in diastolic blood pressure nor the mechanism was
clear, a more detailed subanalysis of data related to hypertension was
performed.

Hypertension and Echocardiography Substudies

Concern regarding a 7-mm Hg mean increase in diastolic blood pressure is justifiable because this is the range of blood pressure change
which is associated with long-term differences in stroke mortality. The
number of patients in the Canadian Multicentre Study is too small to
allow useful comment on mortality, and data relating to long-term outcome will have to be obtained from larger trials with longer follow-up.

An analysis of factors thought likely to influence the development of
hypertension was undertaken. Overall, despite the increase in mean
diastolic blood pressure, there was no significant difference in the incidence of severe hypertension (defined as a diastolic blood pressure of
≥ 110 mm Hg or a hypertension-related seizure) in rHuEpo-treated patients compared to control (14 percent vs. 13 percent; $P > 0.1$). Patients
receiving rHuEpo were more likely than placebo patients to develop severe hypertension if they had a previous history of hypertension ($P =
0.037$) or had previously received a transplant ($P = 0.049$). There was
a significant interaction among the occurrence of severe hypertension,
treatment (erythropoietin or placebo), and the presence or absence of
native kidneys ($P = 0.002$). In erythropoietin-treated patients, the incidence of severe hypertension in previously untransplanted patients
with native kidneys in place was 21.4 percent compared to 5.7 percent
in other erythropoietin-treated patients.

There was a significant correlation ($r = 0.42$; $P < 0.001$) between
the rise in hemoglobin during the first 5 weeks of rHuEpo therapy and
the change in diastolic blood pressure during the same period. No similar relationship was seen for systolic blood pressure. There was no correlation between change in hemoglobin and change in diastolic blood
pressure between weeks 0 and 17 of rHuEpo therapy.

At the conclusion of the randomized study, placebo patients were begun on rHuEpo therapy in a dose of 50 units/kg intravenously three
times per week after hemodialysis. Despite a mean increase of 7 mm
Hg in diastolic blood pressure during the first 4 months of rHuEpo therapy, no correlation was found between changes in diastolic blood pressure and change in hemoglobin between weeks 0 and 5. However, the
mean increase in hemoglobin was lower (11 g/litre in these patients

Table 14.9. The Effect of rHuEpo on Left Ventricular Mass

	Baseline	Follow-up	P
Hemoglobin (g/litre)	63 ± 8	114 ± 15	0.0001
Diastolic blood pressure (mm Hg)	76 ± 12	81 ± 9	0.01
Body weight (kg)	65.8 ± 13	66.3 ± 13	0.33
LV mass (g)	253 ± 77	215 ± 71	0.0004
LV end-diastolic diameter (cm)	5.5 ± 0.6	5.1 ± 0.6	0.003
Mean wall thickness (cm)	0.99 ± 0.1	0.96 ± 0.1	0.32
LV end-diastolic volume (ml)	173 ± 60	138 ± 48	0.005

Note: Clinical data and left ventricular (LV) size measurements at baseline and follow-up for 22 patients receiving rHuEpo. Data are given as means ± SD.

compared to 19 g/litre between 0 and 5 weeks in patients from the randomized portion of the study).

No permanent clinical sequelae based on weekly clinical observation over the total duration of follow-up occurred secondary to hypertension throughout the study. This cannot, however, be taken as a guarantee that long-term problems will not occur. One important marker of the long-term consequences of hypertension, left ventricular hypertrophy, was assessed from serial three-dimensional and M-mode echocardiograms.

The change in left ventricular mass was assessed in rHuEpo-treated patients who had maintained a 30 g/litre or greater increase in hemoglobin for a minimum of 6 months (14). The results are summarized in Table 14.9. Left ventricular mass fell significantly ($P < 0.004$) during rHuEpo therapy by a mean of 15 percent. In patients with the most severe left ventricular enlargement (left ventricular mass > 210 g), a 20 percent decrease in left ventricular mass occurred during rHuEpo therapy ($P < 0.001$). Patients whose left ventricular mass was <210 g before therapy had no change in left ventricular mass after rHuEpo. Overall, the change in left ventricular mass was related to the change in hemoglobin with a slope of − 1.1 g/g/litre ($2P = 0.03$). The baseline hemoglobin was found by multiple linear regression to be an important determinant of this effect; an equivalent rise in hemoglobin was associated with a greater reduction in left ventricular mass in patients more severely anemic to begin with.

The presence of left ventricular hypertrophy is a powerful, independent predictor of increased mortality in end-stage renal disease (15), and anemia is one of the key determinants of left ventricular hypertrophy (16). The reduction in left ventricular mass after rHuEpo therapy occurred despite the increase in diastolic blood pressure. The net result of rHuEpo therapy, at least in terms of cardiac morbidity and mortality, may at worst be neutral and at best be positive. Further, careful follow-up of larger numbers of patients treated over an extended period is necessary to answer this question.

The Canadian Multicentre Maintenance Study

Study Outline

Ninety-eight of the 99 patients who completed the initial Canadian Multicentre Study (EP86-004) continued therapy in a maintenance protocol (EP88-101) for a further 12 months. Patients previously on placebo began rHuEpo therapy in an open label fashion at a dose of 50 units/kg intravenously three times per week after hemodialysis. The dose of rHuEpo was adjusted to maintain hemoglobin in the range of 105 to 125 g/litre.

Hematologic parameters were measured every 2 weeks, and iron status and serum chemistry were measured every 4 weeks. Quality of life (KDQ) assessment and the 6-minute walk test were performed every 6 months. Data concerning adverse events were recorded at each dialysis.

Results

After 12 weeks of rHuEpo therapy, the hemoglobin value in 31 patients previously receiving placebo (Group 1) had risen to 108.3 ± 17.3 g/litre and was indistinguishable from that in 67 patients initially receiving rHuEpo (Group 2). The mean hemoglobin value remained stable within the target range throughout the remainder of the 52-week study period (Fig 14.6). The dose of rHuEpo at week 52 was 176.6 ± 154.4 units/kg/week in Group 1 and 210 ± 144.4 units/kg/week in Group 2 ($P = 0.43$).

Nineteen patients (3 in Group 1 and 16 in Group 2) each experienced at least one episode of access failure. The mean time to access failure after initiation of rHuEpo therapy was 25.2 ± 19.5 weeks (range, 2 to 78). The cumulative rate of access failure for all patients during rHuEpo therapy was 17 percent (Fig 14.7a). Access failure was more frequent in patients with implanted access (Gortex, Vitagraft, saphenous vein graft), with failures in 46 percent of these compared to only 7 percent of native arteriovenous fistula (Fig 14.7b).

Mean diastolic blood pressure rose from 77 ± 11.2 mm Hg to 81.8 ± 14.7 mm Hg ($P < 0.02$) in Group 1 patients given rHuEpo. The 7-

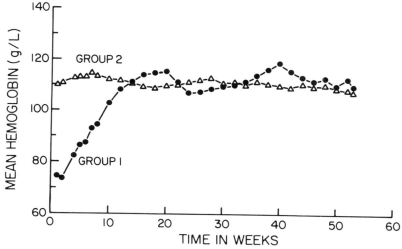

Figure 14.6. EP88-101. The mean hemoglobin for patients previously on placebo (group 1) and patients initially on rHuEpo. By week 12, there was no significant difference in hemoglobin between the groups.

mm Hg increase in mean diastolic blood pressure noted in Group 2 patients during the 6 months of rHuEpo therapy was sustained during the further 12 months of follow-up.

The improvement in the fatigue, depression, and relationships dimensions of the KDQ noted during the first 6 months of rHuEpo therapy in Group 2 patients were sustained during the additional 12 months of follow-up. The KDQ scores of Group 1 patients did not change during the placebo period but improved when patients began rHuEpo (Table 14.10). There was a modest, not statistically significant increase in distance walked in the 6-minute walk test after rHuEpo therapy.

Conclusions

The results of this maintenance study confirmed and extended the results of the 6-month Canadian Multicentre Study (17). Stable hemoglobin concentrations and rHuEpo dose requirements were maintained over a 12- to 18-month period. The only serious clinical consequences were a modest increase in diastolic but not systolic blood pressure and an increased risk of access failure, especially for patients with implanted access.

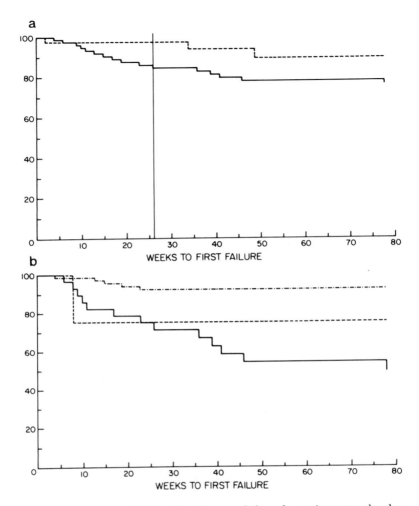

Figure 14.7. a, the cumulative risk of access failure for patients on placebo or rHuEpo during studies EP86-004 and EP88-101. Dashed line indicates the placebo group; solid line, rHuEpo. The vertical line at week 26 indicates the point at which placebo patients began rHuEpo. b, the rate of access failure for patients on rHuEpo by the type of vascular access. Solid line indicates Gortex/Vitagraph/saphenous vein graft (type 1); line of dashes and dots, arteriovenous fistula (type 2); line of hyphens, other. Type 1 vs. type 2: $P = 0.0001$. The statistical analysis is by the life table method.

Table 14.10. Scores for Quality of Life and Exercise Capacity during Long-Term rHuEpo Therapy

	Placebo*				Erythropoietin			
	0 mo	6 mo	12 mo	18 mo	0 mo	6 mo	12 mo	18 mo
KDQ								
Physical	4.2	4.6	4.2	4.5	3.8	5.3†	4.4	4.5
Fatigue	4.5	4.5	5.1	5.0†	4.2	5.2†	5.3†	5.2†
Relationships	5.0	5.0	5.4	5.7†	5.0	5.5†	5.7†	5.7
Depression	5.1	5.1	5.5	5.5	4.8	5.3†	5.4†	5.4†
Frustration	4.9	4.9	5.0	5.1	4.7	4.9	4.9	5.1
Six-minute walk	446	440	464	494	447	486	502	499

*Placebo patients began rHuEpo at 6 months.
†$P < 0.05$ vs. baseline.

Discussion

Studies of erythropoietin in Canada have focused, in general, on long-term safety and efficacy and on the effects of rHuEpo on quality of life in hemodialysis patients. In general, the studies confirm the efficacy of rHuEpo as reported by others (4,5,8,18), with over 90 percent of patients having their anemia corrected to within specified target ranges. The incidence of adverse events has been low in these studies, with the incidence of seizures, in particular, being much less than that reported elsewhere (9,19). There are a number of possible reasons for the low incidence of adverse events.

First, the selection criteria for these Canadian studies completed to date were very stringent. Patients with serious concomitant diseases were excluded. The patients studied probably represent no more than 30 percent of patients with end-stage renal disease currently on dialysis in Canada. Many of the other rHuEpo studies reported have used less stringent selection criteria and may thus have included larger numbers of patients predisposed to problems such as seizure or hypertension. However, a search of published data on rHuEpo fails to identify any specific factors that predict the likelihood of seizure during rHuEpo therapy, apart from the rapidity of hematocrit rise.

A second factor that may have contributed to the low adverse event rate is the low rate of rise of hematocrit. In the Canadian Multicentre Study, the hematocrit was raised by about 1 to 1.5 percent weekly, with the rHuEpo dose being reduced if the hemoglobin value exceeded 125 g/litre or the hematocrit exceeded 35 percent. In this way, the rapid rates of hematocrit rise reported in association with seizures in other studies were avoided (4,8,19).

Finally, the failure to detect an increased rate of seizure in rHuEpo-treated compared to placebo-treated patients may simply indicate that there is no real seizure risk associated with rHuEpo therapy. Data concerning the incidence of seizures in hemodialysis populations are hard to come by. However, data from the Canadian Hemodialysis Morbidity Study suggest an annual rate of seizures of 4.3 percent for non-rHuEpo-treated patients. Thus, the incidence of seizures in rHuEpo-treated patients in the Canadian Multicentre Study and in most other studies, including the European Multicentre Study (18), is close to the expected incidence for non-rHuEpo-treated patients.

With respect to hypertension, data from the Canadian Multicentre Study are similar to those from the European (18) and U.S. (20) multicenter studies. Canadian patients experienced a statistically significant increase in diastolic blood pressure despite an overall increase in antihypertensive medication prescriptions. The clinical significance of this blood pressure rise cannot be determined because of the small sample size and the relative infrequency of relevant outcomes such as stroke, angina, or myocardial infarction. Data from the echocardiographic study of these patients (14), however, suggest that, in the short term at least, correction of anemia has a beneficial effect on left ventricular remodeling, despite the increase in diastolic blood pressure.

Others reported a similar beneficial effect on ventricular mass during rHuEpo therapy in patients who did not experience an overall increase in diastolic blood pressure (21). Both the Canadian study (14) and that of London et al. (21) involved patients who were or had been hypertensive before rHuEpo therapy. Satoh et al. (22) reported their observations on hemodynamic function after rHuEpo administration to nonhypertensive subjects with normal cardiac function. These patients experienced a significant reduction in left ventricular end-diastolic diameter and wall stress after rHuEpo therapy, along with a reduction in the previously increased cardiac output. These data were interpreted as indicating that correction of anemia by rHuEpo therapy suppressed the hyperdynamic circulation required to maintain tissue oxygenation.

The effect of rHuEpo on blood pressure in hemodialysis patients thus seems to be a short-term increase in the severity of diastolic hypertension, which is offset by favorable changes in tissue oxygenation that permit a reduction in cardiac size and work and a reduction in ventricular hypertrophy. The long-term effects of the persistent elevation in diastolic blood pressure remain uncertain. Careful follow-up of the larger numbers of patients currently beginning therapy with rHuEpo is necessary to follow any trends in long-term cardiovascular morbidity and mortality. Collection of these data will be difficult and may be best achieved by modification of existing registry databases such as the European Dialysis and Transplant Association (EDTA) registry or the Canadian Renal Failure Registry.

Of some concern is the apparent increased rate of access problems and difficulty in maintaining the extracorporeal hemodialysis circuit in patients receiving rHuEpo. Access failure was significantly more common in rHuEpo-treated patients compared to controls in the Canadian Multicentre Study (13). The rate of access failure (14.1 percent) was similar to that reported in the European (14.7 percent) and U.S. (11.7 percent) studies. When patients were followed for 12 to 18 months, the rate of access failure climbed to 21 percent, with the risk of access failure being much higher for implanted access (e.g., graft) compared to native arteriovenous fistulas (51 vs. 7 percent).

Data concerning long-term patency rates of hemodialysis access for non-rHuEpo-treated patients are relatively scarce. Churchill (23) reported probabilities of graft or fistula clotting of 24.5 percent and 8.5 percent, respectively, after 12 months of follow-up of non-rHuEpo-treated hemodialysis patients. Thus, if the hematocrit rise associated with rHuEpo therapy does make access failure more probable, this increased risk seems largely confined to patients with grafts. This is consistent with the observation that most access failures in the U.S. study occurred in grafts (20). More data are required to define the risk factors for access failure during rHuEpo therapy and to identify therapies.

The Canadian Multicentre Study demonstrated a statistically and clinically significant improvement in aspects of quality of life related to physical functioning (13). Of perhaps more surprise were the significant improvements in the depression and relationships dimensions of the KDQ. These improvements were mirrored in the improvements noted in the sickness impact profile, a general health questionnaire.

These data are consistent with observations made by others (24,25). Evans et al. reported improvement in both subjective and objective measurements of a wide range of quality-of-life variables, including energy and activity levels, well being, sexual function, health status, and functional ability (24). They were unable to identify any specific changes in work and employment status. Delano reported similar results in a smaller group of patients (25). Many other studies reported subjective improvements in quality of life after rHuEpo therapy (4,5,8,18,20,26).

An attempt was made in the Canadian Multicentre Study to identify a relationship between hemoglobin change and quality-of-life improvement. Although a statistically significant positive correlation between change in hemoglobin and change in quality of life and exercise capacity was found, the correlation coefficient was modest (13). This suggests that there may be a continuous relationship between hemoglobin increase and quality of life. This observation was not noted previously. However, given the observation that the incidence of access failure was higher in the patients with higher hemoglobin values, the optimal target hemoglobin may be a trade off of benefits (quality-of-life improvement) vs. risks (hypertension and access failure). Data from the Canadian studies suggest that the optimal target hemoglobin might be 105 to 115 g/litre, corresponding to a hematocrit of 0.32 to 0.38.

A number of studies using very different methods documented the subjective and objective improvement in exercise capacity after rHuEpo administration (13,27–30). Increases in maximal workload and tissue oxygenation and enhanced recovery from exercise were all noted. Mayer et al. (28) noted an increase in anaerobic threshold in association with increased oxygen uptake and peripheral oxygen utilization at maximal exercise, after partial correction of anemia. Bocker et al. (27) reported an improvement in work capacity after just 2 months of rHuEpo therapy. Improvement in exercise capacity in the Canadian Multicentre Study paralleled improvement in quality of life (13). As with the Bocker study, the objective improvement in exercise capacity as measured by the modified Naughton stress test was maximal after just 2 months of rHuEpo therapy, by which time mean hemoglobin levels were within the target ranges in each treatment group. This very early objective improvement in exercise capacity correlates well with subjective improvements in physical functioning reported by other authors.

In addition to improvements in general well-being and physical performance, a number of authors reported improvements in appetite and sexual function after rHuEpo therapy (10,24,25,31,32). The number of patients complaining of sexual dysfunction before rHuEpo therapy in the Canadian Multicentre Study was too small to make any useful comment regarding the effect of rHuEpo therapy. However, some investigators have documented an improvement in sexual function after anemia correction with rHuEpo therapy, occurring in association with reduction in hyperprolactinemia (31,32). The mechanism of the improvement in sexual function is not clear at present.

The improvement in appetite noted during rHuEpo therapy may help explain the high incidence of hyperkalemia reported by some authors

(5,8,18). Patients in the Canadian Multicentre Study did not have an increase in serum potassium while on rHuEpo, nor was there an increased frequency of hyperkalemia (defined as a serum potassium of >6.0 mmol/litre).

Shinaberger et al. (33) suggested that the hematocrit increase seen during rHuEpo therapy might adversely affect dialyzer performance, particularly during high flux dialysis. Some authors reported worsened predialysis serum urea, creatinine, potassium, and phosphate values during rHuEpo therapy (5,8,18,34–36). Data from the Canadian Multicentre Study do not indicate any significant changes in predialysis blood chemistry or any systematic changes in dialysis prescription. Other authors (37–40) similarly were unable to confirm an adverse effect of rHuEpo therapy on blood chemistries or dialysis efficiency, at least for small molecules like urea. Shinaberger et al. argued that, although urea clearance may not be affected by high-hematocrit dialysis, clearance of other potential uremic toxins may be and that this will eventually cause an increase in morbidity among dialysis patients (33). This, however, remains speculative at present. Currently, there are no convincing data from published clinical trials of rHuEpo to support the hypothesis that increasing hematocrit has a detrimental effect on dialysis efficiency.

ACKNOWLEDGMENTS

I thank Ortho Pharmaceutical (Canada) Ltd. for their help and support in this study and also give special thanks to the J. W. Johnson Pharmaceutical Research Institute for their support. Thanks goes to all of the principle investigators for their time and hard work involved in this study: Dr. P. E. Barre, Royal Victoria Hospital, Montreal, Quebec; Dr. A. D. Cohen, Victoria General Hospital, Halifax, Nova Scotia; Dr. D. Churchill, St. Joseph's Hospital, Hamilton, Ontario; Dr. P. A. Keown, Vancouver General Hospital, Vancouver, British Columbia; Dr. A. Laupacis, University Hospital, London, Ontario; Dr. H. Mandin, Foothills Hospital, Calgary, Alberta; Dr. J. K. McKenzie, St. Boniface Hospital, Winnipeg, Manitoba; Dr. S. Nadler, Ottawa General Hospital, Ottawa, Ontario; Dr. G. Posen, Ottawa Civic Hospital, Ottawa, Ontario; Dr. J. D. E. Price, University Hospital, British Columbia; Dr. D. Sim, Robarts Research Institute, London, Ontario; Dr. D. Slaughter, Ortho Pharmaceutical, Toronto, Ontario; Dr. R. Werb, St. Paul's Hospital, Vancouver, British Columbia; and Ms. C. Wong, Robarts Research Institute, London, Ontario.

REFERENCES

1. Eschbach JW. Hematologic problems of dialysis patients. In: Drukker W, Parsons FM, Maher JF, eds. Replacement of renal function by dialysis. Boston: Martinus Nijhoff, 1983.

2. Jacobs K, Shoemaker C, Rundersdorf R, et al. Isolation and characterization of genomic and cDNA clones of human erythropoietin. Nature 1985; 313:806–10.

3. Lin FK, Suggs S, Lin CH, et al. Cloning and expression of the human erythropoietin gene. Proc Natl Acad Sci USA 1985;82:7580–4.

4. Winearls CG, Oliver DP, Pippard MJ, Reid C, Downing MR, Cotes PM. Effect of human erythropoietin derived from recombinant DNA on the anemia of patients maintained by chronic hemodialysis. Lancet 1986;2:1175–8.

5. Eschbach JW, Egrie JC, Downing MR, Browne JK, Adamson JW. Correction of the anemia of end-stage renal disease with recombinant human erythropoietin. N Engl J Med 1987;316:73–8.

6. Kindler J, Eckardt KU, Ehmer B, et al. Single dose pharmacokinetics of recombinant human erythropoietin in patients with various degrees of renal failure. Nephrol Dial Transplant 1989;4:345–9.

7. Flaharty K, Besarab A, Vlasses P, Caro J. Pharmacokinetics of human recombinant erythropoietin in ESRD patients [Abstract]. Kidney Int 1990;37: 237A.

8. Casati S, Passerini P, Campise MR, et al. Benefits and risks of protracted treatment with human recombinant erythropoietin in patients having haemodialysis. Br Med J 1987;295:1017–20.

9. Edmunds ME, Walls J, Tucker B, et al. Seizures in haemodialysis patients treated with recombinant human erythropoietin. Nephrol Dial Transplant 1989;4:1065–9.

10. Hart LG, Evans RW. The functional status of ESRD patients as measured by the sickness impact profile. J Chronic Dis 1984;40(Suppl 1):117–30S.

11. Churchill DN, Torrance GW, Taylor DW, et al. Measurement of quality of life in end-stage renal disease: the time trade off approach. Clin Invest Med 1987;10:14–20.

12. Jaeschke R, Singer J, Guyatt G. Health status measurement: ascertaining the minimal clinically important difference. Controlled Clin Trials 1989; 10:407–15.

13. Canadian Erythropoietin Study Group. Association between recombinant human erythropoietin and quality of life and exercise capacity of patients receiving haemodialysis. Br Med J 1990;300:573–8.

14. Silberberg J, Racine N, Barre P, Sniderman AD. Regression of left ventricular hypertrophy in dialysis patients following correction of anemia with recombinant human erythropoietin. Can J Cardiol 1990;6:1–4.

15. Silberberg JS, Barre P, Prichard S, Sniderman AD. Left ventricular hypertrophy: an independent determinant of survival in endstage renal failure. Kidney Int 1989;36:286–90.

16. Silberberg JS, Rahal D, Patton R, Sniderman AD. Role of anemia in the pathogenesis of left ventricular hypertrophy in endstage renal failure. Am J Cardiol 1989;64:222–4.

17. Muirhead N, Wong C (for the Canadian Erythropoietin Study Group). Long term erythropoietin therapy for anemia in hemodialysis patients [Abstract]. Kidney Int 1990;37:312A.

18. Sundal E, Kaeser U. Correction of anemia of chronic renal failure with recombinant human erythropoietin: safety and efficacy of one year's treatment in a European Multicentre Study of 150 haemodialysis-dependent patients. Nephrol Dial Transplant 1989;4:979–87.

19. Brown AL, Tucker B, Baker LRI, Raine AG. Seizures related to blood transfusion and erythropoietin treatment in patients undergoing dialysis. Br Med J 1989;299:1258–9.

20. Eschbach JW, Abdulhadi MH, Brown JK, et al. Recombinant human erythropoietin in anemic patients with end-stage renal disease. Ann Intern Med 1989;111:992–1000.

21. London GM, Zins B, Pannier B, et al. Vascular changes in hemodialysis patients in response to recombinant human erythropoietin. Kidney Int 1989; 36:878–82.

22. Satoh K, Masuda T, Ikedo Y, et al. Hemodynamic changes by recombinant erythropoietin therapy in hemodialysis patients. Hypertension 1990;15: 262–5.

23. Churchill DN. Morbidity in chronic hemodialysis patients—a study of prognosis [Abstract]. Kidney Int 1990;37:291A.

24. Evans RW, Rader B, Manninen DL, and the Cooperative Multicentre EPO Clinical Trial Group. The quality of life of hemodialysis recipients treated with recombinant human erythropoietin. JAMA 1990;263:825–30.

25. Delano BG. Improvements in quality of life following treatment with rHuEPO in anemic hemodialysis patients. Am J Kidney Dis 1989;14:14–8.

26. Lundin AP. Quality of life: subjective and objective improvements with recombinant human erythropoietin. Semin Nephrol 1989;(Suppl 1):22–9.

27. Bocker A, Reimer E, Nonnast-Daniel B, et al. Effect of erythropoietin treatment on O_2 affinity and performance in patients with renal anemia. Contrib Nephrol 1988;66:165–75.

28. Mayer G, Thum J, Cada EM, Stummvoll HK, Graf H. Working capacity is increased following recombinant human erythropoietin treatment. Kidney Int 1988;34:525–8.

29. Nonnast-Daniel B, Creutzig A, Kuhn K, et al. Effect of treatment with recombinant erythropoietin on peripheral haemodynamics and oxygenation. Contrib Nephrol 1988;66:325–32.

30. Robertson HT, Haley R, Guthrie M, et al. Recombinant erythropoietin improves exercise capacity in anemic hemodialysis patients. Am J Kidney Dis 1990;15:325–32.

31. Schaefer RM, Kokot F, Wernze H, Geiger H, Heidland A. Improved sexual function in hemodialysis patients on recombinant erythropoietin: a possible role of prolactin. Clin Nephrol 1989;31:1–5.

32. Bommer J, Kugel M, Schwobel B, Ritz E, Barth HP, Seelig R. Improved sexual function during recombinant human erythropoietin therapy. Nephrol Dial Transplant 1990;5:204–7.

33. Shinaberger JH, Miller JH, Gardner PW. Erythropoietin alert: risks of high hematocrit hemodialysis. Trans Am Soc Artif Org 1988;34:179–84.

34. Zehnder C, Gluck Z, Descoendres C, Uelinger DE, Blumberg A. Human recombinant erythropoietin in anaemic patients on maintenance haemodialysis—secondary effects of the increase in haemoglobin. Nephrol Dial Transplant 1988;3:657–60.

35. Acchiardo S, Moore L, Miles D, Key J, Burk L, Sargen J. Does eryth-

ropoietin treatment change hemodialysis requirements? [Abstract]. Kidney Int 1989;35:237.

36. Mohini R. Clinical efficacy of recombinant human erythropoietin in hemodialysis patients. Semin Nephrol 1989;9(Suppl 1):16–21.

37. Delano BG, Lundin AP, Galonsky R, Quinn-Defaro RM, Rao TKS, Friedman EA. Dialyzer urea and creatinine clearance are not significantly altered in erythropoietin treated maintenance hemodialysis patients. ASAIO Trans 1990; 36:36–9.

38. Schmidt B, Ward RA. The impact of erythropoietin on hemodialyser design and performance. Artif Organs 1989;13:35–42.

39. Casati S, Campise M, Crepaldi M, Lobo J, Graziani G, Ponticelli C. Hemodialysis efficiency after long term treatment with recombinant human erythropoietin. Nephrol Dial Transplant 1989;4:718–20.

40. Zehnter E, Pollok M, Ziegenhagen D, et al. Urea kinetics in patients on regular dialysis treatment before and after treatment with recombinant human erythropoietin. Contrib Nephrol 1988;66:149–55.

Chapter 15

Recombinant Human Erythropoietin (Epoetin Beta) in Patients with End-Stage Renal Disease: United States and Japan

Joseph T. Sobota and Yoshihei Hirasawa

The most exciting development in the treatment of the anemia of end-stage renal disease has been the introduction of replacement therapy with recombinant human erythropoietin (rHuEpo). Human erythropoietin is normally produced in only very limited quantities and thus could not be used for replacement therapy. With the purification of human erythropoietin from urine in 1977 (1) and the subsequent cloning of the human gene and its expression in Chinese hamster ovary cells, however, the production of significant quantities of rHuEpo was made possible (2,3). The results of several clinical trials demonstrated the efficacy of rHuEpo in the treatment of the anemia of end-stage renal disease (4–8).

Epoetin beta (Marogen® Sterile Powder, Chugai-Upjohn, Inc., Rosemont, Illinois) is rHuEpo derived from cloned human fetal liver cells and expressed in Chinese hamster ovary cells (Fig 15.1). Epoetin beta is purified from the spent medium of the Chinese hamster ovary cells by a patented technique that includes reverse-phase high-performance liquid chromatography, which is essential for the isolation of pure, homogeneous glycoprotein.

Carbohydrates represent approximately 40 percent of the human urinary erythropoietin molecule and are essential for its in vivo activity. The carbohydrate moiety of epoetin beta is virtually indistinguishable from that of human urinary erythropoietin (9,10), and the amino acid sequence is identical to that of the naturally occurring hormone (9).

Human erythropoietin (EPO)
_____
(purified from urine)

↓

Preparation of oligonucleotide probes

↓

Hybridization with lambda human genome library

↓

Isolation of clone with human EPO gene

↓

Transfection of clone into COS-1 cells

↓

Single-stranded EPO-specific probes

↓

Hybridization with mRNA from human fetal liver

↓

Isolation of mRNA for EPO gene

↓

Using reverse transcriptase, obtain cDNA for EPO

↓

Transfection into CHO cells

↓

Preparation of epoetin beta from culture supernatant

Figure 15.1. The outline for the preparation of epoetin beta from the human erythropoietin gene. _Source: Adapted from Reference 18_

Epoetin beta is prepared in lyophilized form and supplied in vials containing 3000 or 8000 units. The powder is reconstituted with sterile saline for intravenous administration. Although it does require refrigeration, no evidence of denaturation upon shaking has been observed and, thus, no special handling is required. The specific activity of epoetin beta, as determined by the polycythemic mouse bioassay, is 180 units/μg of erythropoietin polypeptide.

This chapter reviews the results of the clinical studies of the efficacy, safety, and tolerability of epoetin beta in the treatment of anemia of patients with end-stage renal disease in North America and Japan. Although the clinical studies in North America and Japan have many common features, medical practice differs somewhat. For example, the dose ranges of epoetin beta used were selected by the individual investigators to be consistent with the average body weight of the population of that particular country. In addition, differences in diet, genetics, cultural customs, and sensitivities may be reflected in some of the clinical data obtained. The results of these studies demonstrate that, despite these differences, treatment of renal anemia with epoetin beta leads to the improvement of both the anemia and the quality of life of patients with end-stage renal disease.

The Pharmacokinetics of Epoetin Beta

The pharmacokinetics of epoetin beta were studied in normal individuals and in patients with nephric and anephric end-stage renal disease and were found to be similar in all three populations (11). The mean apparent serum half-life of epoetin beta in normal individuals ranges from 4.4 to 11 hours and is related to the dose, as clearance tends to decrease as a function of the dose (12). The dose-dependent plasma concentration of epoetin beta seems to be independent of renal function (13); has a volume of distribution between 40 and 90 ml/kg at doses of 10 to 1000 units/kg, which is consistent with distribution primarily in the plasma (Table 15.1) (12); and is eliminated primarily by nonrenal routes, with less than 5 percent eliminated by the kidney (14).

The role of carbohydrates in the survival of epoetin beta in the plasma is well documented. In one study, epoetin beta was labeled with iodine 125 and injected intravenously into rats (15). As shown in Figure 15.2, the majority of the epoetin beta remained in the circulation for up to 30 minutes. However, when similar experiments were carried out after the enzymatic removal of sialic acid residues from epoetin beta,

Table 15.1. The Pharmacokinetics of Epoetin Beta in Normal Males

	Dose (units/kg)				
	10	50	150	500	1000
N	6	6	6	6	6
Vd_{ss} (ml/kg)	89.05	39.50	49.20	46.47	62.72
	(23.57)	(3.87)	(8.12)	(13.38)	(22.7)
$T_{1/2}$ (h)	4.42	5.34	6.10	8.49	11.02
	(1.18)	(0.52)	(0.88)	(0.83)	(0.03)
Cl (ml/min)	0.57	0.09	0.07	0.07	0.09
	(1.37)	(0.73)	(1.07)	(3.05)	(2.17)

Source: Adapted from Reference 12

Abbreviations: N, number of subjects; Vd_{ss}, volume of distribution at steady state; $T_{1/2}$, serum half-life; Cl, clearance.

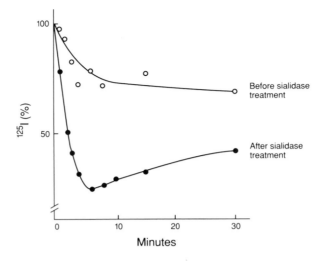

Figure 15.2. The clearance of ^{125}I-epoetin beta and ^{125}I-asialoepoetin beta. ^{125}I-labeled epoetin beta was injected intravenously into rats before (open circles) or after (closed circles) the removal of sialic acid, and the amount of radioactivity in the blood was measured periodically. *Source: Reference 15*

most of the asialoepoetin beta disappeared from the plasma within 6 minutes.

To determine into which organs of the body the ^{125}I-asialoepoetin beta was concentrated, the radioactivity present within four major organs of the rat was analyzed 30 minutes after injection. Nearly 85 percent of the asialoepoetin beta was taken up by the liver. Thus, the carbohydrate configuration of epoetin beta prevents its rapid clearance from the circulation. This finding underscores the importance of the preparatory technique, which provides for the proper glycosylation of this recombinant protein and ensures its pharmacokinetic properties in vivo.

The pharmacokinetics of epoetin may depend on the route of administration. Data obtained from a clinical study of subcutaneous administration of epoetin beta to patients with end-stage renal disease suggest that approximately 50 percent (range, 15 to 96 percent) of the intravenous dose appears in the serum, with a peak concentration observed at approximately 22 hours (13). The serum concentrations are maintained longer after subcutaneous administration than after intravenous administration of similar doses, which suggests that subcutaneous administration may be more physiologic. One study of patients

with end-stage renal disease indicated that the total weekly maintenance dose of epoetin beta can be reduced by 37 percent when converting from intravenous to subcutaneous therapy (16).

Clinical Trials

Phase I studies were carried out in normal individuals; subjects in
the North American Phase II and Phase III trials were nonhospitalized
men and women between the ages of 18 and 80 who had been on
chronic hemodialysis for at least 3 months. Women were either post-
menopausal or receiving oral contraceptives. Each patient was required
to have a baseline hemoglobin concentration of less than 8.5 g/dl and,
if hypertensive, to have been on a stable drug regimen for more than 3
months.

Patients were excluded from the studies if they had a history or evidence of any of the following: anemia from any cause other than end-
stage renal disease, myocardial infarction, seizure disorder, significant
hepatic dysfunction, other hematologic disorders, insulin-dependent
diabetes mellitus with poor glucose control, multiple drug allergies, or
malignancy within the past 5 years. Patients were also excluded if they
had received androgen or immunosuppressive therapy within 1 month
of entry into the study.

Phase I Studies

Two studies were carried out in normal subjects to determine the
safety of epoetin beta. In the Japanese Phase I study (17), 24 normal
adult men, aged 26 to 38 and weighing 55 to 91 kg, were randomly
assigned to four different groups. Each group consisted of six individuals; four received epoetin beta at the same one-dose level, and the
other two received placebo. Epoetin beta was administered at successive doses of 36 units, 360 units, 1800 units (approximately 25 units/
kg), and 3600 units (approximately 50 units/kg). After a particular dose
was shown to be safe by both clinical and laboratory examinations, the
doses of epoetin beta were increased to the next level. The results of
this study showed that individuals who received a single dose of 3600
units had a slight increase in reticulocyte count (within the normal
range) when assessed 4 days after they had received the dose. In addition, there was no evidence of antibody formation against epoetin
beta.

In the North American Phase I study, eight healthy individuals received epoetin beta at single doses of 10 to 1000 units/kg (14). The

Table 15.2. The Design of the North American
Dose-Finding Studies of rHuEpo

Period	Dose (units/kg)
Fixed-dose period (4 wk)	25 or 100 or 200
Dose-adjustment period (16 wk)	50 or 150

Note: Patients who met the criteria for entry into the study were randomized to receive rHuEpo at 25, 100, or 200 units/kg. During the dose-adjustment period, doses were adjusted according to the patient's response (see text).

results of the study showed a dose-related increase in the group mean reticulocyte count, when compared with baseline values (measured 2 to 3 days before the administration of epoetin beta) in individuals receiving at least 150 units/kg.

Phase II Study

The efficacy of treatment with epoetin beta was assessed by changes in hemoglobin, hematocrit, and reticulocyte count and by the number of transfusions of packed red blood cells required.

Hemoglobin Concentration. In North America, 131 patients were entered in the open label, dose-ranging, 20-week study (Study A) (7,18). The design of this study is outlined in Table 15.2. The first 4 weeks constituted a fixed-dose period during which patients received epoetin beta at 25, 100, or 200 units/kg intravenously three times per week after their regular dialysis. This was followed by a 16-week dose-adjustment period during which doses were adjusted to maintain the hemoglobin concentration in the range of 10.5 to 12.5 g/dl.

All groups in this study started at a baseline mean hemoglobin concentration of about 7.1 g/dl. The changes in hemoglobin concentration during the course of the study are shown in Figure 15.3. At the end of the 4-week fixed-dose period, the groups receiving 25, 100, and 200 units/kg of epoetin beta had achieved mean hemoglobin concentrations of 7.83, 8.38, and 9.36 g/dl, respectively.

During the 16-week dose-adjustment period, the mean hemoglobin values of all groups continued to increase progressively in proportion to the doses of epoetin beta administered. However, the different treatment groups reached peak hemoglobin concentrations at different days (Fig 15.3). In addition, although the hemoglobin values rose more quickly in the group receiving 200 units/kg, the values were comparable in the groups receiving 100 and 200 units/kg by day 110 (Fig 15.3). Furthermore, the hemoglobin concentrations of the group treated with 25 units/kg continued to rise throughout the dose-adjustment period to a peak of 9.11 g/dl at day 138 (Fig 15.3). These results suggest that this low dose, over a longer period, is also effective in increasing the hemoglobin concentration.

Hematocrit and Reticulocyte Count. At the end of the fixed-dose period, there were dose-related elevations in the hematocrit; a similar relationship was observed between the dose of epoetin beta and the uncorrected mean reticulocyte count. Peak reticulocyte counts ranged from 4.74 percent on day 12 for the group receiving 100 units/kg to 2.93 percent for the group receiving 25 units/kg and 5.73 percent for the group receiving 200 units/kg at day 22.

Requirements for Transfusion. During the fixed-dose period of this study, the number of units of packed red blood cells transfused per patient per week decreased in the groups receiving epoetin beta at either 100 or 200 units/kg (7,18) (Fig 15.4). During the dose-adjustment period, all treatment groups (25, 100, and 200 units/kg) showed substantial reductions in the frequency of transfusions (Fig 15.4).

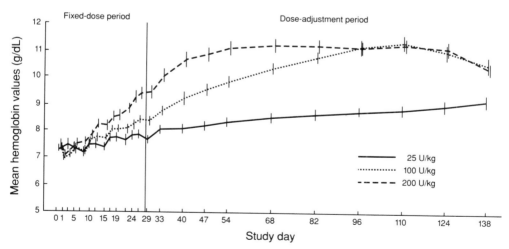

Figure 15.3. The change in the hemoglobin concentration with the dose of rHuEpo and the duration of the treatment. Error bars represent one standard error of the mean.

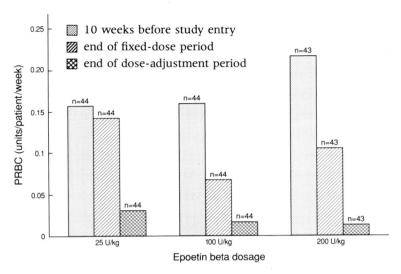

Figure 15.4. The mean number of units of packed red blood cells (PRBC) transfused before and after rHuEpo therapy in a North American dose-finding study. *Source: Adapted from Reference 18*

Phase III Studies

North American Clinical Trials. The results of Study A demonstrated that epoetin beta was very effective in increasing the hemoglobin concentration in a dose-related manner, and double-blind studies were carried out to determine whether the changes in the hemoglobin were due to the treatment with epoetin beta. Two identical multicenter studies (Study B, $N = 115$ [113 patients evaluable for efficacy; all patients evaluable for safety]; Study C, $N = 131$) were conducted, enrolling patients who had never before received epoetin beta (7,8,19). The first 6 weeks were the fixed-dose period; patients received either epoetin beta (100 units/kg) or placebo intravenously three times per week after dialysis. The next 6 weeks were a dose-adjustment period during which the doses could be adjusted depending on the patient's hemoglobin level (Table 15.3).

Hemoglobin Concentration. The mean hemoglobin concentration in the placebo groups of both studies remained essentially unchanged, at about 7 g/dl over the course of the studies, whereas the mean hemoglobin concentration in both groups treated with epoetin beta increased to 11 g/dl.

Hematocrit and Reticulocyte Count. Changes in the hematocrit were consistent with and parallel to the changes in hemoglobin (Fig 15.5) (7,8). Group mean changes from baseline, adjusted by analysis of covariance, showed between-group differences at all study days after the initiation of the treatment. The means at the end of the fixed-dose period and dose-adjustment period, respectively, were 0.48 percent and 1.63 percent for the placebo group and 8.75 percent and 12.77 percent for the group treated with epoetin beta (Study B). Similarly, the mean reticulocyte counts showed significant between-group differences on all study days and increased only in the group receiving epoetin beta.

Changes in Mean Corpuscular Volume and Mean Corpuscular Hemoglobin Concentration. There was no change in the mean corpuscular volume in the placebo group during either the fixed-dose or the dose-adjustment period (8). In the groups treated with epoetin beta, the mean corpuscular volume showed a 2 to 4 percent increase. This increase in the mean corpuscular volume, observed in both groups treated with epoetin beta, may be due to reticulocytosis because the reticulocytes are larger than the mature erythrocytes. An observed 3 percent decrease in the mean corpuscular hemoglobin concentration may be due to a relatively larger increase in the hematocrit compared to the hemoglobin concentration.

Transfusion Requirements. The number of transfusions of packed red blood cells required by patients receiving placebo did not change. In contrast, the patients receiving epoetin beta had a substantially diminished need for transfusions (Fig 15.6) (8). During the 12-week prestudy

Table 15.3. The Design of the North American Placebo-controlled Studies of rHuEpo

Period	Dose (units/kg)
Fixed-dose period (6 wk)	100 or 0 (placebo)
Dose-adjustment period (6 wk)	50 or 100 or 150 or 0 (placebo)

Note: Patients who met the criteria for entry into the study were randomized to receive either 100 units of rHuEpo per kg or placebo. During the dose-adjustment period, doses were adjusted according to the patient's response (see text).

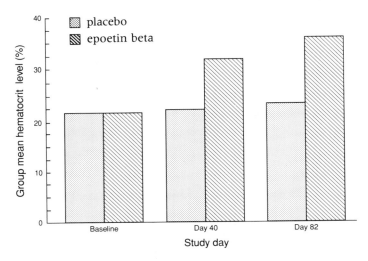

Figure 15.5. The change in the hematocrit in North American placebo-controlled studies. The group mean hematocrit was measured at baseline (day 0), at the end of the fixed-dose period (day 40), and at the end of the dose-adjustment period (day 82). *Source: Adapted from Reference 8*

period, the patients randomized to epoetin beta treatment had required 146 units of packed red blood cells (group total). While these patients were being treated with epoetin beta during the fixed-dose period, however, only 39 units (group total) were required. During the dose-adjustment period, there was a greater reduction in the transfusion requirements (to 5 units), and these transfusions were given to correct postoperative blood loss in two patients. These results demonstrate the virtual elimination of transfusions in patients adequately treated with epoetin beta.

Japanese Trials

In a larger multicenter study in Japan, 179 dialysis patients received placebo or epoetin beta at 1500 units per person (approximately 25 units/kg) or 3000 units per person (approximately 50 units/kg) intravenously three times per week for 8 weeks (20). The results of this study are shown in Figure 15.7. Although the group mean change in hemoglobin concentration at week 8 was -0.19 for the patients receiving placebo, the group mean change in hemoglobin concentration was $+1.83$ and $+2.30$ g/dl for the 1500-unit and 3000-unit treatment groups, respectively. Both the hemoglobin concentration and the reticulocyte count increased in a dose-related manner at week 2, although reticulocyte count did diminish relatively at weeks 4 and 8. The anemia improvement rates (i.e., increment of hemoglobin >1.0 g/dl) were 3.5 percent in the placebo group, 77.6 percent in the 1500-unit dose group, and 83.1 percent in the 3000-unit dose group.

Transfusion Requirements. The numbers of transfusions received by patients treated with placebo and with epoetin beta were compared before and during the treatment period (20). The placebo group received a total of 68.5 units in the 3 months preceding the study and required 35 units during the 8-week treatment period. In the patients receiving 1500 units of epoetin beta, 51 units were transfused during the prestudy period, whereas only 3 units were transfused during the treatment period. Similarly, the 3000-unit treatment group received 55 units of packed red blood cells during the prestudy period and only 11

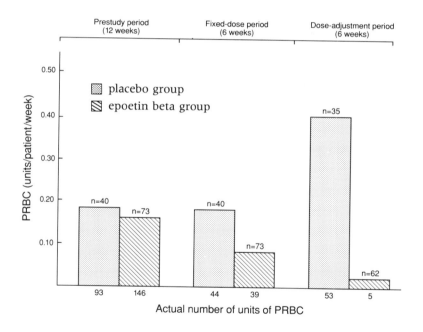

Figure 15.6. The mean number of units of packed red blood cells (PRBC) transfused during the North American placebo-controlled studies. The actual number of units given per group is shown below the bars. *Source: Reference 8*

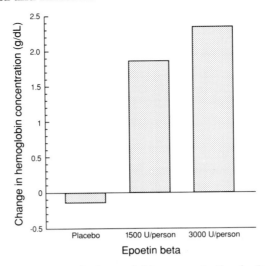

Figure 15.7. The change in the hemoglobin concentration in Japanese multicenter studies. The mean increment of the hemoglobin for each group is shown in grams/decilitre after the 8-week treatment period. *Source: Reference 20. Reprinted by permission of S. Karger, Basel.*

units during the treatment period. These results confirm the efficacy of epoetin beta in the reduction or elimination of the need for transfusions to treat the anemia of end-stage renal disease.

The Quality of Life

To determine how therapy with epoetin beta affected the quality of life, a questionnaire was used to evaluate parameters of well-being during the multicenter placebo-controlled studies in North America (7,8). The quality of life was measured by a "functional activity assessment" questionnaire before entry into the study, at day 40 (the end of the fixed-dose period), and at day 82 (the end of the dose-adjustment period).

Patients treated with epoetin beta reported greater overall satisfaction with life during treatment, in contrast to patients in the placebo group. These responses were judged significantly different from placebo ($P < 0.05$). Similarly, statistically significant responses were seen in the treatment group for the question regarding the overall quality of health during treatment. One question concerned the patients' optimism for the future. The responses at the end of the dose-adjustment period (day 82) showed that the expectations of the patients receiving epoetin beta therapy had increased from baseline, whereas those of the placebo group remained at or below baseline. The difference between the groups on day 82 was also statistically significant ($P < 0.05$). Although several other questions in the quality-of-life assessment did not show significant differences between groups (e.g., number of hours spent daily on housework, self-reliance, motivation, or quality of health expected in the future), these probably reflect the additional medical and social problems in dialysis patients, which may reduce the perceived positive effect of the improving anemia. Despite these additional considerations, however, the patients treated with epoetin beta reported statistically significant ($P < 0.05$) differences in psychologic well-being, overall energy scale, ability to work, and social interaction, reflecting a significant improvement in the quality of life.

Another study was designed specifically to evaluate the effects on the quality of life of long-term treatment with epoetin beta (21). Ninety-one patients receiving maintenance doses of epoetin beta (the mean dose at the time of this study was 218 units/kg/week; the mean duration was 18 months) and 96 patients on maintenance in-center hemodialysis not receiving epoetin beta participated in the study. The quality-of-life parameters measured included global and psychologic well-being, energy, activity levels, appetite, work, and sexual function. When adjusted for covariates (health status and demographics), 16 of 26 parameters were significantly higher ($P < 0.05$) in the patients receiving epoetin beta. All of the remaining measurements were higher for those receiving epoetin beta than for untreated patients, but the differences were not statistically significant.

Nonhematologic Measures of Efficacy

In Japan, exercise tolerance (on nondialysis days) was evaluated in patients treated with epoetin beta (22). The studies involved the evaluation of performance on a treadmill and of cardiac function by echocardiography. Patients were treated with three different doses of epoetin beta: 1500, 3000, or 4500 units. The duration of tolerated exercise increased significantly ($P < 0.001$) from 384 $\pm$ 116 seconds (baseline) to 474 $\pm$ 91 seconds in patients with an increase in hematocrit of more than 6 percent. Concomitantly, significant decreases in the resting pulse rate ($P < 0.05$) and left ventricular volume were also observed. There was also a decrease in cardiac output and stroke volume during treatment with epoetin beta.

Maximal oxygen consumption (Vo_2max), which is often used as an indication of physical work capacity, is at a low level in patients on hemodialysis. Even at the beginning of therapy with epoetin beta, with only a 6 percent increase in hematocrit, the Japanese study noted a statistically significant improvement in Vo_2max (from 22.5 ± 4.2 ml/kg/minute, baseline, to 27.2 ± 6.8 ml/kg/minute; $P < 0.001$), which continued to increase as the hemoglobin rose and then tended to stabilize. Although the patients selected for this study were younger (mean age, 37 years) than those in other studies of the efficacy of epoetin beta, these results nevertheless illustrate improved exercise tolerance in patients on epoetin beta treatment.

Adverse Events

During both the North American and the Japanese multicenter clinical trials, epoetin beta was well tolerated. The most commonly reported adverse events during all studies were hypertension, headache, asthenia, fatigue, clotted arteriovenous access, chest pain, cramps, insomnia, dyspnea, and itching.

Phase II Studies

In the North American fixed-dose study (7,18), the overall percentage of patients who had one or more clinical adverse events, whether or not drug related, was 68 percent in the groups receiving both 25 units/kg and 100 units/kg and was 63 percent in the group receiving 200 units/kg. During the dose-adjustment period, 93 percent of the patients receiving 25 units/kg and 200 units/kg reported adverse events, whereas 88 percent of the patients receiving 100 units/kg reported adverse events during the same period. The adverse experiences reported, however, were usually categorized as "slight" and did not affect the participation of the patients in the study.

In the Japanese fixed-dose studies, the incidence of reported adverse experiences was much lower (20) because only drug-related experiences were classified as adverse. This is in contrast to the North American studies, in which any symptom, no matter how slight and whether or not drug related, was reported. In the Japanese studies, only 15 cases of drug-related adverse events were observed in 162 patients (incidence, 8 percent) treated for 12 weeks on fixed doses of epoetin beta.

In another Japanese study, patients received 1800, 3600, 5400, or 7200 units of epoetin beta. No adverse experience was observed in 25 of the 27 patients (92.6 percent) (11). Two patients each had a fever and a feeling of fatigue, but these problems were considered clinically insignificant.

Placebo-controlled Studies

In the two large, multicenter North American clinical trials, the overall percentage of patients who had one or more adverse experiences during the fixed-dose period was 73 percent in the placebo group and 85 percent in the group receiving epoetin beta; during the dose-adjustment period, 74 percent of the placebo group and 81 percent of the treated group reported adverse events (7,8). The incidence was almost the same for patients receiving placebo, an observation suggesting that the incidence reflects the serious medical situation of patients entered into these studies.

In the Japanese multicenter Phase II placebo-controlled study, the incidence of adverse experiences was only 7.5 percent (23). The differences between the North American and the Japanese studies may be due to the different definitions of adverse experiences.

Certain specific adverse responses—clotting of the arteriovenous access, headache, and hypertension—were noted repeatedly during all studies and are discussed in detail below.

Clotting of the Arteriovenous Access

Clotting of the arteriovenous access was one of the most frequently reported adverse events and was noted in both the North American and the Japanese studies. In one of the North American placebo-controlled studies, 5 percent of the patients in the placebo group and 4 percent of the patients in the epoetin beta group had clotted accesses during the fixed-dose period (8). During the dose-adjustment period, no patient in the placebo group had a clotted graft, whereas 10 percent of the patients on epoetin beta therapy had clotted grafts. The North American studies indicated that there is no relationship between clotting of the arteriovenous access and the rapidity with which the hemoglobin values increase (7,8).

Clotted grafts are a recurrent problem in many patients on hemodialysis. In a study of the long-term survival of the grafts in a general hemodialysis population, 70 percent of the grafts were still patent at 12 months (24). As shown in Figure 15.8, life table analysis of the 1-year survival of the grafts in patients receiving epoetin beta was 71 percent (18), suggesting that the incidence of clotting in patients treated with epoetin beta is similar to that of this general dialysis population. Thus, graft clotting is probably not causally related to the treatment. The re-

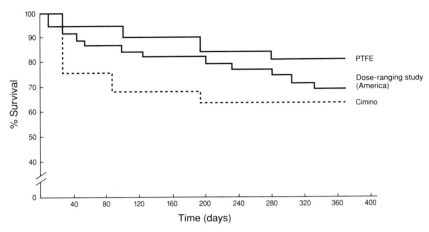

Figure 15.8. A life table analysis of the 1-year survival of arteriovenous access. Cimino indicates Cimino fistula; PTFE, polytetrafluoroethylene graft. *Source: Adapted from Reference 18*

sults of another study that evaluated the incidence of vascular access clotting over a 5.25-year period confirm this finding (25).

There was no relationship among clotting of the arteriovenous access, treatment with epoetin beta, and changes in coagulation function tests (8). The group mean platelet count fluctuated in both the placebo and the treatment groups throughout the course of the study. The prothrombin time was above baseline throughout the study and highest (12.56 seconds) at day 82, the end of the dose-adjustment period. The partial thromboplastin time was unchanged in the placebo group but, by the end of the epoetin beta dose-adjustment period, there was a 5.12-second prolongation from baseline. The fibrinogen concentration did not change from baseline values for either the epoetin beta or the placebo group. The neutrophil, lymphocyte, and eosinophil counts remained at or near baseline levels.

Headache

Headache may be associated with increasing hypertension and should not be ignored. In the North American and Japanese studies, headache was a significant event (7,8,20,23). In the placebo-controlled North American studies, headache occurred in the placebo group in 5 percent of patients during the fixed-dose period and in 3 percent of patients during the dose-adjustment period. In the epoetin beta-treated patients, in contrast, headache occurred in 11 percent during the fixed-dose period and in 10 percent during the dose-adjustment period. Increasing complaints of headache may, however, be associated with the rapidity with which the hemoglobin is rising in response to treatment with epoetin beta, as indicated in Table 15.4.

Hypertension

There was no statistically significant difference in the systolic and diastolic blood pressures between the placebo and the treatment groups in the North American studies on any study day (8). However, hypertension developed during the dose-adjustment period and may be related to the rate of increase in hemoglobin. Table 15.4 shows that patients with a "brisk" increase in hemoglobin had a higher frequency of both headache and hypertension (37 percent). The North American and Japanese studies suggested that the frequency of headache and hypertension may be related to a rapid rate of rise in hemoglobin. The mean time to onset of headache and hypertension suggests that these are probably causally related to the hematopoietic response. Thus, as the rate of increase of hemoglobin is related to the dose of epoetin beta, the dose should be adjusted to induce a modest rate of increase in the hemoglobin and hematocrit.

Seizure

Seizure is not an infrequent occurrence in patients with end-stage renal disease and may in fact occur at a frequency of 5 to 10 percent per year in patients on dialysis. In the North American placebo-controlled studies, during the 12-week fixed-dose period, patients in the treatment group had a seizure frequency of 1.0 percent; the seizure

Table 15.4. The Frequency of Headache and Hypertension and the Rate of Rise of Hemoglobin

| Rate of Rise of Hemoglobin, g/dl/wk | % of Patients Reporting: | | | |
| | Fixed-Dose Period | | Dose-Adjustment Period | |
	Headache	Hypertension	Headache	Hypertension
Slow (0.02–0.2)	11	0	0	0
Moderate (> 0.2–0.4)	9	3	3	3
Brisk (> 0.4–0.6)	13	0	4	4
Rapid (> 0.6)	20	10	20	0

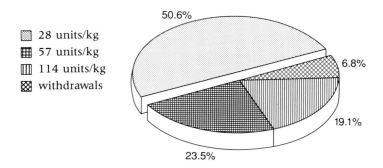

50.6%

- ▒ 28 units/kg
- ▦ 57 units/kg
- ▥ 114 units/kg
- ▩ withdrawals

6.8%

19.1%

23.5%

Figure 15.9. The doses of epoetin beta required for hemoglobin maintenance in Japanese Phase II trials.

frequency was 1.2 percent in the placebo group (8). Some additional seizures occurred during the dose-adjustment period, but the seizures did not necessitate withdrawal from the studies, except where they were cocaine induced (a protocol violation). The North American and Japanese studies showed no significant difference in seizure rate related to the rise in hematocrit.

Dosage Requirements

In the Japanese multicenter studies, epoetin beta was given in fixed doses of 1500 units (approximately 25 units/kg) or 3000 units (approximately 50 units/kg), three times per week, after routine dialysis (20). There was a more rapid hematopoietic effect in the group receiving the 3000-unit dose. At the end of 12 weeks, 50 percent of the patients were maintained at a dose of 1500 units (equivalent to 28.57 units/kg), whereas 23.5 percent of treated patients required 3000 units (57.14 units/kg) and 19.1 percent of the patients required more than 100 units/kg to maintain the hemoglobin concentration in the desired range (Fig 15.9). These studies demonstrate that, although some patients may be more responsive to epoetin beta, all patients treated with epoetin beta can have a rise of hemoglobin of about 0.3 g/dl/week.

In the North American study, patients initially received 25, 100, or 200 units/kg of epoetin beta three times per week in conjunction with their routine dialysis (7,18). Dosages were then adjusted to maintain hemoglobin concentrations in the range of 10.5 to 12.5 g/dl. By day

138 of the study, more than 80 percent of the patients initially receiving 200 units/kg were maintained on doses of less than 75 units/kg; only 20 percent of the patients required maintenance doses greater than 75 units/kg. It is not known why some patients require higher doses to sustain target hematocrit levels of 33 to 36 percent or why some patients respond more rapidly to a particular dose. No correlation has been found between the requirement for a higher maintenance dose and the levels of immunoreactive parathyroid hormone, iron, or aluminum.

The clinical studies suggest that the rapidity of correction of anemia is not related to the patient's well-being. Partial correction of the anemia to hemoglobin levels of 11.5 g/dl and hematocrit values of 35 percent is sufficient to obviate the need for transfusion and substantially improve the patient's quality of life (7). Therefore, a dose of about 50 $\pm$ 25 units/kg three times per week may facilitate a slow correction of the anemia and also allow the patient time to adjust gradually to the increased viscosity of the blood, without hypertension and headache. This point remains to be investigated in future studies.

Results of recent studies indicate that subcutaneous dosing may be as pharmacologically effective as intravenous dosing (13,16). The weekly amount given subcutaneously (in two doses) may be reduced by about 37 percent from the weekly amount given intravenously (in three doses) without a consequent reduction in the effect on hemoglobin level (16). Indeed, patients with end-stage renal disease treated with epoetin beta subcutaneously once or twice a week (total weekly dose of 120 to 200 units/kg) had effective responses (16). Subcutaneous dosing allows self-administration of the hormone and may be more cost-effective; larger clinical studies are necessary to confirm these issues.

Dialysis Prescription

Blood Chemistry Values

Therapy with epoetin beta causes an increase in hematocrit and consequently a decrease in plasma volume, which could affect the efficiency of the dialysis. Therefore, blood urea nitrogen, creatinine, phosphorus, and potassium were measured at baseline and during the placebo and the epoetin beta studies at days 5, 12, 26, 40, 54, and 82 (8). There were no discernible trends in either the placebo or the epoetin beta-treated group; in addition, no significant between-group differences were noted.

The serum potassium levels showed marked fluctuations in both the placebo and the treated groups throughout these studies. These fluctuations are relatively common in patients on chronic dialysis. In several cases, serum potassium concentrations were more than 1.0 meq above the normal range and may have resulted either from improved appetite and increased dietary consumption of potassium as the anemia abated or from decreasing efficiency of the dialysis as the hematocrit increased. These findings emphasize that dietary compliance in dialysis patients must be carefully monitored during treatment with epoetin beta.

Iron Supplementation

Because adequate iron storage is a requisite for the efficacy of epoetin therapy, it is recommended that the transferrin saturation (serum iron divided by iron binding capacity) be at least 20 percent and the serum ferritin be at least 100 ng/ml at the onset of epoetin beta therapy. Intravenous iron must be used if oral iron preparations do not maintain adequate iron stores. In the Japanese studies, oral iron preparations were administered after a mean corpuscular hemoglobin (MCH) of ≤ 28 pg or a serum ferritin of ≤ 100 ng/ml was observed (20). In the North American studies, serum iron and ferritin, which may have been elevated initially because of frequent blood transfusions, decreased during the fixed-dose period. Iron supplementation tended to stabilize these values in the normal range.

Heparin Requirements

Heparin requirements during dialysis may need to be adjusted upward as a consequence of epoetin beta therapy. The increased heparin requirements are a result of the increased hematocrit and blood viscosity (B. S. Spinowitz, J. Arslanian, C. Charytan, R. A. Golden, J. Rascoff, and M. Galler, Impact of epoetin beta on dialyzer clearance and heparin requirements, unpublished data).

Pediatric Studies

The value of epoetin beta for children with the anemia of end-stage renal disease is still being investigated. In a pilot 8- or 12-week study carried out in Japan, 42 children (mean age, 10.6) received epoetin beta (50 or 75 units/kg) two or three times per week after either peritoneal dialysis or hemodialysis (26). Epoetin beta improved renal anemia in 83.3 percent of the patients, and the dose recommended for pediatric patients is 50 units/kg. There was no difference in effectiveness according to sex, age, or originating disease. The quality of life improved substantially as the anemia improved.

A most significant finding of this preliminary study is that the improvement in anemia was not accompanied by either headache or an increase in hypertension. In this study, the number of adverse experiences was very low, probably because these children had less serious comorbidities, such as pre-existing hypertension or cardiac disease.

Conclusion

These clinical studies in North America and Japan demonstrate that epoetin beta is efficacious and safe in the treatment of renal anemia. Routine transfusions of red blood cells are eliminated, and there is a global improvement in the well-being of the patient with end-stage renal disease.

REFERENCES

1. Miyake T, Kung CKH, Goldwasser E. Purification of human erythropoietin. J Biol Chem 1977;252:5558–64.

2. Jacobs K, Shoemaker C, Rudersdorf R, et al. Isolation and characterization of genomic and cDNA clones of human erythropoietin. Nature 1985; 313:806–10.

3. Lin FK, Suggs S, Lin CH, et al. Cloning and expression of the human erythropoietin gene. Proc Natl Acad Sci USA 1985;82:7580–5.

4. Koch KM, Kuhn K, Nonnast-Daniel B, Scigalla P. Treatment of renal anemia with recombinant human erythropoietin. Contrib Nephrol 1988;66.

5. Eschbach JW, Egrie JC, Downing MR, Browne JK, Adamson JW. Correction of the anemia of end-stage renal disease with recombinant human erythropoietin. N Engl J Med 1987;316:73–8.

6. Winearls CG, Oliver DO, Pippard M, Reid C, Downing MR, Cotes PM. Effect of human erythropoietin derived from recombinant DNA on the anemia of patients maintained by chronic hemodialysis. Br Med J 1986;295:1017–20.

7. Sobota JT. Recombinant human erythropoietin in patients with anemia due to end-stage renal disease: U.S. multicenter trials. Contrib Nephrol 1989; 76:166–78.

8. Simpson K. Placebo-controlled trials of epoetin beta in patients with renal anemia. Health Sci Rev 1991 (in press).

9. Sasaki H, Bothner B, Dell A, Fukuda M. Carbohydrate structure of erythropoietin expressed in Chinese hamster ovary cells by a human erythropoietin cDNA. J Biol Chem 1987;262:12059–76.

10. Fukuda M. Biochemistry of erythropoietin: role of the carbohydrate. Health Sci Rev 1991 (in press).

11. Hirasawa Y, Hirashima K, Ogura Y, et al. The effect of a single dose of

recombinant human erythropoietin on renal anemia in patients undergoing hemodialysis. Rinsho Toseki (Jpn J Clin Dial) 1989;5:453–60.

12. Flaharty KK, Caro J, Erslev A, et al. Pharmacokinetics and erythropoietic response to human recombinant erythropoietin in healthy men. Clin Pharmacol Ther 1990;47:557–64.

13. Flaharty KK, Besarab A, Vlasses PH, Caro J. Pharmacokinetics of recombinant human erythropoietin (H-rEPO, Marogen™) in ESRD patients [Abstract]. Kidney Int 1990;37:237.

14. Flaharty KK, Vlasses PH, Caro J, et al. Clinical pharmacology of single doses of human recombinant erythropoietin in healthy men [Abstract]. Am Soc Clin Pharmacol Ther 1989;45(2):135.

15. Fukuda MN, Sasaki H, Lopez L, Fukuda M. Survival of recombinant human erythropoietin in the circulation: the role of carbohydrates. Blood 1989;73:84–9.

16. Besarab A, Vlasses P, Caro J, Flaharty K, Medina F, Scalise R. Subcutaneous (SC) administration of recombinant human erythropoietin (H-rEPO) for treatment of end-stage renal disease anemia [Abstract]. Kidney Int 1990; 37:236.

17. Uji Y, Hirashima K, Hirasawa Y, et al. A Phase I study of recombinant human erythropoietin in healthy volunteers: single dose study. Shinryo To Shinyaku (New drugs Physicians) 1989;26:1–28.

18. Spinowitz BS. Dose-finding clinical trial of epoetin beta for anemia of end-stage renal disease. Health Sci Rev 1991 (in press).

19. Bennett WM. A multicenter clinical trial of epoetin beta for anemia of end-stage renal disease. J Am Soc Nephrol 1991;1:990–8.

20. Suzuki M, Hirasawa Y, Hirashima K, et al. Dose-finding, double-blind, clinical trial of recombinant human erythropoietin in Japanese patients with end-stage renal disease. Contrib Nephrol 1989;76:179–92.

21. Deniston OL, Luscombe FA, Buesching D, Richner RE, Spinowitz BS. Effects of long-term epoetin beta therapy on the quality of life of hemodialysis patients. ASAIO Trans 1990;36:M157–60.

22. Tsutsui M, Suzuki M, Takahashi Y, Hirasawa Y, Matsushita C, Nomura M. Correction of renal anemia by recombinant human erythropoietin: effects on exercise tolerance and cardiac function. Rinsho Touseki (Jpn J Clin Dial) 1989;5:1945–53.

23. Hirasawa Y, Hirashima K, Arakawa M, et al. A multi-center, double-blind, active drug controlled, Phase III clinical trial of recombinant human erythropoietin (Chugai EPOCH) using mepitiostane as a comparative drug to evaluate the clinical safety and efficacy of EPOCH in hemodialysis patients with renal anemia. Zin To Touseki (Kidney Dial) 1989;27:171–84.

24. Palder SB, Kirkman RL, Whittemore AD. Vascular access for hemodialysis. Ann Surg 1985;202:235–9.

25. Besarab A, Medina F, Musial E, et al. Recombinant human erythropoietin does not increase clotting in vascular accesses. ASAIO Trans 1990; 36:M749–53.

26. Kitagawa T, Ito K, Komatsu Y, et al. The clinical studies of recombinant human erythropoietin (epoetin) in children with renal anemia. Contemp Dial Nephrol November 1990:40–5.

Chapter 16

Recombinant Human Erythropoietin (Epoetin Alfa and Beta) in Patients on Hemodialysis: Western Europe

Christopher G. Winearls, E. Sundal,
H. Stocker, K. J. Boughton,
and J. Bommer

The testing of recombinant human erythropoietin (rHuEpo) in Europe was first planned in 1984 by P. Mary Cotes, of the Clinical Research Centre in Harrow, England, and Nowell Stebbing, then of Amgen, as a collaborative project. Later this and the subsequent clinical trials of the Amgen rHuEpo, now designated epoetin alfa (Epogen [Amgen], Eprex [Cilag]), were organized by the Cilag Company, which had obtained the rights to development in Europe. Soon after, the rHuEpo produced by the Genetics Institute and designated epoetin beta (Recormon) was tested in Europe by the Boehringer-Mannheim Company. This chapter reviews the major completed trials undertaken by clinical investigators working with these two recombinant erythropoietins.

The London-Oxford Pilot Study (1–4)
Christopher G. Winearls

The London-Oxford pilot study was planned to test whether the administration of rHuEpo would reverse the anemia of uremia and thus included a number of investigations to characterize this anemia and provide information on the effect of rHuEpo on various measurements of erythropoiesis. At that time there was absolutely no information on the intravenous dosages likely to be effective; therefore, the protocol allowed a wide range of dosages to be used.

Eleven hemodialysis patients without confounding clinical problems

291

or additional causes of anemia were selected to enter the clinical protocol. This involved pharmacokinetic, erythrokinetic, and bone marrow progenitor studies before and after a therapeutic effect of rHuEpo had been obtained. Four additional patients were later recruited for an evaluation of safety and efficacy.

After a 2-week run-in period, a treatment schedule of escalating dosages of rHuEpo was started. In all except the first patient, who received 3 units/kg, the starting dose was 12 units/kg given intravenously as a bolus at the end of each hemodialysis treatment three times per week. The dose was doubled every 2 weeks until a response, defined as an increase in hemoglobin of more than 2 g/dl above the baseline concentration or the maximum reached after blood transfusion, was attained. Thereafter, the dose was adjusted to maintain a hematocrit of 35 to 40 percent. Because changes in the dosage were made at intervals that were too short for the effect of a particular dose to become apparent, the dosages reached exceeded the true requirement that emerged during the maintenance phase. Thus, all patients received higher doses during the early phase of treatment than they subsequently required for maintenance. All 15 patients responded, and the need for transfusions was abolished in the 4 who had previously been dependent on regular blood transfusion.

Pharmacokinetic Studies

Pharmacokinetic studies were performed when the first dose was administered and then again when the patients had reached a maintenance phase. The interval between the two studies varied from 96 to 378 days. The pharmacokinetic profiles were compatible with a single-order exponential elimination curve. The $T_{1/2}$ values were 2.3 to 7.3 hours (mean, 4.9 hours) in the first study and 3.2 to 5.2 hours (mean, 4.21 hours) in the second. The second study was performed when there had been an expansion of the erythron, so it seems that the size or activity of the erythroid marrow is not a major determinant of the elimination of erythropoietin from the circulation. Estimates of the turnover of endogenous erythropoietin derived from the basal concentrations of endogenous erythropoietin, the volume of distribution, and the elimination constant were similar at the two study times, suggesting that reversal of anemia does not suppress endogenous erythropoietin production. Furthermore, the endogenous erythropoietin turnover of the anephric patients was not obviously different from that of the patients retaining their failed kidneys. The near simultaneous measurement of the erythron transferrin uptake and the erythropoietin turnovers before and after the response to treatment allowed a comparison of the relation between the availability of erythropoietin and the size of the erythron. It can be seen from Figure 16.1 that the size of the erythron was related to the availability of erythropoietin (endogenous only before treatment and the sum of endogenous and exogenous during treatment).

Erythrokinetics

As expected, the total red cell volume was below normal before treatment (mean, 8.9 ml/kg for the transfusion-dependent patients and 14.1 ml/kg in the seven nontransfused patients) and increased after treatment to 24.2 ml/kg and 26 ml/kg, respectively. These increases in red cell volume were accompanied by reciprocal changes in plasma volume, so the blood volume was barely changed (Fig 16.2).

Red cell survival in the seven nontransfused patients was only modestly shortened before treatment and was not altered by treatment (Fig 16.2). In the four transfusion-dependent patients, red cell survival was much shorter than normal, but this could be explained in three by the shorter survival of the transfused cells. After treatment, red cell survival in these three was similar to that in the nontransfused group, which argues against a short red cell life-span as the explanation for their more severe anemia and transfusion dependence. The fourth transfusion-dependent patient had a short red cell survival even after treatment. This may account for her relatively high rHuEpo maintenance dose requirement (300 units/kg/week to maintain a hemoglobin of 9.9 g/dl). There was, however, no overall correlation between red cell life-span and maintenance dose requirement. The erythron transferrin uptake, an accurate measure of erythroid marrow activity, was derived from the plasma iron turnover and the saturation of the total iron-binding capacity. Before-treatment values for erythron transferrin uptake were subnormal in all but one case, and after treatment an overall twofold increase was observed (Fig 16.2).

Erythroid Progenitor Studies

The response of bone marrow erythroid progenitors to rHuEpo treatment was studied in nine of the subjects. Bone marrow aspiration from the iliac crest was performed before and during treatment (16 hours after the last administration of rHuEpo). After treatment, the number of bone marrow burst-forming units-erythroid (BFU-E) fell to a mean of 24.5 percent of the pretreatment values, but there was no significant change in the numbers of colony-forming units-erythroid (CFU-E). The surprising decrease in BFU-E may be explained by depletion of this compartment by erythropoietin-driven maturation to CFU-E without a commensurate replenishment from the pluripotential stem cell pool.

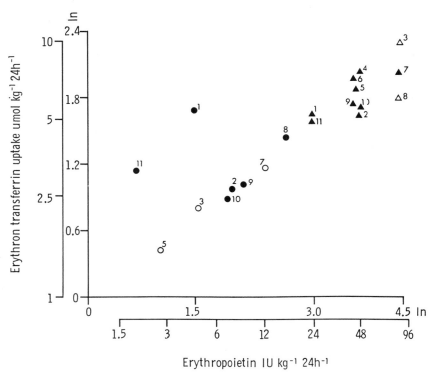

Figure 16.1. The relation between the availability of erythropoietin and erythron transferrin uptake. The availability of erythropoietin before treatment is plotted as the turnover of endogenous plasma erythropoietin in nephric (closed circles) and anephric (open circles) subjects. The availability of erythropoietin at a new steady state during treatment with rHuEpo is plotted as the sum of the turnover of endogenous plasma erythropoietin and exogenous rHuEpo administered intravenously (thrice-weekly dose × 3:7) (closed triangles). When the second erythrokinetic and pharmacokinetic studies were carried out at different doses of rHuEpo, the dose at the time of the erythrokinetic study was used to derive the availability of erythropoietin (open triangles). Individual subjects are identified by numbers on the figure. A logarithmic transformation was used on both axes. ln, natural logarithm.
Source: Reference 2. Reprinted by permission of Oxford University Press.

The equally surprising failure to change of the numbers of CFU-E would then have to be explained by self-renewal and replenishment by BFU-E keeping the size of this compartment constant. The mitotic rate (percentage of cells in S phase) was examined using the tritiated thymidine suicide technique and showed an increase from 45.2 to 68.4 percent for

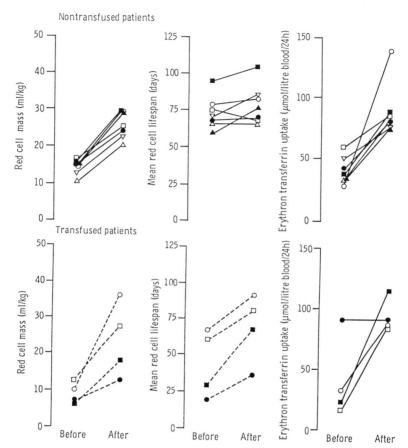

Figure 16.2. The effect of treatment with rHuEpo on red cell mass, mean red cell life span, and erythron transferrin uptake. The values before treatment and at a new steady state after 85–185 days of treatment are shown for non-transfused patients (upper panel), 2 (closed circles), 3 (open circles), 7 (closed squares), 9 (open squares), 10 (open triangles), and 11 (open inverted triangles), and for transfused patients (lower panel), 1 (closed circles), 4 (open circles), 5 (closed squares), and 6 (open squares). *Source: Reference 2. Reprinted by permission of Oxford University Press.*

CFU-E and from 16.4 to 45.1 percent for BFU-E. In a search for serum inhibitors of erythropoiesis in these patients, comparisons of cultures of their bone marrow with either fresh autologous serum or pooled normal human serum were made. Although human serum supports the growth of CFU-E less well than does fetal calf serum, no difference was observed between patient serum and control serum in the growth of either CFU-E or BFU-E.

Clinical Aspects

This cohort of patients were among the first to receive rHuEpo in Europe and have now been followed for 2 to 4 years. Eight remain on rHuEpo, six have received successful transplants, and one died after a massive gastrointestinal hemorrhage. There was no tendency for the doses to increase with time, and the requirements were similar to those observed in the large multicenter trials. Apart from the episode of hypertensive encephalopathy in the first patient, there have been no major complications or adverse events attributable to treatment. Four patients suffered vascular access failure requiring surgical intervention; in each case, however, there were pre-existing anatomic problems or additional factors such as dehydration. Six patients described "flu-like" symptoms after the intravenous administration of rHuEpo. These symptoms were tolerable but uncomfortable, were relieved by the prior administration of acetaminophen, and tended to diminish with time when lower doses of rHuEpo were administered slowly. (See Table 16.1.)

The European Multicenter Study of rHuEpo (Epoetin Alfa) in 169 Patients on Hemodialysis (5–8)*

E. Sundal, H. Stocker, and K. J. Boughton

In 1986, when the study described here was planned, Phase I results were available, but there were few clinical data on the use of rHuEpo. There was a need for a large multicenter trial to provide sufficient data

*The investigators were J. Bariety, Hôpital Broussais, Paris, France; J. Bommer, I. Medizinische Universitätsklinik, Heidelberg, Germany; B. Canaud, Hôpital Lapeyronie, Montpellier, France; B. G. Danielson, University Hospital, Uppsala, Sweden; H. Kreis, Hôpital Necker, Paris, France; S. Lamperi, Ospedale San Marino, Genoa, Italy; P. Michielsen, Gasthuisberg Hospital, Leuven, Belgium; C. Ponticelli, Ospedale Maggiore Policlinico, Milan, Italy; K. Rhyner, University Hospital, Zurich, Switzerland; R. M. Schaefer, Medizinische Universitätsklinik, Würzburg, Germany; C. Toussaint, Hôpital Erasme, Brussels, Belgium; D. Verbeelen, Free University Hospital, Brussels, Belgium; and C. Zehnder, Kantonsspital Aarau, Switzerland.

Table 16.1. Long-Term Outcome in 15 Patients Entered into the London-Oxford Pilot Study

Patient	Duration of Treatment (mo)	Status	Hemoglobin, g/dl	Dose, units/ kg/week	Adverse Events during Study
1	50	ON	9.9	300	Hypertensive encephalopathy
2	48	ON	8.7	180	Cancer prostate
3	48	ON	13.0	114	Access failure
4	48	ON	12.2	133	Access failure, flu syndrome
5	41	Transplant	13.4	155	Flu syndrome
6	47	ON	11.2	123	Access failure
7	28	Dead	13.4	348	GI hemorrhage
8	39	Transplant	8.5	210	—
9	27	Transplant	11.3	75	Flu syndrome
10	33	Transplant	12.0	150	Flu syndrome
11	39	ON	10.8	120	—
12	31	ON	11.0	185	—
13	18	Transplant	10.2	150	Flu syndrome, hyperkalemia
14	16	Transplant	11.9	300	Hypertension, hyperkalemia
15	24	ON	10.5	100	Flu syndrome
		Median	11.1	152	
		Range	8.5–13.4	75–300	

on efficacy and safety for the registration of the drug in Europe. Although the efficacy of rHuEpo in the treatment of renal anemia is now proven, published reports of such trials include comparatively few patients and raise a number of important questions about dosage and long-term safety.

The results of the Cilag European multicenter study in patients on regular hemodialysis, an interim report of which has been published (5), have therefore been updated and reviewed. This study generated data on long-term efficacy ($n = 126$) and safety ($n = 169$) in a relatively large number of patients.

Patients and Methods

Entrance criteria required that the patients, aged 18 to 70 years, had anemia exclusively caused by end-stage renal disease, with hematocrits of less than 30 percent and no other major concomitant clinical abnormalities. In particular, patients with uncontrolled hypertension were excluded. Regular (three times per week) hemodialysis for at least 3 months was required. The patients remained on their regular medication throughout the study, but those on corticosteroids and immunosuppressant therapy were excluded.

The study was designed as an open label, nonrandomized trial. The dose regimen was selected from very limited data available from pilot studies. All patients were started at a dose of 24 units/kg intravenously three times per week for a minimum of 2 weeks. The dose was doubled if the mean of the last week's three hemoglobin determinations was less than 10 percent higher than the baseline hemoglobin. Further dose escalations up to a maximum of 768 units/kg three times per week were initially allowed. During the course of the study, however, it became evident that it was unnecessary to exceed a dose of 192 units/kg three times per week, and the protocol was amended accordingly.

Responders were defined as patients experiencing an increase in hemoglobin of more than 2 g/dl (at any dose) above their individual baseline value. When this goal had been achieved, the patients were transferred to maintenance therapy, but further dose increments were allowed to "titrate" the hemoglobin into the arbitrarily defined optimal range of 10 to 12 g/dl ("full response"). Thereafter, the individual weekly dose was adjusted by altering either dose or frequency. Oral iron supplements at doses of up to 200 mg of elemental iron per day were prescribed unless there was evidence of iron overload.

A number of laboratory investigations—including testing of serum for the presence of IgG rHuEpo antibodies (as measured by radioimmunoprecipitation assay)—were performed at regular intervals. The relationship of any adverse reaction to rHuEpo administration was described by the investigator.

The statistical analysis was mainly descriptive as this was an open study, but several formal significance tests were performed and interpreted in an explorative way (i.e., without combining them in a multiple test procedure). The following three areas were highlighted: (a) monitoring efficacy over time, (b) defining appropriate dose regimens to achieve target hemoglobin concentrations, and (c) establishing the long-term safety profile of the drug.

Results

The demographic data of the study population are summarized in Table 16.2. The age distribution was highly variable among participating

Table 16.2. Demographic Data (with Median, Minimal, and Maximal Values)

Patient number	169
Sex	
Male	83 (49%)
Female	86 (51%)
Age, years	50 (18–74)
Body weight (kg)	
Male	62 (34–115)
Female	56 (33–94)
Kidney state	
Nephric	107
Nonfunctioning graft	41
Bilateral nephrectomy	21
Duration of hemodialysis treatment, months	51 (1–252)
Patients with need of transfusions during past 3 mo	12
Baseline hemoglobin at study entrance (g/dl)	7.07 (2.60–9.58)
History of arterial hypertension	90 (53%)
Baseline erythropoietin level, units/litre	18 (1–186)

centers; in fact, the median varied from 28 to 63 years. One 74-year-old patient was included because he was otherwise acceptable.

Mean and median baseline hemoglobin values were dependent upon the duration of hemodialysis; patients treated for longer than 5 years ($n = 75$) had a mean of 6.8 g/dl and those treated for less than 1 year ($n = 30$) a mean of 7.7 g/dl ($P < 0.001$, Mann-Whitney test). The remaining patients ($n = 64$) had a mean between these extremes (7.1 g/dl). Only 12 patients were transfusion dependent in the sense that they required at least 1 unit of blood every 3 months.

A total of 90 patients had a history of hypertension; however, only 1 of them had a diastolic value exceeding 100 mm Hg at study entrance. The mean basal erythropoietin level for 162 patients (data from 7 missing) was 20.5 mU/ml ± 21.7 (SD); there was no difference with regard to duration of dialysis treatment.

Table 16.3 lists the different reasons for which patients dropped out. The 43 patients represent 25.4 percent of the population originally recruited.

Efficacy. For different reasons 6 patients had to be excluded from the efficacy analysis. Of the 163 remaining patients, all but 8 were respond-

Table 16.3. Distribution of
Reasons for Discontinuation

Reason	n
Personal	4
Adverse drug experience	8
Intercurrent illness	4
Treatment failure	1
Renal transplant	26
Total	43

ers within 16 weeks of therapy, and all but 1 were responders after 30 weeks of observation. Ninety percent of the patients responded at doses of ≤192 units/kg three times per week. The only nonresponder was a 60-year-old man with the adult variant of polycystic renal disease who had a baseline hemoglobin of 8.8 g/dl and a corresponding erythropoietin serum level of 33 mU/ml. Reticulocyte response was adequate (increment from 2 to 5.7 percent), and serum ferritin dropped from 19 ng/ml to less than 10 ng/ml, but his hemoglobin never exceeded 9 g/dl in spite of his receiving rHuEpo, 192 units/kg three times per week for 6 weeks. This may be attributed to inadequate iron replacement.

For the "full response" analysis, 161 patients were eligible; in 90 percent the hemoglobin reached the target of more than 10 g/dl within 16 weeks. After an observation period of 42 weeks, only 2 patients had not responded, the previously described iron-deficient patient and one with no obvious reason for the poor response. He started therapy with a baseline hemoglobin of 6.2 g/dl and a basal erythropoietin serum level of 18 mU/ml. In spite of adequate iron stores (ferritin, >1000 ng/ml), he achieved a maximal hemoglobin of only 8.3 g/dl after 5 months of treatment at a dose of rHuEpo of 192 units/kg three times per week.

The response/time relationship is shown in Figure 16.3. Three subpopulations were constructed with regard to their baseline hemoglobin: hemoglobin of <6 g/dl ($n = 22$), hemoglobin of 6 to 8 g/dl ($n = 81$), and hemoglobin of >8 g/dl ($n = 23$). As can be seen, the response curves for the three groups run in parallel (i.e., the rate of hemoglobin increase is quite similar regardless of baseline hemoglobin concentration).

In some patients the increase in peripheral reticulocyte count appeared as early as after one or two injections; in the pooled population, however, the response became evident only after 1 to 2 weeks. The absolute reticulocyte count almost tripled during the course of therapy (from 38×10^{12}/litre to 100×10^{12}/litre). In general, the hemoglobin response became evident about 1 week after the reticulocyte increase. The hematocrit and red blood cell count reflected the pattern of hemoglobin. During the period of rHuEpo dose escalation to achieve response, the mean serum ferritin concentration fell from 397 ng/ml to 255 ng/ml.

An analysis of variance (ANOVA) on the dose response examined the following factors: the investigator, patients' age and weight, renal disease, duration of dialysis treatment, and ferritin concentrations. This analysis revealed that the investigator was the most powerful factor ($P < 0.01$) and that the others did not influence the response.

A total of 126 patients have been followed for at least 1 year. As soon as they had qualified as full responders, the dose regimens were individualized. Figure 16.3 shows that the hemoglobin concentration could be maintained within the predefined optimal range (10 to 12 g/dl) throughout the entire observation period of the year.

As shown in Figure 16.4, the median weekly dose could be substantially reduced after approximately 10 weeks of treatment (i.e., after the patients started to qualify as full responders). After the 4th month, however, the required dose remained more or less stable for all sub-

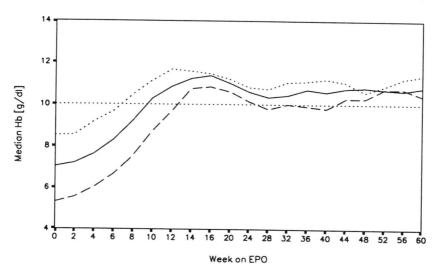

Figure 16.3. The median hemoglobin concentration could be titrated into a range of 10–12 g/dl regardless of the initial baseline levels.

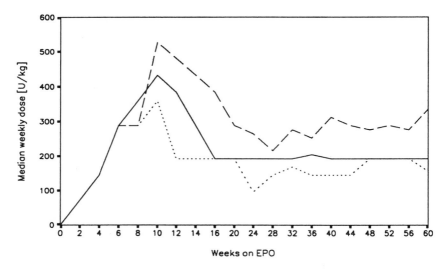

Figure 16.4. The median weekly dose that is required to maintain the hemoglobin in the arbitrarily defined optimal range appears to be different according to baseline levels of hemoglobin: a low initial hemoglobin requires a greater dosage of rHuEpo than does a high initial hemoglobin.

groups of patients. When considering the median weekly dose by patient subgroup during the last 12 weeks of the 1 year of treatment, the differences among groups were statistically significant ($P < 0.01$; Kruskal-Wallis test): when baseline hemoglobin was less than 6 g/dl ($n = 22$), the maintenance dose was 250 to 300 units/kg/week; when baseline hemoglobin was 6 to 8 g/dl ($n = 81$), the median weekly dose was approximately 200 units/kg; and when baseline hemoglobin was more than 8 g/dl ($n = 23$), the median dose was 150 to 200 units/kg/week.

In none of the subgroups was there loss of efficacy of rHuEpo over time. The median hemoglobin decreased to levels below 10 g/dl at different times during the study, but this reduction was usually intentionally induced by the investigators who, for different reasons, chose to achieve a new individual "optimal" hemoglobin level.

By the 52nd week of therapy, the whole weekly dose was given as one single administration in 34 patients, as two administrations in 70, and as three administrations in 20 patients. When rHuEpo was discontinued for some reason, the hemoglobin concentration dropped by approximately 0.4 g/dl/week.

The erythropoietin levels at baseline were not statistically significantly different among the three subgroups of patients ($P > 0.01$). During the 1-year treatment the mean level increased from 20.5 ± 21.7 mU/ml to 37.3 ± 60.4 mU/ml ($P < 0.01$, Wilcoxon test). The increase was least obvious in the patients with high baseline hemoglobin values (Table 16.4). This variation may be explained by dose differences and the timing of blood sampling.

Safety. The patient incidence rate of adverse drug experiences reported over time is summarized in Table 16.5. When considering any kind of report, the incidence was highest during the first 3 months (70 percent). It declined steadily thereafter, reaching 39 percent during the last 3 months.

This pattern was also reflected in the occurrence of hypertensive events. The patient incidence rate for the whole study was 34 percent; however, when looking separately at each of the five sequential time periods of 3 months, the corresponding incidence rates for the total study duration of 15 months were 18 percent, 14 percent, 11 percent, 5 percent, and 5 percent. Only 41 of the 57 patients who experienced such problems were among the 90 with a known history of hypertension. In most cases the blood pressure elevation could be rapidly controlled by drugs or the adjustment of dry weight. In only one patient did treatment have to be discontinued because of intractable hyperten-

Table 16.4. Erythropoietin Serum Concentrations

	Week of Treatment	n	Erythropoietin Serum Concentration, mU/ml		
			Mean $\pm$ SD	Median	Range
All patients	0	121	20.5 ± 21.7	18	1–186
	52	111	37.3 ± 60.4	28	1–508
Hb* < 6	0	20	16.7 ± 12.9	15	2–41
	52	22	37.1 ± 50.4	30	1–237
6 ≤ Hb ≤ 8	0	78	22.2 ± 25.4	18	1–186
	52	71	40.0 ± 69.9	28	2–509
Hb > 8	0	23	18.1 ± 11.4	18	4–46
	52	18	27.3 ± 14.7	29	4–63

*Hb, hemoglobin.

Table 16.5. The Incidence of Adverse Experiences

Time Period	Total Number of Patients	Adverse Experience	
		Number of Patients	%
1–3 mo	169	118	70%
4–6 mo	160	83	52%
7–9 mo	152	76	50%
10–12 mo	138	64	46%
13–15 mo	130	51	39%
All periods	169	152	90%

sion. The mean blood pressure of the study population did not change over time. It seemed that there was no relationship between the rate of hemoglobin increase and the occurrence of hypertensive episodes during the rHuEpo dose escalation period. On the contrary, the rate of hemoglobin increase was slightly lower in the patients suffering hypertensive problems (Table 16.6).

Five patients presented with hypertensive encephalopathy and/or seizures (Table 16.7). One patient suffered hypertensive encephalopathy with and another without seizures. One patient with a history of epilepsy (but without anticonvulsive drug treatment for 2 years) suffered a grand mal seizure when his hemoglobin had increased from 6.9 to 10.0 g/dl within 3 months; the incident was not associated with hypertension. Another patient experienced generalized convulsions after 2½ hours on dialysis without blood pressure problems and with a hemoglobin of 6.9 g/dl. A further patient (with a history of epilepsy) suffered a seizure after 16 months of treatment when his hemoglobin was 10.8 g/dl and his blood pressure was normal.

A total of 28 patients (17 percent) had clotting problems with their vascular access. Although this complication seemed to occur in access sites that were already anatomically compromised, most of these patients had experienced a clinically significant increase in hematocrit at the time of the event. Problems with the extracorporeal circuit occurred in 19 patients (11 percent); only in 14, however, was the problem related to clotting. Most episodes resolved with no treatment or an increase of the heparin dose.

Mean and median serum creatinine values at baseline ($n = 126$) were 993 μol/litre and 962 μol/litre, respectively. After 1 year of treatment the corresponding values were 1063 μol/litre and 1067 μol/litre; the difference from baseline was statistically but not clinically significant ($P < 0.001$).

The slight increase in serum potassium concentrations (mean, 5.25 to 5.49 mmol/litre; median, 5.2 to 5.4 mmol/litre) was statistically significant ($P = 0.006$). There was also a statistically significant increase ($P < 0.001$) in serum phosphate concentration during the 1-year treatment period (mean, 1.71 to 1.92 mmol/litre; median, 1.64 to 1.91 mmol/litre), but the serum calcium values remained stable throughout the study. No increase in serum bilirubin levels was observed.

The mean platelet counts increased from 209,000 at baseline to 238,000 after 1 year; the corresponding median values were 205,000 and 227,000. The difference from baseline was statistically significant ($P < 0.001$) at all evaluation points (i.e., each month). At no time was any patient's count outside the normal range.

There was also a slight but statistically significant increase in white

Table 16.6. The Incidence of Hypertensive Episodes in Relation to Rate of Hemoglobin Increase

Treatment Period	Hemoglobin Increase, g/dl/week	
	Hypertensive Episode	No Hypertensive Episode
Weeks 0–4	0.08	0.14
	($n = 7$)	($n = 162$)
Weeks 5–8	0.24	0.27
	($n = 10$)	($n = 155$)
Weeks 9–12	0.27	0.30
	($n = 22$)	($n = 142$)

Table 16.7. Patients with Hypertensive Encephalopathy and/or Seizures

Patient Number	History of Epilepsy	Hypertension at Event	Seizure	Encephalopathy	Hemoglobin at Event	Month of Treatment
403	+	−	+	?	7.6	3
413	+	−	+	−	10.8	16
416	−	−	+	−	6.9	2
602	−	+	−	+	11.7	8
953	−	+	+	+	10.0	6

blood cells ($P = 0.03$). However, both the baseline mean value (6300) and the end-point mean (6500) were well within the normal range.

One patient suffered palpebral edema 15 hours after the last rHuEpo administration and was therefore withdrawn from the study. Another patient had an eosinophilia (maximum, 38 percent) of unknown origin. Pretreatment values had been 10 to 15 percent. A further patient who experienced repeated pruritus after drug administration had a maximal eosinophil count of 13 percent.

A peculiar possible adverse drug reaction was an attack of acute intermittent porphyria in a patient whose disease had been clinically silent for 37 years. Two other patients had cutaneous eruptions classified as "pseudo porphyria cutanea tarda" after more than 1 year of treatment; the exanthema disappeared spontaneously under continuous rHuEpo treatment.

A total of 11 patients experienced a flulike syndrome after the rHuEpo injection, but coexistent back or limb pain was not present in all of them. Thus, these symptoms did not quite conform with the original description of Winearls et al. (1).

The other side effects recorded during this study represented the usual category of symptoms frequently encountered in hemodialysis patients. Neither physical examination nor electrocardiography revealed changes attributable to treatment.

No antibodies to rHuEpo were detected in any patient during the entire observation period.

Twenty-six patients received kidney transplants during the 1-year duration of the study. Three further patients received renal allografts after termination of the formal study. Because these patients were still treated with rHuEpo, they have been included in the survey as well. Baseline median hemoglobin was 7.0 g/dl (range, 4.9 to 9.6), and the median had increased to around 11 g/dl at the time of transplantation. The median hemoglobin value reached a maximum of 13 g/dl 6 months later and was approximately 12.8 g/dl after 1 year of follow-up.

The numbers were too small to establish whether there was any effect of rHuEpo treatment on early transplant function, rejection, or survival.

Discussion

This study provides further evidence that regular intravenous administration of rHuEpo will effectively alleviate or correct the anemia in the majority of dialysis-dependent patients. This beneficial effect can be achieved regardless of the initial hemoglobin concentration, but the time required to achieve full correction of anemia depends on the magnitude of the correction required.

If the patient is iron-replete, it is relatively easy to titrate the hemoglobin concentration into the range of 10 to 12 g/dl. One of the two nonresponders had severely depleted iron stores, but the reticulocyte response of 5.7 percent indicates that he also may have had occult bleeding. It is therefore crucial to assess the iron status before and during rHuEpo therapy and to give iron supplements if necessary.

The analysis of variance showed that the response depended only on the investigators (who, for different reasons, tended to keep their patients on low doses longer than required by the protocol). Once started, rHuEpo treatment must be continued to keep the hemoglobin concentration at a chosen level. When the drug is withdrawn, the hemoglobin concentration declines by approximately 0.4 g/dl/week.

The optimal dose for each patient must be established by dose titration. In the present study the intervals between dose adjustments during the dose-escalating period were too short to define the appropriate starting dose regimen. However, later studies (data on file, Cilag AG Research) suggested that 50 units/kg three times per week for 4 weeks is the optimal starting dose and the model treatment dose for most patients; this dose regimen induces a hemoglobin increase of approximately 1 g/dl/month. Further dose increments in steps of 25 units/kg should depend on the initial response.

It remains to be established whether there is a relationship between the frequency of application and the weekly dose necessary to maintain the target hemoglobin level because those parameters were not independently varied. The total weekly dose required to maintain stable hemoglobin levels seems to be different when related to the severity of the anemia (i.e., the dose requirements are greater when baseline hemoglobin is low). There is no loss of rHuEpo efficacy over a treatment period of 1 year. The statistically significant increase in erythropoietin serum levels observed in this study (Table 16.4) presumably reflects a slight accumulation of the drug, although this would not be predicted from the pharmacokinetic data.

Although experimental work suggests that there is an association between hematocrit increase and elevation of blood pressure (9), the present study did not detect any association between the rate of hematocrit increase and the occurrence of hypertensive problems. Nevertheless, 57 patients—16 of them without a history of hypertension—experienced worsening hypertension requiring the institution of or an increase in antihypertensive medication.

Such elevations of blood pressure may lead to hypertensive encephalopathy associated with seizures (1,10,11). The present study indicated that not all seizures in hemodialysis patients are associated with hypertension (Table 16.7) and that seizures may occur when the patient is hypotensive. There is no reason to believe that rHuEpo per se provokes epileptic activity because (a) radiolabeled rHuEpo does not penetrate into the central nervous system of rats, (b) the drug does not potentiate metrazole-induced seizures in mice, and (c) rHuEpo has no effect on electroencephalography in normal volunteers under conditions of sleep, hyperventilation, and photic stimulation (data on file, Ortho Pharmaceutical Corp.).

There may be an increased risk of clotting of the extracorporeal circuit, as 19 patients (11.2 percent) encountered such problems. The clotting can be managed by increasing the heparin dose during dialysis, but in most cases no action is necessary.

Thrombosis of the vascular access requiring active intervention was noted in 28 patients (17 percent). As not all of them had clinically significant elevation of hematocrit at the time of event, the hematocrit increase presumably is not the sole causal factor. In fact, this complication tended to occur in access sites that were already anatomically compromised.

The present study also noted a slight increase in the platelet count, albeit within the normal range. This may be due to stimulation of erythropoietin receptors on megakaryocytes. However, iron deficiency may also cause an increase in platelet count. One participating center (12) reported that the bleeding time shortens (a measure of platelet-endothelial interaction) after treatment with rHuEpo. This is, however, not caused by the drug per se, as similar changes also occur after a regular blood transfusion.

No clinically significant changes in creatinine and potassium concentrations occurred, although these may have been obscured by changes in dialysis and diet instituted by the physicians. Although dialyser creatinine clearance would be expected to decrease as hematocrit increases (13), available reports suggest that, when changes do occur, they are not clinically significant (14). These changes can easily be managed through altered dialysis prescription or dietary advice (15).

The potential of rHuEpo to cause allergic reactions has been recognized but did not seem to be a major clinical problem. A patient with palpebral edema suggested an allergic reaction, but this was not confirmed. Recurrent hives after second and third exposures to rHuEpo were also noted in two normal volunteers, although there was no evidence of immunologic sensitization (data on file, Ortho Pharmaceutical Corp.).

The pathogenesis of the flulike syndrome after rHuEpo administration is obscure. Winearls et al. (1) drew attention to "bone pain associated with flu-like symptoms" in 4 of 10 patients, whereas the present study observed this phenomenon in only 11 of 169 patients (6.5 percent). In the 2 patients who repeatedly experienced bone pain after bolus injections of rHuEpo, this adverse reaction was apparently no longer a problem when the injection duration was extended to 1 or 2 minutes.

The patient with recurrence of acute intermittent porphyria after the disease had been clinically silent for 37 years is interesting because the attack could theoretically have been caused by increased heme synthesis. Two cases of rash consistent with porphyria cutanea tarda were not considered to be related to rHuEpo. The influence of rHuEpo on porphyrin metabolism was studied in normal volunteers (data on file, Ortho Pharmaceutical Corp.); in spite of a marked increase in erythropoiesis, there was no evidence of increased porphyrin synthesis based on 24-hour collections of porphobilinogen, δ-aminolevulinic acid, coproporphyrin, and uroporphyrin.

The results of the follow-up examinations of the 29 patients who received renal transplants after having reached a hemoglobin concentration of at least 10 g/dl suggest that rHuEpo treatment has no untoward effect on the outcome of transplantation.

In summary, the safety evaluation at 1 year showed no unexpected findings. Adverse reactions were most frequently reported during rHuEpo dose escalation when hematocrit was increasing. Thereafter, the figures steadily declined. None of the patients developed antibodies to rHuEpo. The activity of the drug was remarkably consistent, and no evidence of drug resistance developed. As the risks of treatment can now easily be identified and managed, the risk/benefit ratio of rHuEpo therapy is quite acceptable.

The German Multicenter Trials of rHuEpo (Epoetin Beta) (16–20)*
J. Bommer

In 1987, the first German multicenter study of rHuEpo (Boehringer-Mannheim) was started in 95 adult, nontransfused patients with he-

*Participants: J. Bahlman, Hannover; C. P. Baldamus, Köln; J. Bommer, Heidelberg;

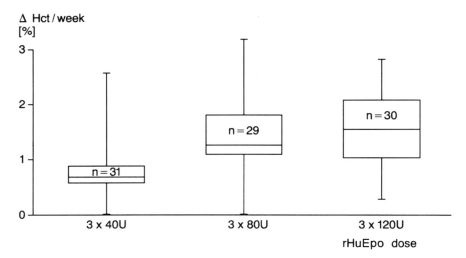

Figure 16.5. The increase in hematocrit (volume % per week) (median, interquartile, and total range) under rHuEpo therapy with 40, 80, and 120 units per kg three times per week.

matocrit levels of less than 27 percent who had been on hemodialysis for more than 5 months. The exclusion criteria were infections or chronic inflammatory disease, epilepsy, folate or vitamin B_{12} deficiency, aluminum overload, and poorly controlled hypertension. The patients were randomized to three treatment groups and received fixed doses of rHuEpo: 40, 80, or 120 units/kg intravenously three times per week until a target hematocrit of 30 to 50 percent was reached. If the target was not reached by 12 weeks, the dose was increased to 80 or 120 units/ kg three times per week.

A dose-dependent response was observed, with a median weekly increment in hematocrit of 0.6 percent at 40 units/kg, 1.34 percent at 80 units/kg, and 1.64 percent at 120 units/kg (Fig 16.5) (16). However, the weekly increment in hematocrit varied markedly within each of the dose groups, ranging from less than 0.2 percent per week to more than 2 percent per week, illustrating the remarkable differences in responsiveness in individual patients.

In 1988, a study of the treatment of adult transfusion-dependent he-

H. J. Gurland, Hannover; G. A. Jutzler, Homburg/Saar; K. M. Koch, Hannover; M. Moltzahn, Berlin; H. H. Neumayer, Berlin; E. Quellhorst, Hann. Münden; W. Schoeppe, Frankfurt; H. J. Sieberth, Aachen.

modialysis patients was undertaken in 11 German dialysis centers. The patients had to have received more than 3 units of blood during the preceding 6 months at a hematocrit of less than 28 percent, and the serum ferritin had to be more than 700 μg/litre. The two dose groups were 80 units/kg and 120 units/kg three times per week.

After 3 months of treatment, 95 percent of the patients no longer required transfusions; the response was, as in the nontransfused patients, dose dependent. The median weekly increment in hematocrit was 1.0 percent at a dose of 80 units/kg and 1.2 percent at 120 units/kg. The median rate of rise in hematocrit at the same dose of rHuEpo was lower in the transfused patients than in the nontransfused ones, suggesting a higher dose requirement for this more anemic group. The maintenance doses of the transfused group were higher (40 units/kg three times per week) when compared to the nontransfused patients (30 units/kg three times per week). Although the patients were unselected, they were not randomized, nor were they treated in the same dialysis units; therefore, statistical comparisons between the groups would not have been reliable. The same variability in response to rHuEpo was observed in these transfused patients as had been seen in the nontransfused cohort.

In both trials a number of factors seemed to modify the erythropoietic response to rHuEpo. These included inadequate iron supplements, intercurrent infections, blood loss, cytotoxic agents, previously unrecognized malignant disease, chronic inflammatory conditions, and malnutrition, but not hyperparathyroidism (17). Nevertheless, these factors were still not able to explain all of the interindividual variation in response.

Adverse Events

The adverse reactions observed in both of these German multicenter studies were similar to those reported in other trials. In the first trial an increase in blood pressure was observed after treatment in 21 of 45 (47 percent) patients who were hypertensive or whose blood pressure had been controlled by drugs before entry. Of the patients with normal blood pressure, 6 of 45 (13 percent) developed hypertension, giving an overall incidence of hypertension as an adverse event of 30 percent. Increases in blood pressure were most frequently observed during the period when the anemia was being reversed and were related more to the change in the hematocrit than to the dose of rHuEpo (Table 16.8).

Seventeen episodes of fistula thrombosis occurred in 9 of 85 nontransfused patients, and there were six episodes in the 55 transfused

Table 16.8. Increase of Blood Pressure during
rHuEpo Therapy

Erythropoietin Dose, units/kg/wk	n	Patients with ↑ BP
3 × 40	32	8/32 (25%)
3 × 80	29	10/29 (34%)
3 × 120	30	16/30 (53%)
Hematocrit Increase per Week	n	**Patients with ↑ BP**
< 0.75%	27	7/27 (25%)
0.75–1.5%	32	9/32 (43%)
> 1.5%	32	17/32 (53%)

patients over the 12 to 18 months of observation. As there are no data on the background incidence of this problem, it is impossible to say whether this represents an excess.

There was a dose-dependent increase in platelet counts of about 20 percent during the correction phase. Although counts fell during the maintenance phase, they remained above the pretreatment level. There was an increase in the heparin requirements during dialysis from a median of 7500 units pretreatment to 8850 units during rHuEpo treatment.

Increases in predialysis concentrations of plasma potassium, phosphate, and, to a lesser extent, blood urea were observed, and these required appropriate adjustments to diet and the use of phosphate binders (18). These changes can be explained by the increases in food intake and a modest decrease in dialyzer clearance resulting from the increase in hematocrit. The latter seems to play a minor role, for the creatinine concentrations were remarkably constant.

In the transfused group, the changes in the ferritin concentrations during the correction period in the groups receiving 80 units/kg and 120 units/kg were 31 percent and 35 percent respectively. The reductions in transferrin saturation were 46 percent and 60 percent.

In the trial of nontransfused patients, one patient died of a myocardial infarct after 6 months of treatment. Four patients were withdrawn from the study because of blood pressure (two with hypertensive crises and two because of failure to control blood pressure). In one patient, rHuEpo was stopped for a few weeks after a cardiac arrest, and another developed a subdural hematoma after a fall.

In the trial of treatment in transfused patients, 6 of 55 died during the course of the study. Three of the deaths were from heart failure, one was from bladder cancer, one was from a subdural hematoma, and one followed a myocardial infarct possibly related to rHuEpo treatment. Three patients were withdrawn from the study: one with Wegener's granulomatosis, one with malaise and headache, and one with generalized eczema and fever.

Comparison of Maintenance Dose Schedules

After the target hematocrit had been achieved, a reduced dose of rHuEpo (15 units/kg three times per week) was given to 50 of the non-transfused dialysis patients. In one center the dose of rHuEpo was kept constant at 40, 80, or 120 units/kg, but the frequency was reduced to one or two injections per week according to the hematocrit (mean number of administrations per week, 1.9) (21). In both groups, the median hemoglobin levels were comparable during the late maintenance period (Fig 16.6). The median dose per week, however, was approximately 20

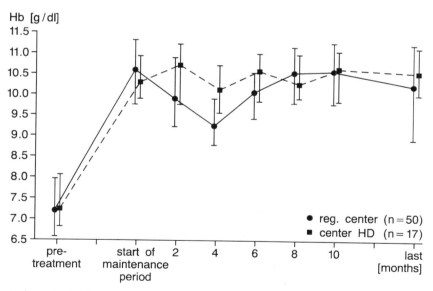

Figure 16.6. The median and interquartile range of hemoglobin levels under rHuEpo therapy using different frequencies of intravenous injection (regular center 3 times per week, Heidelberg center 1–3 times per week, average 2 times per week).

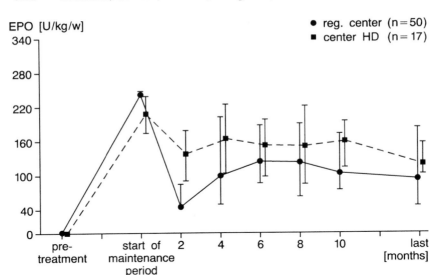

Figure 16.7. The median and interquartile range of the rHuEpo dosage required to obtain the serum hemoglobin levels shown in Figure 16.1 if different frequencies of intravenous injection were used (regular center 3 times per week, Heidelberg center 1–3 times per week, average 2 times per week).

percent higher in the patients receiving less frequent administrations (Fig 16.7). Given what is known of the pharmacokinetics of intravenously administered rHuEpo, this finding suggests that efficacy is greater if administration is more frequent.

In a comparison of the efficacy of intravenous and subcutaneous administration of rHuEpo, 16 patients who had been receiving intravenous treatment for over a year were switched to subcutaneous treatment. Figure 16.8 shows that hematocrit decreased slightly after the start of subcutaneous treatment but later increased to levels comparable to those observed during intravenous administration. In response to previous observations (22), the dose was reduced by 50 percent if the subcutaneous route was to be used. Figure 16.9 shows that the maintenance dose of rHuEpo given subcutaneously two times per week was 50 to 60 percent of the requirement if the drug was given intravenously. The subcutaneous route was well tolerated by all patients apart from the occasional small hematomas observed in a heparinized patient who received the injection at the end of dialysis. Several patients complained about the additional injections but were prepared to tolerate them for medical and financial reasons.

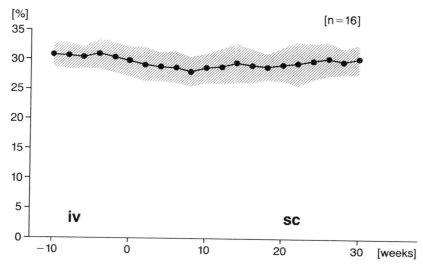

Figure 16.8. Hemoglobin levels under intravenous or subcutaneous rHuEpo therapy. Mean = closed circles. Standard deviation = shaded area.

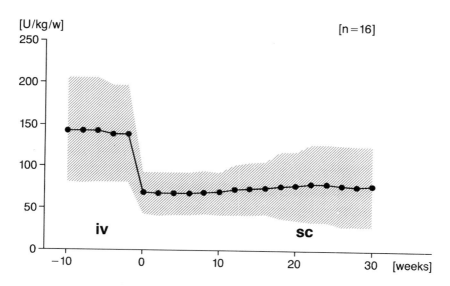

Figure 16.9. The maintenance dosage of rHuEpo given intravenously or subcutaneously to obtain the hematocrit levels shown in Figure 16.4. Mean = closed circles. Standard deviation = shaded area.

The data from these German trials confirm the efficacy of rHuEpo in reversing the anemia of renal failure and give some guidance to the probable maintenance doses and how they can be reduced by the use of the subcutaneous route. Other authors have reported the efficacy of subcutaneous rHuEpo (22–25).

Further Clinical Trials

The Cilag Company has coordinated two further multicenter trials of rHuEpo for which preliminary analyses have been performed. The first was an open label multicenter trial in 137 transfusion-dependent hemodialysis patients (the patients had hemoglobin concentrations of 7 g/dl and had required 3 units of blood during the previous 4 months). The starting dose was 100 units/kg three times per week, aiming for a target of 10 to 12 g/dl. Of 120 evaluable patients, 112 reached this target and no longer needed transfusions. Ten patients experienced seizures; in the majority of these, the event was related to hypertension. The median maintenance dose was 200 units/kg/week.

The second trial tested a dose regimen that would effect a slow correction of anemia. A total of 1167 patients were treated with 50 units/kg three times per week, and adjustments of 25 units/kg were allowed at monthly intervals, aiming for a target hemoglobin of 10 to 12 g/dl. Of evaluable patients, 53 percent reached the target and 81 percent had a rise in hemoglobin of more than 2 g/dl by 12 weeks. The median maintenance dose was ~200 units/kg/week, with higher doses required by the more anemic subjects. The incidence of hypertensive events seems to have been lower than in the previous trials, but the rate of seizures per patient month at risk has not yet been analyzed.

Additional large trials were performed by investigators working with Boehringer-Mannheim and include a placebo-controlled study the results of which are expected in 1991.

REFERENCES

1. Winearls CG, Oliver DO, Pippard MJ, Reid C, Downing MR, Cotes PM. Effect of human erythropoietin derived from recombinant DNA on the anaemia of patients maintained by chronic haemodialysis. Lancet 1986;2:1175–8.

2. Cotes PM, Pippard MJ, Reid CDL, Winearls CG, Oliver DO, Royston JP. Characterisation of the anaemia of chronic renal failure and the mode of its correction by a preparation of erythropoietin (r-HuEPO). An investigation of

the pharmacokinetics of intravenous r-HuEPO and its effect on erythrokinetics. Q J Med 1989;70:113–37.

3. Reid CDL, Fidler J, Oliver DO, Cotes PM, Pippard MJ, Winearls CG. Erythroid progenitor cell kinetics in chronic haemodialysis patients responding to treatment with recombinant human erythropoietin. Br J Haematol 1988; 70:375–80.

4. Stevens JM, Forman EW, Oliver DO, et al. 18–24 months follow-up of chronic haemodialysis patients receiving recombinant human erythropoietin [Abstract]. Nephrol Dial Transplant 1989;3:501.

5. Sundal E, Kaeser U. Correction of anaemia of chronic renal failure with recombinant human erythropoietin: safety and efficacy of one year's treatment in a European multicentre study of 150 haemodialysis-dependent patients. Nephrol Dial Transplant 1989;4:979–87.

6. Casati S, Passerini P, Campise MR, et al. Benefits and risks of protracted treatment with human recombinant erythropoietin in patients having haemodialysis. Br Med J 1987;295:1017–20.

7. Bommer J, Alexiou C, Muller-Bühl U, Eifert J, Ritz E. Recombinant human erythropoietin therapy in haemodialysis patients—dose determination and clinical experience. Nephrol Dial Transplant 1987;2:238–42.

8. Zehnder C, Blumberg A. Human recombinant erythropoietin treatment in transfusion dependent anemic patients on maintenance hemodialysis. Clin Nephrol 1989;31:55–9.

9. Neff MS, Kim KE, Persoff M, Oneseti G, Swartz C. Hemodynamics of uremic anemia. Circulation 1971;43:867–83.

10. Eschbach JW, Egrie JC, Downing MR, Browne JK, Adamson JW. Correction of the anemia of end-stage renal disease with recombinant human erythropoietin. Results of a combined Phase I and II clinical trial. N Engl J Med 1987;316:73–8.

11. Edmunds ME, Walls J, Tucker B, et al. Seizures in haemodialysis patients treated with recombinant human erythropoietin. Nephrol Dial Transplant 1989;4:1065–9.

12. Moia M, Mannucci PM, Vizzotto L, Casati S, Cattaneo M, Ponticelli C. Improvement in the haemostatic defect of uraemia after treatment with recombinant human erythropoietin. Lancet 1987;2:1227–9.

13. Wolfinden C, Hoenich NA, Kerr DNS. Effect of haematocrit on the clearance of small molecules during haemodialysis. Int J Artif Organs 1983;6:127–30.

14. Stivelman J, Van Wyck D, Kirlin L, Ogden D. Use of recombinant erythropoietin with high flux dialysis does not worsen azotemia or shorten access survival [Abstract]. Kidney Int 1988;33:239.

15. Walczyk MH, Golper TA. Correction of anemia of end-stage renal disease with recombinant human erythropoietin [Letter]. N Engl J Med 1987; 317:249.

16. Pollok M, Bommer J, Gurland HJ, et al. Effects of recombinant human erythropoietin treatment in end-stage renal failure patients. Contrib Nephrol 1989;76:201–11.

17. Kühn K, Nonnast-Daniel B, Grützmacher P, et al. Analysis of initial resistance of erythropoiesis to treatment with recombinant human erythropoietin. Results of a multicenter trial in patients with end-stage renal disease. Contrib Nephrol 1988;66:94–103.

18. Grützmacher P, Bergmann M, Weinreich T, Nattermann U, Reimers E,

Pollok M. Beneficial and adverse effects of correction of anaemia by recombinant human erythropoietin in patients on maintenance haemodialysis. Contrib Nephrol 1988;66:104–13.

19. Samtleben W, Baldamus CA, Bommer J, Fassbinder W, Nonnast-Daniel B, Gurland HJ. Blood pressure changes during treatment with recombinant human erythropoietin. Contrib Nephrol 1988;66:114–22.

20. Bommer J, Kugel M, Schoeppe W, Brunkhorst R, Samtleben W, Scigalla P. Dose-related effects of recombinant human erythropoietin on erythropoiesis. Results of a multicenter trial in patients with end-stage renal disease. Contrib Nephrol 1988;66:85–93.

21. Bommer J, Samtleben W, Koch KM, Baldamus CA, Grützmacher P, Scigalla P. Variations of recombinant human erythropoietin application in hemodialysis patients. Contrib Nephrol 1989;76:149–58.

22. Bommer J, Ritz E, Weinreich T, Bommer G, Ziegler T. Subcutaneous erythropoietin [Letter]. Lancet 1988;2:406.

23. Stevens JM, Strong CA, Oliver DO, Winearls CG, Cotes PM. Subcutaneous erythropoietin and peritoneal dialysis [Letter]. Lancet 1989;1:1388–9.

24. Eschbach JW, Kelly MR, Haley RN, Abels RI, Adamson JW. Treatment of the anemia of progressive renal failure with recombinant human erythropoietin. N Engl J Med 1989;321:158–63.

25. Granolleras C, Branger B, Beau MC, Deschodt G, Alsabadani B, Shaldon S. Experience with daily self-administered subcutaneous erythropoietin. Contrib Nephrol 1989;76:143–8.

Chapter 17

Recombinant Human Erythropoietin (Epoetin Alfa) in Patients with Predialysis Renal Failure

Brendan P. Teehan, Miles H. Sigler,
Robert I. Abels, and Joan M. Brown

Anemia is virtually always present in patients with chronic renal failure. Although the correlation between the level of azotemia and the hemoglobin concentration is relatively poor, anemia tends to progress as azotemia advances, and typically the hemoglobin concentration falls to 10 g/dl or less at serum creatinine concentrations of greater than 3 mg/dl. In contrast, the correlation between the mass of red cells labeled with chromium 51 and the serum creatinine level is somewhat better; red cell mass is reduced by about one half at a creatinine value of 3 mg/dl, and only one third of the red blood cell mass remains at a serum creatinine level of 8 to 10 mg/dl (1). The important point is that there is a major reduction in red cell mass and, therefore, oxygen-carrying capacity long before dialysis is necessary. This fact has important consequences for anemic patients with chronic renal insufficiency.

Many potential causes for the anemia of chronic renal failure have been cited. These include circulating inhibitors of bone marrow red cell progenitors (2), decreased red cell life-span (3), increased gastrointestinal blood loss due to the platelet defect typical of renal failure (4), and inadequate erythropoietin response (5). The question of circulating inhibitors was carefully addressed by Segal et al. (6). They showed that serum or plasma from patients with advanced renal failure supported autologous marrow erythroid and nonerythroid colony growth in vitro just as well as did normal serum or plasma. They also demonstrated that there was no difference in serum erythropoietin levels between severely anemic renal failure patients and normal controls, indicating that the inability of the failing kidney to secrete adequate erythropoietin is the major cause of anemia in these patients. Moreover, some studies (1) suggested that this markedly blunted erythropoietin response may be present at serum creatinine levels as low as 3 mg/dl. In fact, serum erythropoietin levels are comparable (about 20 mU/ml) in predialysis patients (mean creatinine, 6 mg/dl) and patients on hemodialysis. Finally, an increasing number of clinical studies has shown that the anemia of chronic renal failure responds in a dose-dependent fashion to the administration of exogenous recombinant human erythropoietin (7–11), suggesting that inhibitors of erythropoiesis, whatever their role may be (12), are subordinate to inadequate erythropoietin secretion from the failing kidneys.

The Physiologic Consequences of Anemia in Predialysis Patients

Although the anemia of chronic dialysis patients, especially those on hemodialysis, is recognized as severe and often transfusion-dependent, the anemia of patients with renal failure who are not yet on dialysis (i.e., predialysis patients) has traditionally been considered mild or moderate in severity and generally not requiring therapy. The relationship between hemoglobin concentration and exercise capacity in healthy volunteers was recently reviewed (13,14), but there are relatively few studies that have attempted to quantify the physiologic deficits in predialysis patients which may be due to anemia (7,10,15). The results of these latter studies are summarized in Table 17.1. On treadmill or bicycle ergometry testing, predialysis patients demonstrate poor exercise tolerance, decreased maximal oxygen uptake, earlier appearance of anaerobic threshold, and increased symptoms of tissue ischemia (angina and claudication). In addition, there is a marked reduction in single-breath carbon monoxide-diffusing capacity, consistent with the degree of anemia. Although limited in number, these studies strongly suggest that the anemia seen in predialysis patients is symptomatic and may be associated with reduced work capacity and, therefore, diminished quality of life.

Before the availability of recombinant human erythropoietin (rHuEpo), anemia in predialysis patients was treated only rarely and then usually because of major debilitating symptoms such as angina or profound weakness. Therapeutic options were limited to transfusions and oral or parenteral androgens. Repeated transfusions were associated with the

Table 17.1. Physiological Deficits in Predialysis Patients

	Clyne et al. (15)	Lim et al. (10)	Teehan et al. (1)	Normal Values
N	20	7	10	
Age (yr)	43	50	62	—
Serum creatinine (mg/dl) or GFR* (ml/min)	11*	6.2	5.1	0.8–1.2
Hematocrit (%)	32	27	25	38–46
Vo$_2$max (ml/kg/min)	—	16.0	13.5	27
Vo$_2$ at anaerobic threshold (ml/kg/min)	—	9.2	—	22–24
Maximal exercise testing	—	—	3.9	7.7
Anemic symptoms during EKG stress testing (%)	90	—	80	0
D$_L$CO (%)	—	—	60	100

Abbreviations: Vo$_2$max, maximal oxygen consumption; Vo$_2$, oxygen consumption; EKG, electrocardiogram; D$_L$CO, carbon dioxide diffusing capacity of the lung.
*GFR, glomerular filtration rate.

risk of iron overload, transmission of a variety of viral infections (hepatitis B and C and cytomegalovirus), and the development of cytotoxic antibodies that might preclude successful transplantation in the future. Use of oral or parenteral androgens has been characterized by a hematopoietic response that may be not only delayed, often over several months, but also unpredictable. Moreover, the use of these agents is associated with varying degrees of hepatotoxicity, including hepatoma in the extreme case. Cloning of the erythropoietin gene and production of large quantities of the recombinant hormone opened a new chapter in the treatment of anemia in patients with chronic renal failure.

The Pharmacokinetics of rHuEpo

Detailed pharmacokinetic studies of rHuEpo were conducted in normal volunteers, dialysis patients, and predialysis patients. The pharmacokinetic profile of rHuEpo administered intravenously to dialysis and predialysis patients (serum creatinine about 6 mg/dl) is very similar. After intravenous administration of rHuEpo to predialysis patients, a dose-dependent peak serum level is documented one-half hour after drug administration. Thereafter, serum levels of rHuEpo fall off in a monoexponential manner. The half-life of rHuEpo after a single intravenous administration is 7.69 ± 1.11 hours; the half-life then declines

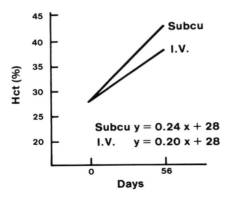

Figure 17.1. A comparison of hematocrit (Hct) related to subcutaneous (Subcu) vs. intravenous (I.V.) rHuEpo, 100 units/kg, given three times per week. The difference between the slopes of the two lines is not significant at $P < 0.05$.

to 4.60 ± 0.28 (SD) hours after multiple administrations of rHuEpo (10). The reasons for this reduction in rHuEpo half-life after multiple administrations are unclear, but it may be related to increased utilization by an expanded pool of erythroid precursors (burst-forming units-erythroid [BFU-E] and colony-forming units-erythroid [CFU-E]) induced by rHuEpo therapy. The volume of distribution of intravenously administered rHuEpo is approximately equal to the plasma volume. As might be anticipated from the plasma half-life kinetics, the area under the time-concentration curve (AUC) after a single intravenous bolus injection is nearly twice as high as that after multiple doses.

Subcutaneous dosing of rHuEpo results in a peak serum level approximately 12 to 24 hours after drug administration. The peak serum level of rHuEpo in normal volunteers after subcutaneous dosing is approximately 5 percent of that observed after intravenous dosing. The AUC at 48 hours after subcutaneous dosing is about 15 percent of the corresponding AUC at 48 hours after intravenous dosing. After attaining peak serum levels following subcutaneous dosing, serum levels of rHuEpo decline slowly, suggesting a repositorylike effect (16).

Despite the lower, more sustained serum levels observed after subcutaneous dosing compared to intravenous dosing, available evidence suggests that rHuEpo is at least as effective by the subcutaneous route as by the intravenous route of administration. For example, rHuEpo, 100 units/kg intravenously or subcutaneously three times per week in predialysis patients induces a rate of rise of hematocrit of 0.20 and 0.24 percentage points per day, respectively (Fig 17.1). The results of intravenous rHuEpo at three dose levels vs. subcutaneous dosing at 100 units/kg three times per week in 131 patients are summarized in Table 17.2.

Clinical Studies

Several studies (1,9,10,17) have now confirmed in predialysis patients what Eschbach et al. (8) and Winearls et al. (7) demonstrated earlier in hemodialysis patients, namely, that there is a dose-dependent increase in hematocrit after therapy with rHuEpo. The largest of these clinical trials was a double-blind, placebo-controlled, multicenter study carried out by the United States Erythropoietin Study Group (17). One hundred seventeen patients were enrolled in three rHuEpo dosing groups: 150 units/kg, 100 units/kg, and 50 units/kg, each given intravenously three times per week. The hematocrit responses in the three treatment groups were then followed for 8 weeks. The fourth group was given placebo intravenously three times per week for 2 months and was then started on rHuEpo therapy on an open label basis. The dose-response curves for the four treatment groups are summarized in Figure 17.2. The daily rate of rise in the hematocrit is equal to the slope of each line. The 150-unit/kg dose was twice as effective, on the average, as the 50-unit/kg dose. It is apparent, therefore, that higher doses of erythropoietin yield proportionately higher rates of rise in the hematocrit, but a threefold increase in dose increases the rise in hematocrit only by a factor of two. Similar results were noted in hemodialysis patients treated with erythropoietin (8). In fact, the dose-response curves are almost identical for predialysis patients and hemodialysis patients, at

Table 17.2. Intravenous vs. Subcutaneous Recombinant Human Erythropoietin Correction of Anemia

Dose	% Anemia Correction	Rate of Rise of Hematocrit/Day	Mean Week at Completion*
Intravenous			
150 units/kg (N = 30)	87	0.26	6.3
100 units/kg (N = 28)	64	0.20†	7.4
50 units/kg (N = 28)	46	0.13	8.5
Subcutaneous			
100 units/kg (N = 45)	58	0.24†	7.7

*Completion of study: point at which patient reached target hematocrit or completed study requirement (intravenous treatment, 8 weeks; subcutaneous treatment, 12 weeks).
†Not significantly different.

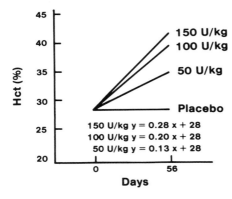

Figure 17.2. The rates of rise of the hematocrit (Hct) at the three dose levels of rHuEpo given intravenously, three times per week, vs. placebo.

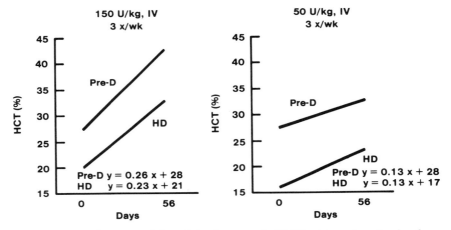

Figure 17.3. The rates of rise of the hematocrit (HCT) at two dose levels of rHuEpo, 50 units/kg and 150 units/kg, given intravenously, three times per week, in predialysis (Pre-D) and hemodialysis (HD) patients. *Source: Data from Reference 8*

least for the dose levels of 50 units/kg and 150 units/kg given three times per week, intravenously (Fig 17.3). Thus, for a typical renal failure patient (hemodialysis or predialysis) receiving 50 units of erythropoietin per kg intravenously three times per week, it would take 76 days or about 2.5 months to increase the hematocrit by 10 percentage points. Using a similar schedule but a higher dose (150 units/kg), the same goal could be achieved in 38 days for a predialysis patient and in 43 days for a hemodialysis patient. The similarities in the dose-response curves between these two patient populations suggest that the relative uremic milieu has no significant effect on the erythopoietic effect of this hormone.

Both the dosing schedule and the route of administration in this study were based on previous experience with hemodialysis patients and on the practical reality that during these early trials the recombinant hormone was available in only relatively large dose volumes (i.e., 3 to 5 ml), which precluded comfortable subcutaneous dosing. More recently, concentrated preparations have been introduced, and limited data are available for comparison between the two routes.

The three phases characteristic of treatment with rHuEpo are shown in Figure 17.4. These are the induction or restoration phase, a period of dose adjustment, and then the maintenance phase. In the example used in Figure 17.4, the hematocrit was restored to the 40 percent range with 50 units of rHuEpo per kg given intravenously three times per week. As the hematocrit rose above 40 percent, the dose was adjusted downward by reducing both the dose and the frequency of dosing. As the hematocrit fell back to the target range (36 to 38 percent), the dose was gradually increased until a stable maintenance value was reached, in this case, 50 units/kg given subcutaneously once per week. In a large multicenter study (18) of predialysis patients ($N = 105$), the hematocrit was restored and initially maintained with intravenous dosing and then

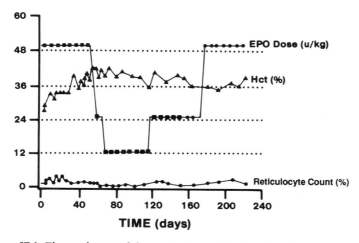

Figure 17.4. Three phases of dose adjustment during the rHuEpo treatment (circles, once per week; squares, three times per week) of anemia in predialysis patients. EPO, erythropoietin; u, units; Hct, hematocrit.

the route was changed to subcutaneous dosing for the extended maintenance phase. Initially, the median hematocrit was maintained at 38 percent at 150 units/kg/week given intravenously, but during the extended maintenance phase the median hematocrit was 36 percent at a median weekly dose level of 75 units/kg/week given subcutaneously.

It is clear, however, that these regimens are arbitrary and derived from the traditional hemodialysis schedule. Endogenous daily erythropoietin production has been estimated at 2 IU/kg/24 hours (19). It may be more rational, therefore, to use a small daily dose, analogous to the use of insulin. This approach was explored by Granolleras et al. (20). Four chronic hemodialysis patients were treated with intravenous erythropoietin three times per week to restore the hematocrit to 36 to 38 percent. The route and frequency were then changed to subcutaneous and daily, respectively. At the conclusion of this study, the target hematocrit was maintained by only 30 percent of the previous intravenous maintenance dose. In contrast, Graf et al. (21) in a larger study failed to show any difference between intravenous and subcutaneous routes in the restoration or maintenance dose. Daily dosing was not used during the maintenance phase, however. Nevertheless, these preliminary studies suggested that a variety of dosing schedules may be explored. Ultimately, a timed-release parenteral preparation of the hormone would seem to be the ideal dosage form for the maintenance phase. This might allow dosing at weekly or even monthly intervals.

During the long-term maintenance phase of one study (1), 4 of 22 patients no longer required rHuEpo to maintain the target hematocrit in spite of stable or worsening renal failure. An extreme example of this phenomenon is illustrated in Figure 17.5. A year after rHuEpo was stopped, the hematocrit remained in the target range while renal function deteriorated and maintenance dialysis was started. There was no evidence of renal cysts or tumor by computed tomographic scanning. Unfortunately, endogenous erythropoietin levels were not measured before or after rHuEpo therapy. There are several possible explanations for this rHuEpo "escape." The proliferation of red blood cell precursors typical of the marrow after rHuEpo therapy coupled with enhanced oxygen delivery to the marrow may result in a greater responsiveness to the low endogenous production of erythropoietin. Alternatively, renal disease may damage the renal oxygen-sensing mechanism more than the erythropoietin-producing cells such that erythropoietin production is low and independent of hematocrit. Once the marrow is restored after rHuEpo therapy and oxygen delivery to the marrow is normalized by

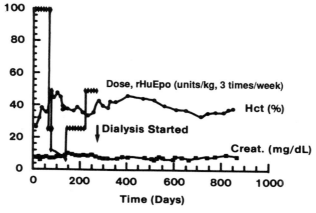

Figure 17.5. Erythropoietin "escape." This chart shows the data of one of four predialysis patients who initially required rHuEpo for the correction of anemia but later maintained a hematocrit (Hct) in the target range (<36 percent) after rHuEpo was discontinued. Creat. indicates creatinine.

increased circulating hemoglobin, the increased pool of red blood cell precursors may become responsive to low endogenous levels of erythropoietin production. Whatever the cause of this phenomenon, it may have important consequences for a small but significant fraction of predialysis patients treated with rHuEpo.

The Hematologic Response to rHuEpo Therapy

The earliest clinical hematologic response is an increase in the percentage of circulating reticulocytes (see Fig 17.4). Earlier, more subtle changes in ferrokinetics were demonstrated by Eschbach et al. (8). Typically, the reticulocyte count increases to 3 to 6 percent and may remain at this level for 2 to 3 weeks. The increase in reticulocyte count is followed by a perceptible rise in hematocrit, usually in less than 1 week, and then the reticulocyte count gradually falls to the normal range. As indicated in Figure 17.4, there may be small fluctuations of both the hematocrit and the reticulocyte count during the period of dose adjustment.

Hemoglobin Electrophoretic Studies

The distribution of hemoglobin species produced after rHuEpo therapy at the dose levels used in predialysis patients was also studied. Hemoglobin electrophoresis was carried out at baseline and again at target hematocrit in seven patients treated with 50, 100, or 150 units/kg intravenously three times per week (22). On these regimens, there was a significant increase in only hemoglobin A concentration, 9.1 to 11.5 g/dl ($P < 0.001$). Hemoglobin A_2 and F levels remained unchanged.

The Target Hematocrit in Predialysis Patients

The target or ideal hematocrit for these patients has not been determined, but values between 36 and 40 percent have generally been recommended (23). In contrast to these recommendations is the approved Food and Drug Administration label which suggests a target hematocrit of 30 to 33 percent and a maximal level of 36 percent. The basis for this recommendation is empiric. In part it reflects the concern that higher values are associated with hypertensive events, increased blood viscosity, and possibly a higher frequency of thrombotic events. In addition, objective physiologic benefits were demonstrated in these patients when the hematocrit was increased only modestly, from a baseline mean of 28 percent to a mean of 36 to 38 percent (see below). Finally, the elevated red blood cell levels of 2,3-diphosphoglycerate typical of anemia in general (24) and of uremic anemia in particular seem to be sustained after rHuEpo therapy in both short- and long-term studies (25). The oxygen dissociation curve for hemoglobin shifts to the right as renal failure advances due to these changes in intracellular phosphate moieties; therefore, oxygen transport and release are improved and it is possible that a lower level of hemoglobin is "adequate" in this population of patients (26).

Chromium 51 Studies during rHuEpo Therapy

The relative changes in red cell mass, plasma volume, and total blood volume in predialysis patients treated with rHuEpo have been elucidated by chromium 51 studies. Two studies (1,10) measuring these variables ($N = 28$) before starting rHuEpo and again at peak hematocrit were reported. Stone et al. (9) reported on ^{51}Cr-labeled red blood cell mass at baseline and at peak hematocrit. These studies are summarized in Table 17.3. Red blood cell mass increased by 48 percent after rHuEpo therapy. For each 1.2-percentage point rise in hematocrit, there was a 1-ml/kg increase in red blood cell mass. It can be estimated that in the average patient about 160 g of new hemoglobin was synthesized as the hematocrit was restored to normal. As red blood cell mass increased, plasma volume decreased; therefore, total blood volume did not change significantly. ^{51}Cr-labeled red blood cell half-life increased toward the

Table 17.3. Chromium 51 Studies after rHuEpo* Therapy

	Normal Values	Pre-rHuEpo	At Peak Hct	% Change
RBC mass (ml/kg)	23–32	12.8	18.9	+48
Plasma volume (ml/kg)	28–39	41.6	38.1	−8
Total blood volume (ml/kg)	53–70	53.9	56.9	+5
^{51}Cr-labeled RBC half-life (d)	25–32	22.5	24.6	+9

Abbreviations: Hct, hematocrit; RBC, red blood cell.
*Dose = 100 units/kg, intravenously or subcutaneously three times per week.

lower limit of normal (25 days), but this estimate of red blood cell life-span in these acute studies may be skewed because a large fraction of the red cell mass (48 percent) was recently released from the bone marrow. Nevertheless, Eschbach (27) found a significant increase in ^{51}Cr-labeled red cell half-life in dialysis patients studied as late as 6 months after rHuEpo treatment was started.

Physiologic Studies after rHuEpo Therapy

Bicycle and treadmill ergometry as well as electrocardiogram stress testing and echocardiography were used to assess the physiologic effect of correcting the hematocrit in predialysis patients (1,10). During the ergometry studies, the following parameters were measured: maximal oxygen uptake (Vo$_2$max), duration of exercise, and Vo$_2$ at anaerobic threshold. Electrocardiogram stress testing used the Naughton or modified Bruce protocol. All studies were obtained at baseline and were repeated at peak hematocrit, which was usually achieved at 8 to 12 weeks of therapy. Baseline values are given in Table 17.1. Echocardiographic data are not shown because no change was noted throughout the studies. Percentage of change from baseline for each of the other parameters is shown in Table 17.4. The largest changes occurred in two critical aspects of work capacity, i.e., maximal oxygen uptake and duration of exercise. The difference in Vo$_2$max between the two studies (9 vs. 35 percent) is unclear, but the percentage of change in hematocrit (36 vs. 42 percent) was greater in the study that also showed the larger increase in Vo$_2$max. The percentage of increase in Vo$_2$max bears a direct linear relation to the increase in red blood cell mass after treatment with rHuEpo (1).

Electrocardiographic stress testing failed to show any change in ST segment patterns (1). The reasons for stopping the test were of interest, however. Evidence of tissue ischemia (angina or claudication) was the

Table 17.4. Physiologic Changes after rHuEpo* Therapy

	Change from Baseline, %	P Value
Hct[†]	+42	< .001
Hct[‡]	+36	< .005
Vo_2max[†]	+35	< .01
Vo_2max[‡]	+9	< .002
Vo_2 at anaerobic threshold[‡]	+8	< .02
Duration of exercise[†]	+77	< .04

Abbreviations: Hct, hematocrit; Vo_2max, maximal oxygen consumption.
*Dose = 100 u/kg, I.V. or S.C. 3 ×/wk
[†]Data from Reference 1.
[‡]Data from Reference 10.

reason for stopping the test in 4 of 10 subjects at baseline. In spite of a 62 percent increase in duration of electrocardiogram stress testing in this subset of patients, however, none experienced tissue ischemia at peak hematocrit. Testing was stopped because of fatigue. The remaining six subjects achieved a mean 23 percent increase in duration of electrocardiogram stress testing, but the reasons for stopping were unchanged (dyspnea and/or fatigue). Because there was no effort at training between baseline and peak hematocrit, the increased duration of exercise was attributed to the increase in hematocrit. The fact that the increased duration of exercise was not statistically significant ($P = 0.33$) was due to a large scatter in the data (1 to 168 percent) and a small sample size ($N = 10$).

The reduction in carbon monoxide diffusing capacity typical of anemia is also present in the anemia of predialysis patients (Table 17.1). At a hemoglobin level of 8 g/dl, the carbon monoxide diffusing capacity is reduced to approximately 60 percent of normal. Predialysis patients were studied at baseline and again at peak hematocrit. After treatment with rHuEpo, the carbon monoxide diffusing capacity increases as a linear function of the rise in hemoglobin concentration (Fig 17.6). When this response is compared to those in a group of patients with mixed anemias (28) and in subjects with normal hemoglobin levels, the slope of the line is similar, but the line is shifted slightly to the left, suggesting a somewhat higher affinity for carbon monoxide in the hemoglobin of predialysis patients.

Studies of the Quality of Life

In addition to the objective physiologic studies reviewed above, several studies (17,29,30) used subjective measures to evaluate quality of life, energy level, and work capacity in both short-term (8 to 12 weeks) and long-term (6 month) studies. These results were based on a self-administered questionnaire in which patients responded, on a 100-mm visual analogue scale, to the questions: What is your ability to do work, compared to last week? What is your energy level, compared to last week? In each case, the results were compared to those in placebo controls.

In general, these parameters not only improved with correction of anemia but also tended to improve further with sustained correction of anemia (i.e., hematocrit of 40 percent for males and 35 percent for females). In one 8-week study (17), work capacity and energy level increased significantly in all patients with corrected anemia. In this short-term study, however, correction of anemia was a function of rHuEpo dose; anemia was corrected in 87 percent of those given 150 units/kg, in 64 percent of those given 100 units/kg, and in 46 percent of those given 50 units/kg intravenously three times per week. As a result, only 24 percent of the patients rated their ability to do work as very good to excellent after therapy. In the 6-month follow-up study of these patients, the number of patients claiming good to excellent work capacity almost doubled (44 percent). A similar percentage (42 percent)

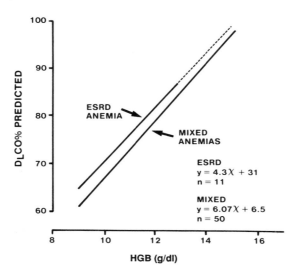

Figure 17.6. A comparison of the diffusing capacity of the lung for carbon monoxide ($d_L CO$) in predialysis anemia patients ($n = 11$) treated with rHuEpo vs. a group of subjects with mixed anemias ($n = 28$) or normal hemoglobin (HGB) concentrations. ESRD, end-stage renal disease. *Source: Data from Reference 28*

of those on placebo during the earlier study also evaluated their work capacity as good to excellent after 6 months of active therapy (18). In another short-term (12-week), fixed-dose (100 units/kg, three times per week) study (30) comparing rHuEpo-treated patients ($N = 45$) to placebo-treated controls ($N = 48$), there was a significant improvement ($P < 0.05$) in subjective sense of well-being, energy level, and ability to do work in treated patients, compared to controls. At least 234 predialysis patients have now been treated with rHuEpo in the combined American and European trials. The annualized mortality rate in this group was 16.6 percent for the rHuEpo-treated patients and 32.9 percent in the placebo group. Because the total number of deaths was relatively small ($N = 16$) and the duration of the placebo period was short (12 weeks), however, a statistically significant conclusion cannot be drawn from these observations.

Finally, there are a number of potential benefits of rHuEpo therapy which are not easily quantified. These include avoiding transfusions (and the consequences thereof, including HLA sensitization, hepatitis, etc.), avoiding androgen therapy, and delaying the start of maintenance dialysis therapy. Because the decision to start dialysis is often based on the appearance of "symptomatic azotemia," and because correction of anemia usually minimizes the symptoms associated with advancing azotemia, it is not surprising that these patients may not be started on dialysis quite as early as they might be if anemia is not corrected. Each of these factors has an economic dimension. Sheingold (31) attempted to evaluate and place a dollar value on these variables and then arrive at a benefit-cost ratio for the use of rHuEpo in the anemia of predialysis patients. The model assumed that only 20 percent of predialysis patients would be treated with rHuEpo. Sheingold concluded that the elimination of red blood cell transfusions (and related morbidity) and androgen therapy, as well as delay of the start of dialysis therapy (by a mean of 3.7 months for each patient), would result in savings of 30 to 70 percent above costs. The potential net benefit amounted to $15 to 37 million per year for the U.S. predialysis population.

Hypertension

Hypertension and hypertensive encephalopathy were reported in the earliest clinical trials of rHuEpo in hemodialysis patients (7,8) but not in volunteers with normal renal function. Severe hypertension was also reported in animal models of chronic renal insufficiency treated with rHuEpo (32). In the earliest large ($N = 117$) study of rHuEpo in predialysis patients (17), hypertension was almost universal in this population: 92 percent in patients treated with active drug and 94 percent in those on placebo. This study focused only on the restoration phase of therapy, i.e., the period during which the hematocrit increases to a target value, in this case 38 to 43 percent. In addition to a placebo control group, three dose levels of rHuEpo were used: 50, 100, and 150 units/kg, three times weekly, given intravenously. Teehan et al. noted that hypertensive events were more common at the higher dose levels (150 units/kg). They also noted that the incidence of hypertensive events seemed to increase with increasing rates of rise of hematocrit, up to 0.3 percentage points per day. The mean rate of rise in hematocrit in patients who experienced a hypertensive event was 0.23 percentage points per day, compared to 0.19 percentage points per day in those who did not experience a hypertensive event. This difference was not statistically significant, but it is generally agreed (23) that a cautious, slow rise in hematocrit (<0.2 percentage points per day) is a safe, appropriate therapeutic goal in these patients. It has also been recommended that blood pressure should be well controlled and carefully followed during the restoration phase of rHuEpo therapy. Ideally, blood pressure should be <140/90 mm Hg before rHuEpo therapy is started and therapy should be interrupted if blood pressure is >160/90.

Of the 117 patients enrolled in this study, 95 entered a long-term maintenance study (18). Hypertension was present in 51 percent and was the most common adverse event reported. However, there was no significant change in mean systolic or diastolic pressure throughout this study for the group as a whole. This seems to reflect the fact that hypertensive events are sporadic and probably followed by adjustments in antihypertensive therapy or rHuEpo therapy. In a subsequent multi-center study (30) using subcutaneous rHuEpo (100 units/kg, three times per week) in predialysis patients, both the incidence of hypertensive events and the frequency of adjustment of antihypertensive therapy were followed. In this double-blind, placebo-controlled study, there was no significant difference in the incidence of hypertensive events in treated patients (42 percent), compared to the placebo group (31 percent). In addition, there was no difference in the rate of rise of hematocrit (0.23 percentage points per day) in rHuEpo-treated patients for whom hypertensive events were reported, compared to those patients for whom no hypertensive events were reported (0.25 percentage points per day). Adjustments in antihypertensive therapy (usually an increase in dose) were comparable in both the treated and the placebo groups. Nevertheless, there was a higher incidence of diastolic blood pressure readings greater than 95 mm Hg in the rHuEpo-treated patients compared to the placebo-treated patients (51 percent vs. 27 percent, $P <$ 0.05), suggesting that rHuEpo-induced correction of anemia may be related to an increased risk of hypertension. Anecdotal reports also suggest that allowing the hematocrit to rise excessively may induce hypertensive events. This is probably related to an increase in whole blood viscosity and peripheral vascular resistance. On the basis of these results, it has been suggested that the dose of erythropoietin should be adjusted so that the rate of rise of hematocrit does not exceed 0.20 percentage point per day. This can be reliably achieved at an initial dose of 50 units/kg/day, in which case the median rate of rise of hematocrit is 0.13 percentage point per day.

The mechanism of hypertension in predialysis patients treated with rHuEpo has not been thoroughly evaluated. The interplay of hematocrit, whole blood viscosity, and peripheral vascular resistance may be relevant to the development of increased hypertension in rHuEpo patients. Increases in hematocrit are associated with increases in whole blood viscosity above baseline values in erythropoietin-treated predialysis diabetic patients (33). At high shear rates, increasing the hematocrit from 20 to 40 percent may produce a 10-fold or more increase in whole blood viscosity (34). Based on Poiseuille's equation, the resistance to flow will increase in direct proportion to blood viscosity if other terms in the equation remain constant. The baroreceptor-mediated change in cardiac output in response to this increased resistance to flow (expressed as increased vascular resistance) will determine the final peripheral resistance and, hence, the arterial blood pressure. If the cardiac output does not fall in parallel with the rise in peripheral vascular resistance, the arterial pressure will be elevated. Studies in hemodialysis patients revealed no significant changes in the renin-angiotensin-aldosterone axis, plasma catecholamines, or vasopressin (35) as the hematocrit was restored to the normal range. In a study that anticipated this question (i.e., the relationship between hypertension and increased hematocrit in end-stage renal disease patients) by nearly 20 years, Neff et al. (36) used invasive cardiovascular monitoring to measure mean arterial pressure, cardiac output, plasma volume, and peripheral vascular resistance while giving transfusions to hemodialysis patients until the hematocrit reached normal levels. Plasma volume was controlled by ultrafiltration and, as the hematocrit rose, Neff et al. noted a progressive rise in mean arterial pressure while cardiac output decreased and peripheral vascular resistance increased. They concluded that restoration of the hematocrit abolished the compensatory vasodilatation typical of anemia. Similar changes were noted during the correction of anemia in euvolemic animals (37). As indicated above, several studies (1,10) failed to show a change in total blood volume in predialysis patients treated with rHuEpo. Thus, the hypertensive response to normalizing the hematocrit in these patients seems to be vasoconstrictor-mediated, not volume-mediated. From a therapeutic perspective, these studies suggest that vasodilator drugs (in contrast to diuretics or β-blockers) may be the preferred agents for treating hypertension in these patients. The potential beneficial effects of angiotensin-converting enzyme inhibitors on residual renal function in this patient population (38) should also be considered (see below).

Residual Renal Function

Maintaining stable renal function or minimizing the rate of progression of renal failure is a major therapeutic goal in patients with chronic renal insufficiency. Because anemia may have some protective effect in this regard (32), the use of rHuEpo in predialysis patients has raised questions. In fact, based on sound physiologic reasoning, a strong case can be formulated for the hypothesis that an increase in hematocrit should result in an accelerated loss of renal function in predialysis patients. For example, if filtration fraction (FF) equals glomerular filtration rate (GFR) divided by renal plasma flow (RPF) (i.e., $FF = GFR/RPF$) and RPF equals the product of renal blood flow (RBF) times $1 - Hct$ (i.e., $RPF = RBF (1 - Hct)$), then $GFR = FF \times RBF(1 - Hct)$, and glomerular filtration rate should decrease as hematocrit increases. Alternatively, glomerular filtration rate may be temporarily maintained by an increase in filtration fraction, perhaps accomplished by increased efferent arteriolar resistance or an increase in glomerular capillary permeability. Actually, filtration fraction varies directly with hematocrit (37–39). These latter changes, however, are known to be associated with accelerated glomerular sclerosis in animal models of advanced renal insufficiency (40).

Following this line of reasoning, Garcia et al. (32) studied several aspects of glomerular function: single-nephron glomerular filtration rate, transcapillary hydraulic pressure ultrafiltration coefficient, and degree of glomerular sclerosis in the 5/6 nephrectomy rat model treated with rHuEpo. Parallel studies were carried out on control azotemic anemic rats not receiving rHuEpo. In the treated animals, compared to controls, there was a significant increase in hematocrit (50 vs. 27 percent) and transcapillary hydraulic pressure (34 vs. 58 mm Hg) but a significant decrease in both single-nephron glomerular filtration rate (88 vs. 72 nl/min) and ultrafiltration coefficient (109 vs. 36 pl (s·mm Hg)). The incidence of glomerular sclerosis was more than twice as high in the rHuEpo-treated rats compared to those that remained anemic (32 percent vs. 13 percent of glomeruli). However, blood pressure was not controlled in this study, and treated rats developed severe elevations of mean arterial pressure, compared to anemic controls (166 vs. 123 mm Hg). Because hypertension is a major independent risk factor in the progression of renal disease, this study failed to answer the question of the effects, if any, of rHuEpo on the progression of renal disease. This study has also been criticized for a methodologic flaw. Because human recombinant erythropoietin was used in a rat model, antigen-antibody complex formation may have contributed to the accelerated renal disease in the treated animals. No immunologic studies (anti-erythropoietin antibodies, serum complement levels, immunofluorescent microscopy, or electron microscopy) were performed in this investigation; therefore, the question of an immune mechanism contributing to the results is unresolved.

In contrast to these laboratory investigations, clinical studies to date have failed to show acceleration of progression of renal disease in human subjects. Typically, these studies used relatively crude estimates of renal function, such as serum creatinine, creatinine clearance, or the reciprocal of serum creatinine (1/Scr) vs. time (17,18). In the first of these studies, 117 patients were divided into four treatment groups (50, 100, and 150 units/kg, three times per week, and placebo) and were followed for 3 months. There was no significant difference in serum creatinine and creatinine clearance among the four groups during this relatively brief study. In a subset ($N = 83$) of this group of patients, historical data allowed a comparison of 1/Scr for the 12 months preceding and 12 months following rHuEpo therapy (Fig 17.7). There was a tendency toward improvement in this parameter, but the change in slope was not statistically significant. In a subsequent study (30,41), anemic predialysis patients were treated with rHuEpo, 100 units/kg, subcutaneously three times per week. Historical creatinine values were available in 71 patients for 12 months before starting rHuEpo. These patients were then followed for another 12 months after therapy was started. The reciprocal of serum creatinine was calculated and followed during both periods (before and during rHuEpo therapy). The relationship of the reciprocal of serum creatinine vs. time for this group of patients is shown in Figure 17.8. Once again, the slope tended to improve after the institution of therapy, but the difference between slopes of the two lines (before and after starting rHuEpo) was not significant. Serum creatinine and creatinine clearance were also followed in this study, and

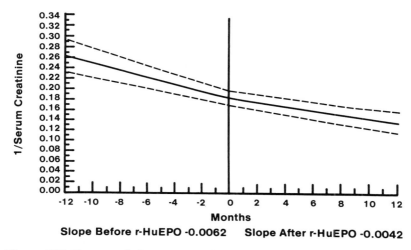

Slope Before r-HuEPO -0.0062   Slope After r-HuEPO -0.0042

Figure 17.7. The rate of change in renal function, as measured by the reciprocal of serum creatinine vs. time for 83 patients for 12 months before and after starting intravenous rHuEpo at three dose levels (50, 100, and 150 units/kg, three times per week). The difference between the slopes is not statistically significant at $P < 0.05$.

no significant difference was found between the treatment and placebo groups.

These studies, comprising 154 patients, in which renal function was studied for up to 12 months, contrast sharply with the animal studies cited above (32). Nevertheless, the physiologic basis for the animal studies and the precision of the experimental techniques used in these studies sound a credible note of caution for clinicians. If the results of these studies can be extrapolated to humans, it would seem that control of blood pressure is essential if acceleration of renal failure is to be avoided. The careful selection of antihypertensive therapy using vasodilators and angiotensin-converting enzyme inhibitors and careful adjustments of rHuEpo dosing may be critical to preserving renal function.

Because creatinine clearance and the reciprocal of serum creatinine vs. time are considered relatively unreliable measures of renal function (42), the current studies may not provide convincing clinical evidence for the safe use of rHuEpo in the treatment of anemia in predialysis patients. This question, however, will soon be answered. A placebo-controlled, double-blind, multicenter trial of rHuEpo in the treatment of anemia in chronic renal failure using [125I]iothalamate as a measure

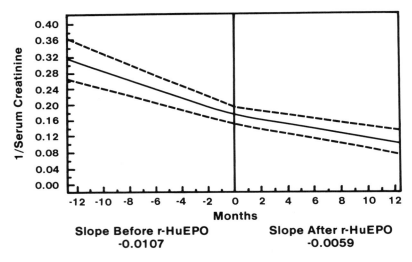

Slope Before r-HuEPO
-0.0107

Slope After r-HuEPO
-0.0059

Figure 17.8. The rate of change in renal function, as measured by the reciprocal of serum creatinine vs. time for 71 patients for 12 months before and after starting subcutaneous rHuEpo at 100 units/kg, three times per week. The difference between the slopes is not statistically significant at $P < 0.05$.

of glomerular filtration rate is currently under way. The results of this study should provide the definitive answer to the question of whether rHuEpo therapy accelerates the rate of progression of renal failure in humans with advanced renal insufficiency. While awaiting these results, the large body of clinical data suggests that the treatment of anemia in predialysis patients with rHuEpo does not accelerate the progression of renal failure when blood pressure is carefully monitored and controlled.

Resistance to rHuEpo Therapy

Several factors may result in a blunted or absent therapeutic response to rHuEpo. Absolute or relative iron deficiency is common, and serum ferritin often falls, sometimes precipitously once therapy is under way. A majority of patients require oral or parenteral iron during the restoration phase. Iron studies should be obtained before rHuEpo is started and iron supplements should be given if serum ferritin is below 100 ng/ml. Folic acid and vitamin B_{12} deficiencies are rare. Intercurrent illness (infection, inflammation), trauma, or surgery results in a marked reduction in the dose-response curve for rHuEpo. A threefold increase in dose (or more) may be required to maintain a given hematocrit after surgery or infection. Instead of "wasting" large amounts of this drug during such periods, it may be wiser to revert to the judicious use of transfusions until these catabolic states have been resolved. Metabolic bone disease may also impair the response to rHuEpo. Aluminum overload may delay the response to therapy, but hyperparathyroidism without marrow fibrosis does not diminish the therapeutic effect of rHuEpo (43).

Summary and Conclusion

Recombinant human erythropoietin is a major therapeutic advance in the treatment of the anemia of chronic renal failure. After rHuEpo therapy, there is a dose-dependent rise in hematocrit. As the hematocrit approaches normal, chromium 51 studies indicate an increase in red blood cell mass, a decrease in plasma volume, a stable total blood volume, and an increase in red blood cell half-life. A reduction in dose is often necessary once a target hematocrit has been achieved. Iron stores may be rapidly depleted, and this may result in a blunted therapeutic response. As anemia is corrected, there is both objective and subjective improvement, including increased exercise capacity, increased maximal oxygen uptake, normalization carbon monoxide-diffusing capacity, decreased evidence of tissue ischemia (angina, claudication), and an improved sense of well-being. Hypertension is common in predialysis patients before and during rHuEpo therapy. The mechanism of hypertension during rHuEpo seems to be related to reversal of the anemia-induced vasodilatation. An element of elevated cardiac output has not been rigorously excluded. Several multicenter studies in humans in which blood pressure was carefully monitored failed to confirm a single animal study that showed enhanced progression of renal failure after rHuEpo therapy. The apparent increase in seizures noted in dialysis patients has not been observed in predialysis patients.

REFERENCES

1. Teehan BP, Sigler MH, Brown JM, et al. Hematologic and physiologic studies during correction of anemia with recombinant human erythropoietin in predialysis patients. Transplant Proc 1989;21(no. 6, Suppl 2):1–5.
2. Radtke HW, Rege AB, LaMarche MB, et al. Identification of spermine

as an inhibitor of erythropoiesis in patients with chronic renal failure. J Clin Invest 1981;67:1625–9.

3. Joske RA, McAlister JM, Prankerd TAJ. Isotope investigations of red cell production and destruction in chronic renal disease. Clin Sci 1956;15:511.

4. Gafter U, Bessler H, Malachi T, et al. Platelet count and thrombopoietic activity in patients with chronic renal failure. Nephron 1987;45:207–10.

5. McGonigle RJ, Wallin JD, Shadduck RK, et al. Erythropoietin deficiency and inhibition of erythropoiesis in renal insufficiency. Kidney Int 1984;25: 437–44.

6. Segal GM, Eschbach JW, Egrie JC, et al. The anemia of end-stage renal disease: hematopoietic progenitor cell response. Kidney Int 1988;33:983–8.

7. Winearls CG, Oliver DO, Pippard MJ, et al. Effect of human erythropoietin derived from recombinant DNA on the anemia of patients maintained by chronic hemodialysis. Lancet 1986;2:1175–8.

8. Eschbach JW, Egrie JC, Downing MR, et al. Correction of the anemia of end-stage renal disease with recombinant human erythropoietin. N Engl J Med 1987;316:73–8.

9. Stone WJ, Graver SE, Krantz SB, et al. Treatment of the anemia of predialysis patients with recombinant human erythropoietin: a randomized, placebo-controlled trial. Am J Med Sci 1988;296:171–9.

10. Lim VS, DeGowin RL, Zavala D, et al. Recombinant human erythropoietin treatment in pre-dialysis patients. Ann Intern Med 1989;110:108–14.

11. Eschbach JW, Abulhadi M, Brown JK, et al. Recombinant human erythropoietin in anemic patients with end stage renal disease. Ann Intern Med 1989;111:992–1000.

12. Kushner DS, Beckman BS, Fisher JW. Do polyamines play a role in the pathogenesis of the anemia of end-stage renal disease? Kidney Int 1989;36: 171–4.

13. Woodson RD. Hemoglobin concentration and exercise capacity. Am Rev Respir Dis 1984;129(Suppl):S72–5.

14. Celsing F, Svedenhag J, Pihlstedt P, et al. Effects of anaemia and stepwise-induced polycythaemia on maximal aerobic power in individuals with high and low haemoglobin concentrations. Acta Physiol Scand 1987;129: 47–54.

15. Clyne N, Jogestrand T, Lins LE, et al. Factors limiting physical working capacity in predialysis patients. Acta Med Scand 1987;222:183–90.

16. Kampf D, Kahl A, Eckardt KU, et al. Intraindividual comparative pharmacokinetics of recombinant human erythropoietin (r-HuEPO) after IV and SC administration in CRF patients [Abstract]. Proc Eur Dial Transplant Assoc 1989;26:203.

17. Teehan BP, Krantz S, Abraham P, et al. Double-blind placebo controlled study of the therapeutic use of recombinant human erythropoietin for anemia associated with chronic renal failure in predialysis patients. Am J Kidney Dis (in press).

18. Data on file at R. W. Johnson Pharmaceutical Research Institute, 1989, protocol no. G86-053.

19. Eckardt KU, Bauer C. Erythropoietin in health and disease. Eur J Clin Invest 1989;19:117–27.

20. Granolleras C, Branger B, Deschodt B, et al. Daily self administered subcutaneous erythropoietin: the optimal form of EPO for ESRD patients [Abstract]. Proc Eur Dial Transplant Assoc 1989;26:200.

21. Graf H, Barnas U, Loibl F, et al. Subcutaneous versus intravenous administration of recombinant erythropoietin: a prospective study of effectiveness and side effects [Abstract]. Proc Eur Dial Transplant Assoc 1989;26:200.

22. Data on file at R. W. Johnson Pharmaceutical Research Institute, 1987, protocol no. G86-011.

23. Fisher JW, Bommer J, Teehan BP, et al. Statement on the clinical use of recombinant erythropoietin in anemia of end-stage renal disease: NKF position paper. Am J Kidney Dis 1989;25:163–9.

24. Goodford PJ, Norrington FE, Paterson RA, et al. The effect of 2,3-diphosphoglycerate on the oxygen dissociation curve of human haemoglobin. J Physiol (Lond) 1977;273:631–45.

25. Maxwell AP, Douglas JF, Afrasiabi M, et al. Erythropoietin pharmacokinetics and red cell metabolism in haemodialysis patients [Abstract]. Proc Eur Dial Transplant Assoc 1989;26:207.

26. Keown PA. Recombinant human erythropoietin: from concept to clinic. Dial Transplant 1988;17:629–32.

27. Eschbach JW. The anemia of chronic renal failure: pathophysiology and the effects of recombinant erythropoietin. Kidney Int 1989;35:134–48.

28. Blumenthal WS, Johnston RF, Kauffman LA. The effect of anemia on pulmonary diffusing capacity with derivation of a correction equation. Am Rev Respir Dis 1970;102:965–9.

29. Data on file at R. W. Johnson Pharmaceutical Research Institute, 1988, protocol no. G86-125.

30. Data on file at R. W. Johnson Pharmaceutical Research Institute, 1989, protocol no. H87-054.

31. Sheingold SH. Costs and benefits of recombinant human erythropoietin therapy for anemia associated with pre-dialysis chronic renal failure. Washington, D.C.: Battelle Medical Technology and Policy Research Center, 1990; report BHARC-013/89/059.

32. Garcia DL, Anderson S, Rennke H, et al. Anemia lessens and its prevention with recombinant human erythropoietin worsens glomerular injury and hypertension in rats with reduced renal mass. Proc Natl Acad Sci USA 1988;85:6142–6.

33. Brown CD, Friedman EA. Stable renal function and benign course in azotemic diabetics treated with erythropoietin (EPO) for one year [Abstract]. Kidney Int 1989;35:190.

34. Dormandy JA. Clinical significance of blood viscosity. Ann R Coll Surg Engl 1970;47:211–8.

35. Paganini E, Thomas T, Fouad F, et al. The correction of anemia in hemodialysis patients using recombinant human erythropoietin (rHuEPO): hemodynamic effects [Abstract]. Kidney Int 1988;24:204.

36. Neff M, Kim K, Persoff M, et al. Hemodynamics of uremic anemia. Circulation 1981;43:876–83.

37. Murray JF, Gold P, Johnson L. The circulatory effects of hematocrit variations in normovolemic and hypervolemic dogs. J Clin Invest 1963;42:1150–9.

38. Keane WF, Anderson S, Mattias A, et al. Angiotensin converting enzyme inhibitors and progressive renal insufficiency. Ann Intern Med 1989;111:503–16.

39. Simchon S, Chen RYZ, Carlin RD, et al. Effects of blood viscosity on

plasma renin activity and renal hemodynamics. Am J Physiol 1986;250:F40–F46.

40. Hostetter TH, Meyer TW, Rennke HG, et al. Chronic effects of dietary protein in the rat with intact and reduced renal mass. Kidney Int 1986;30:509–17.

41. Data on file at R. W. Johnson Pharmaceutical Research Institute, 1989, protocol no. H87-055.

42. Levey AS, Perrone RD, Madias NE. Serum creatinine and renal function. Annu Rev Med 1988;39:465–90.

43. Hollomby DJ, Muirhead AB, Hodsman PE, et al. The role of aluminum and PTH in erythropoietin resistance in hemodialysis patients [Abstract]. Kidney Int 1990;37:301.

Recombinant Human Erythropoietin (Epoetin Alfa and Beta) in Patients on Ambulatory Peritoneal Dialysis

Iain C. Macdougall, Judith M. Stevens,
Rowland T. Hughes, R. David Hutton,
Gerald A. Coles, and John D. Williams

The majority of patients with end-stage renal failure suffer from moderate to severe anemia. After the start of dialysis, the hematocrit will often spontaneously improve and tends to do so to a greater degree with continuous ambulatory peritoneal dialysis (CAPD) than with hemodialysis; several studies reported a significant increase in red cell mass during the first few months of the former treatment (1–3). Consequently, the need for regular transfusions is relatively uncommon in patients on CAPD. However, a minority of patients continue to have a degree of anemia sufficient to impair effort tolerance and quality of life. The exact proportion of patients who would benefit from erythropoietin is unknown. In Cardiff, of 127 adults on CAPD for more than 3 months, 28 had a hemoglobin value of less than 8.0 g/dl and 50 had levels of 8.1 to 10.0 g/dl. Depending on the exact criteria used for prescribing erythropoietin, this means that up to 61 percent of CAPD patients might be suitable for this hormone treatment. Because the number of patients receiving this type of dialysis worldwide is increasing, there is a considerable potential for erythropoietin therapy.

Early studies with erythropoietin were concerned solely with hemodialysis subjects and utilized intravenous dosing. Clearly, this route of administration is impractical for CAPD subjects, and two alternative routes, intraperitoneal and subcutaneous, have been investigated. Experiments in rabbits suggested that significant quantities of erythropoietin would be absorbed when given intraperitoneally, even in the presence of dialysate (4), but subsequent investigations in CAPD patients failed to confirm this. The relative bioavailability of intraperitoneal erythropoietin administered with the dialysate compared to the same dose administered intravenously ranged from 2.5 to 8.5 percent (5–8), indicating that intraperitoneal administration would require higher doses than would intravenous administration and thus would be more expensive.

After subcutaneous dosing, plasma levels of erythropoietin rise after 2 hours and peak at 12 to 24 hours (5–7,9). Subsequently, levels slowly decline, but at 96 hours they are still higher than baseline values (5). The bioavailability of subcutaneous erythropoietin expressed as a percentage of the same dose administered intravenously has varied from 10 percent (6) to 49 percent (7), but the majority of studies report values of approximately 20 percent (5,10,11).

These findings suggested that subcutaneous administration of erythropoietin two or three times per week could provide an increase in the concentration of erythropoietin in the serum of sufficient magnitude and duration to maintain the stimulus for increased red cell production and is therefore likely to be an effective mode of administration. One further consideration was whether the mode of dialysis itself would affect the dose of the hormone. It was thus reassuring to find that losses of erythropoietin in the dialysate after intravenous administration were less than 3 percent and could, for practical purposes, be ignored (5,6).

With this knowledge, our centers have studied the treatment of anemia with subcutaneous erythropoietin in CAPD patients. The remainder of this chapter describes the results, clinical benefits, and problems encountered.

The Cardiff Study

Fifteen patients, 3 male and 12 female, were investigated. They had all been on CAPD for a minimum of 20 months. Their ages ranged from 23 to 74 years, and the renal disease was glomerulonephritis in 3, pyelonephritis in 3, hypertension in 2, postpartum in 2, obstructive uropathy in 1, and of undetermined cause in 4. Each patient had a hemoglobin concentration of less than 8.0 g/dl. All patients had a ferritin value of more than 24 μg/litre, and none had vitamin B_{12} or folate depletion. Causes of anemia other than renal failure were excluded. Patients continued with their usual CAPD regime and received ferrous sulfate, 200 to 600 mg daily.

Recombinant human erythropoietin (rHuEpo) (epoetin beta; Boehringer-Mannheim) was dissolved in sterile water and injected subcutaneously at one or two sites on the upper arms so that the volume administered was a maximum of 1 ml at any one site. The starting dose was 60 units/kg twice weekly. This was increased to three times per week if no response had occurred after 4 weeks of therapy. Further adjustments were made as necessary. The target hemoglobin was 10 to 12 g/dl, and the desired rate of rise was 1 g/dl/month.

The Oxford-Hammersmith Clinical Research Centre Study

Sixteen patients, 9 male and 7 female, were studied. They had been on CAPD for a mean period of 32.8 months (range, 3.5 to 92). Their ages ranged from 25 to 74 years, and the primary diagnosis was glomerulonephritis in 4, hypertension in 3, vascular disease in 3, cortical necrosis in 1, polycystic disease in 1, pyelonephritis in 2, diabetes in 1, and amyloidosis in 1. The starting hemoglobin value was 9.0 g/dl or less (mean ± SD, 7.2 ± 0.9). Patients continued their usual CAPD regime, and 9 were taking oral iron supplements. Causes of anemia other than renal failure were excluded, but 1 patient with the β-thalassemia trait and 1 with homozygous α-thalassemia 2 were included in the study. Both had achieved normal hemoglobin concentrations in the past after renal transplantation.

rHuEpo (epoetin alfa; Ortho) was administered as a single dose in the upper thigh. The starting dose was initially 150 units/kg three times per week, which three patients received. Because the rate of rise of hemoglobin in these patients was too rapid, all others were commenced on 100 units/kg three times per week. In each patient, the dose of rHuEpo was adjusted so that the hemoglobin concentration achieved and maintained for a period of at least 4 weeks was initially 11 to 11.5 g/dl and was then 13 to 13.5 g/dl.

Hematologic Response

Of the 15 individuals treated in the Cardiff study, 10 achieved a hemoglobin value of more than 10 g/dl within 16 weeks and were classified as good responders (Fig 18.1). Four of the remaining 5 individuals had an increase in their hemoglobin concentration but failed to reach the target level. Two of these 4 had persistent infection, 1 was found to have marrow fibrosis probably due to secondary hyperparathyroidism,

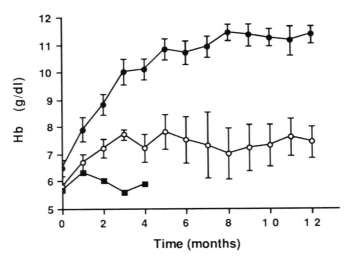

Figure 18.1. The response of hemoglobin (Hb) to rHuEpo treatment in the Cardiff patients on continuous ambulatory peritoneal dialysis. Closed circles indicate the mean values of the 10 good responders; open circles, mean values of the 4 poor responders; closed squares, hemoglobin values of the 1 nonresponder.

and 1 patient died suddenly after 3 months of treatment. The remaining patient showed no response at all despite a severalfold increase in rHuEpo dosage over a 3-month period. She was subsequently found to have liver metastases from a carcinoma of the breast removed 3½ years previously and died a few weeks later.

Fifteen of the 16 patients at the Oxford-Hammersmith Clinical Research Centre had a rise of hemoglobin of at least 2 g/dl. Fourteen subjects achieved the first target of 11.0 to 11.5 g/dl, and 7 reached the final target hemoglobin concentration of 13.0 to 13.5 g/dl. The patient with no response had a pyrexia of unknown origin and was withdrawn from the study after 10 weeks of therapy. Two subjects had impaired responses. One was found to be homozygous for α-thalassemia 2 and also had osteomyelitis. The other had a satisfactory initial rise in hematocrit, but this subsequently fell; the response to rHuEpo returned with a rise to 12 g/dl only after removal of infected pins from an old fracture site.

Dosage of rHuEpo

In the Cardiff study, the initial dosage was 120 units/kg/week. The final maintenance dosage in the good responders was 60 to 240 units/

kg/week, with 6 of the 10 patients receiving 120 units/kg/week. During the Oxford-Hammersmith Clinical Research Centre trial, the median dosage required to maintain a hemoglobin concentration of 11.0 to 11.5 g/dl was 75 units/kg/week, with a range of 37.5 to 375 ($N = 14$). The median dosage necessary to maintain the final target concentration of 13.0 to 13.5 g/dl was 150 units/kg/week, with a range of 75 to 300 units/kg ($N = 7$).

Results

Iron Status

Intravenous iron was given to the Cardiff patients when the transferrin saturation fell below 20 percent. A total of 17 doses of 2 ml of iron dextran (100 mg of elemental iron) each were administered to 12 patients. Increased doses of oral iron were prescribed to the Oxford-Hammersmith Clinical Research Centre patients when the ferritin value fell below 100 μg/litre. One individual was unable to tolerate ferrous sulfate by mouth, however, and her hemoglobin response improved with parenteral iron therapy. Another patient responded slowly to oral iron and was therefore given intravenous treatment.

White Cell and Platelet Counts

In neither study were there significant changes in the white cell or platelet count.

Ferrokinetic Data

Red cell and plasma volumes were measured in the patients at Oxford-Hammersmith Clinical Research Centre using ^{51}Cr-labeled red cells and ^{59}Fe-labeled transferrin (12). Of 15 patients who were studied before rHuEpo administration, 9 were restudied at a hemoglobin concentration of 11 to 11.5 g/dl and 6 underwent a third study at a hemoglobin of 13 to 13.5 g/dl.

Before rHuEpo, red cell volumes were subnormal (mean, 10.5 ml/kg, $n = 15$). When the hemoglobin concentration had increased to 11 to 11.5 g/dl, the mean red cell volume was 16.2 ml/kg ($n = 9$) and at 13 to 13.5 g/dl it was 20.4 ml/kg ($n = 6$) (Fig 18.2). There was a reciprocal fall in plasma volume at each stage so that total blood volume remained unchanged.

Erythron transferrin uptake, a measure of marrow activity (14), was also assessed in the same patients. When the hemoglobin concentration had reached 11 to 11.5 g/dl, the erythron transferrin uptake had increased in six patients, was unchanged in two, and had fallen in one.

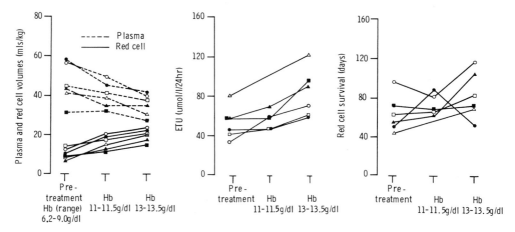

Figure 18.2. Changes in erythrokinetics with rHuEpo treatment in the Oxford-Hammersmith Clinical Research Centre patients on continuous ambulatory peritoneal dialysis. Left panel, changes in individual plasma (dashed lines) and red cell (solid lines) volumes; center panel, changes in erythron transferrin uptake (ETU); right panel, changes in red cell survival. Hb, hemoglobin. *Source: Reference 13*

All six individuals studied at a hemoglobin concentration of 13 to 13.5 g/dl showed an increase in erythron transferrin uptake (Fig 18.2).

In the six patients studied on three occasions, red cell survival had not significantly changed at a hemoglobin concentration of 11 to 11.5 g/dl but, when retested at a hemoglobin concentration of 13 to 13.5 g/dl (after 36 to 62 weeks), mean red cell survival had significantly increased compared to the pretreatment value (mean increase at 20 days and a 95 percent confidence interval, 1 to 39 days) (Fig 18.2).

Biochemical Changes

Both studies serially recorded urea, creatinine, electrolyte, and phosphate levels in plasma. No significant changes were seen in any of the patients.

Peritoneal Function

Eight of the Cardiff patients were studied with a peritoneal equilibration test (15) before rHuEpo therapy and after reaching the target hemoglobin concentration. There were no significant changes in ultrafiltration volume, plasma/dialysate creatinine ratios, or 0- to 4-hour dialysate glucose concentration ratios. Peritoneal creatinine clearance was measured in the Oxford-Hammersmith Clinical Research Centre trial. In comparison with preerythropoietin treatment values, no significant changes were found at hemoglobin concentrations of 11.0 to 11.5 g/dl or 13.0 to 13.5 g/dl.

Cardiovascular Effects

Taking the two studies together, a total of 4 previously normotensive individuals required antihypertensive therapy and 12 patients already on treatment had to increase the dose of their drugs. As a consequence, no statistically significant changes were seen in mean systolic or diastolic pressures in the groups as a whole.

Despite these observations, the Oxford-Hammersmith Clinical Research Centre patients were found to have a decrease in mean cardiothoracic ratio from 0.51 preerythropoietin to 0.48 at a hemoglobin concentration of 11.0 to 11.5 g/dl ($P < 0.007$) and to 0.47 at a level of 13.0 to 13.5 g/dl ($P < 0.02$). Seven of the Cardiff patients had formal exercise testing before erythropoietin treatment and after the hemoglobin concentration reached 10.0 g/dl. They had a significant increase in exercise duration ($P < 0.001$) and maximal oxygen consumption ($P < 0.01$).

Adverse Effects

There were three deaths during the trials, but none of these was thought to be due to rHuEpo therapy. One patient had transient myalgia, and another had occlusion of a popliteal artery, which resolved on heparin therapy despite continuation of rHuEpo treatment.

Discussion

Our studies show that subcutaneous administration of rHuEpo to subjects on CAPD is effective in correcting the anemia associated with end-stage renal disease. The dosage regimes chosen by our centers were different, one starting with a low dose and increasing as necessary and the other deliberately commencing with a high dose to achieve an early boost to the hemoglobin concentrations. Despite these differences, the final maintenance doses necessary to keep the hemoglobin at approximately 11 g/dl were similar in the two patient groups. It has been demonstrated that subcutaneous administration of rHuEpo is more efficient than intravenous administration (16), so it was not surprising to find that, to maintain the same concentration of hemoglobin, our CAPD patients generally required less rHuEpo than did hemodialysis patients receiving rHuEpo intravenously. An alternative to subcutaneous administration two or three times per week which merits further evaluation is daily low-dose subcutaneous rHuEpo. This may permit a further reduction in the total amount of rHuEpo required to maintain an adequate concentration of hemoglobin (17).

Our studies suggest that starting doses of 40 to 60 IU/kg two or three times per week are ideal, whereas higher doses, particularly those of 100 IU/kg or more three times per week, may induce a rise in hemoglobin concentration at a rate that would considerably increase the risk of hypertension and seizures.

Intraperitoneal administration of rHuEpo is effective (18), but high doses are necessary and, although it is a convenient method of administration, it cannot be considered for regular use. Perhaps the only indication is for subjects on intermittent peritoneal dialysis as it has been suggested that the bioavailability of erythropoietin is markedly increased when given into a dialysate-free abdomen (19). It seems unlikely, however, that this method will be superior to the subcutaneous route.

Iron supplementation is frequently required in hemodialysis patients during rHuEpo therapy, partially because of continued blood loss but mainly because of the iron requirement of the expanding erythron (20). Many of our CAPD patients also required additional iron to maintain the increase in erythroid activity. We suggest that biochemical parameters of iron status, including ferritin and percentage of saturation of the total iron-binding capacity, should be serially measured in all patients treated with rHuEpo. This should stop the development of functional iron deficiency, which, in our experience, is a relatively common cause of an inadequate response to treatment (21).

The increase in erythron transferrin uptake in the patients in the Oxford-Hammersmith Clinical Research Centre study as they received increasing doses of rHuEpo supports evidence that erythroid activity is directly related to the availability of erythropoietin (12).

An improvement in red cell survival during treatment with rHuEpo has not been a consistent finding. In CAPD patients treated for 2 months (22) and in hemodialysis patients treated for 4 to 7 months (12) or for 5 months (23), red cell survival did not alter significantly. However, in hemodialysis patients treated for longer periods (24), the red cell survival showed a significant increase, suggesting that the effect may be related to duration of treatment. The mechanism of this effect of treatment with rHuEpo is unclear, but it seems possible that correction of the hemostatic defect of uremia (25) may contribute by reducing occult gastrointestinal losses, which may be greater than normal in patients on hemodialysis (26).

It has been suggested that hemodialysis patients receiving rHuEpo have a tendency to higher plasma potassium and/or phosphate levels, possibly due to the increased viscosity reducing the efficiency of the dialyser. It was therefore important to find no changes in any biochemical parameter in the CAPD patients despite the rising hematocrit. In addition, it was gratifying that no changes in peritoneal function were found. Steinhauer et al. (27) reported an increase in net ultrafiltration volume during rHuEpo therapy. The discrepancy with our findings is as yet unexplained.

Important improvements in cardiorespiratory function are seen with rHuEpo treatment in hemodialysis patients (28–30). The current studies confirm that these beneficial results apply equally to CAPD patients. The reduction in cardiothoracic ratio probably reflects in part a fall in left ventricular mass (30). The latter is reported to be an independent risk factor for dialysis patients (31), and we hope that its decrease will be followed by an improved prognosis. The increases in exercise duration and oxygen consumption represent the direct effect of the increase in oxygen-carrying ability of the blood as the hematocrit rises.

Hypertension remains the most serious side effect of rHuEpo therapy. Half of our patients needed to start or increase antihypertensive medication. It is clearly important that blood pressure be monitored closely during treatment with this hormone, irrespective of the mode of renal replacement therapy.

True resistance to erythropoietin is said to be rare (32). However, two of our patients failed to respond, one because of previously undiagnosed carcinomatosis and the other as a result of a pyrexia of unknown origin. Of more importance was the fact that several of our patients had impaired responses because of infection. This emphasizes the importance of looking for iron deficiency, infection, or occult malignancy before considering an increase in the dose of rHuEpo in any patient who fails to have an adequate response to treatment.

Conclusion

Subcutaneous rHuEpo is effective in correcting the anemia associated with end-stage renal disease when administered to patients on CAPD. As with hemodialysis patients, it is important to monitor blood pressure and iron status to minimize side effects and maximize the efficiency of this form of hormone-replacement therapy.

ACKNOWLEDGMENTS

We are grateful to Boehringer-Mannheim and Ortho Pharmaceutical Corporations for supplies of recombinant human erythropoietin and for financial support.

REFERENCES

1. DePaepe MBJ, Schelstraete KHG, Ringoir SMG, Lameire NH. Influence of continuous ambulatory peritoneal dialysis on the anaemia of end-stage renal disease. Kidney Int 1983;23:744–8.
2. Summerfield GB, Gyde DHB, Forbes AMW, Goldsmith HJ, Bellingham AJ. Haemoglobin concentration and serum erythropoietin in renal dialysis and transplant patients. S and J Haematol 1983;30:389–400.
3. Saltissi D, Coles GA, Napier JAF, Bentley P. The haematological response to continuous ambulatory peritoneal dialysis. Clin Nephol 1984;22:21–7.
4. Bargman JM, Breborowicz A, Rodela H, Somboles K, Oreopoulous DG. Intraperitoneal administration of recombinant human erythropoietin in uremic animals. Perit Dial Int 1988;8:249–52.
5. Macdougall IC, Roberts DE, Neubert P, Dharmasena AD, Coles GA, Williams JD. Pharmacokinetics of recombinant human erythropoietin in patients on continuous ambulatory peritoneal dialysis. Lancet 1989;1:425–7.
6. Boelaert JR, Schurgers ML, Malthys EG, et al. Comparative pharmacokinetics of recombinant erythropoietin administered by the intravenous, subcutaneous and intraperitoneal routes in continuous ambulatory peritoneal dialysis patients. Perit Dial Int 1989;9:95–8.
7. Kampf D, Kahl A, Passlick J, et al. Single dose kinetics of recombinant human erythropoietin after intravenous, subcutaneous and intraperitoneal administration. Contrib Nephrol 1989;76:106–11.
8. Gahl GM, Passlick J, Pustelnick A, et al. Intraperitoneal versus intravenous recombinant human erythropoietin in stable CAPD patients [Abstract]. Presented at the EDTA annual meeting, Gothenburg, 1989:199.
9. Hughes RT, Cotes PM, Oliver DO, et al. Correction of the anaemia of chronic renal failure with erythropoietin: pharmacokinetic studies in patients on haemodialysis and CAPD. Contrib Nephrol 1989;76:122–30.
10. Neumayer HH, Brockmoller J, Fritschka E, Roots I, Scigalla P, Wattenberg M. Pharmacokinetics of recombinant human erythropoietin after SC administration and in longterm IV treatment in patients on maintenance hemodialysis. Contrib Nephrol 1989;76:131–42.
11. Salmonson T, Danielson BG, Wikstrom B. Pharmacokinetics and pharmacodynamics of recombinant erythropoietin after SC and IV administration [Abstract]. Presented at the EDTA annual meeting, Gothenburg, 1989:210.
12. Cotes PM, Pippard MJ, Reid CDL, Winearls CG, Oliver DO, Royston JP.

Characterization of the anaemia of chronic renal failure and the mode of its correction by a preparation of human erythropoietin (r-HuEPO): an investigation of the pharmacokinetics of intravenous erythropoietin and its effects on erythrokinetics. Q J Med 1989;70:113–37.

13. Hughes RT, Cotes PM, Pippard MJ, et al. Subcutaneous administration of recombinant human erythropoietin to subjects on continuous ambulatory peritoneal dialysis: an erythrokinetic study. Br J Haematol 1990;75:268–73.

14. Cazzola M, Pootrakul P, Huebers HA, Eng M, Eschbach J, Finch CA. Erythroid marrow function in anemic patients. Blood 1987;69:296–301.

15. Twardowski ZJ, Nolph KD, Khanna R, et al. Peritoneal equilibration test. Perit Dial Bull 1987;7:138–47.

16. Eschbach JW, Kelly MR, Haley NR, Abels RI, Adamson JW. Treatment of the anemia of progressive renal failure with recombinant human erythropoietin. N Engl J Med 1989;321:158–63.

17. Granolleras C, Branger B, Beau MC, Deschodt G, Alsabadanic B, Shaldon S. Experience with daily self-administration subcutaneous erythropoietin. Contrib Nephrol 1989;76:143–8.

18. Frenken LAM, Coppers PJW, Tiggeler RGWL, Koene RAP. Intraperitoneal erythropoietin [Letter]. Lancet 1989;2:1495.

19. Kromer G, Solf A, Ehmer B, Kaufmann B, Quellhorst E. Single dose pharmacokinetics of recombinant human erythropoietin comparing intravenous, subcutaneous and intraperitoneal administration in IPD patients [Abstract]. Kidney Int 1990;37:33.1.

20. Eschbach JW, Egrie JC, Downing MR, Browne JK, Adamson JW. Correction of the anaemia of end-stage renal disease with recombinant human erythropoietin. N Engl J Med 1987;316:73–8.

21. Macdougall IC, Hutton RD, Cavill I, Coles GA, Williams JD. Poor response to treatment of renal anaemia with erythropoietin corrected by iron given intravenously. Br Med J 1989;229:157–8.

22. Macdougall IC, Cavill I, Davies ME, Hutton RD, Coles GA, Williams JD. Subcutaneous recombinant erythropoietin in the treatment of renal anaemia in CAPD patients. Contrib Nephrol 1989;76:219–26.

23. Zehnder C, Blumberg A. Human recombinant erythropoietin treatment in transfusion dependent anemic patients on maintenance haemodialysis. Clin Nephrol 1989;31:55–9.

24. Eschbach JW. The anemia of chronic renal failure: pathophysiology and the effects of recombinant erythropoietin. Kidney Int 1989;35:134–48.

25. van Geet C, Hauglustaine D, Verresen L, Vanrusselt M, Vermylen J. Haemostatic effects of recombinant erythropoietin in chronic haemodialysis patients. Thromb Haemost 1989;61:117–21.

26. Rosenblatt S, Lifschitz M, Welch R, Fadem S, Stein J. Gastrointestinal blood loss and iron deficiency in patients on chronic haemodialysis [Abstract]. Kidney Int 1977;12:488.

27. Steinhauer HB, Lubrick-Birkner I, Dreyling KW, Horl WH, Schollmeyer P. Increased ultrafiltration after erythropoietin induced correction of renal anaemia in patients on continuous ambulatory peritoneal dialysis. Nephron 1989;53:91–2.

28. Mayer G, Thum J, Cade EM, Stummvoll HK, Graf H. Working capacity is increased following recombinant human erythropoietin treatment. Kidney Int 1988;34:525–8.

29. London GM, Zius B, Pannier B, et al. Vascular changes in hemodialysis

patients in response to recombinant human erythropoietin. Kidney Int 1989; 36:878–82.

30. Macdougall IC, Lewis NP, Saunders MJ, et al. Long-term cardiorespiratory effects of the partial correction of renal anaemia by recombinant human erythropoietin. Lancet 1990;335:489–93.

31. Silberberg JS, Barre PE, Prichard SS, Sniderman AD. Impact of left ventricular hypertrophy on survival in end-stage renal disease. Kidney Int 1989; 36:286–90.

32. Eschbach JW, Downing MR, Egrie JC, Browne JK, Adamson JW. USA multicenter clinical trial with recombinant human erythropoietin (Amgen). Contrib Nephrol 1989;76:160–5.

Chapter 19

Recombinant Human Erythropoietin (Epoetin Beta) in Children with Renal Anemia: Western Europe

Paul Scigalla

Renal anemia is more serious in children than in adults and is largely responsible for the reduced physical stamina of children with end-stage renal failure (1). The transfusion requirement of end-stage renal failure in children is higher than that of adults (2). Transfusions can arrest the reduced stamina, which is usually accompanied by impaired memory and power of concentration. Disadvantages of these polytransfusions are the formation of cytotoxic antibodies (1,3) (which renders kidney transplantation more difficult or even impossible), the transmission of infections (such as non-A, non-B hepatitis or AIDS), or iron overload (which may lead to chronic liver damage and to myocardial or endo-crinologic disturbances) (4).

The growth of children with end-stage renal failure is usually in-hibited. The pathogenesis of this growth retardation is multifactorial, but anemia is assumed to be one of the factors (5–8). This indicates the medical necessity of correcting renal anemia. Until a few years ago, renal anemia could be treated only by the administration of cobalt (9) or androgens (10,11), by the optimization of the hemodialysis regi-mens, or by blood transfusion. Recombinant human erythropoietin (rHuEpo) now also offers the possibility of a causative treatment of ane-mia in uremic children.

On the basis of previous experience with rHuEpo in the therapy of renal anemia in adults, children with end-stage renal failure were treated with rHuEpo in a European multicenter trial launched in Jan-uary 1988. The objectives of this clinical trial were and remain (a) to investigate the influence of rHuEpo therapy on the transfusion require-

Table 19.1. Centers Participating in Clinical Trials of rHuEpo, with the Number of Patients and the Investigators

Center	Number of Patients	Investigator
Berlin	11	Zoellner
Cologne	4	von Lilien
Essen/Moers	10	Bonzel
Frankfurt/Main	1	Dippell
Freiburg	2	Leititis
Hamburg	1	Schwarke
Hanover	10	Offner
Heidelberg	3	Müller-Wiefel
Lille	3	Foulard
Marburg	2	Gordjani
Münster	6	Bulla
Nancy	4	Andre
Nantes	3	Guyot
Paris	8	Loirat
	9	Bensman
Reims	2	Roussel
Rouen	6	Landthaler
Strasbourg	6	Geisert
Toulouse	5	Barthe
Zurich	4	Leumann

ment of children with end-stage renal failure, (*b*) to investigate the possibility of reducing the iron overload of children with end-stage renal failure by stimulating erythropoiesis through rHuEpo, (*c*) to investigate the influence of rHuEpo therapy on children's linear growth, and (*d*) to investigate the tolerance of rHuEpo in long-term therapy.

This chapter summarizes the experiences of 100 patients from 20 pediatric nephrology centers throughout Western Europe. At the time of interim evaluation (March 15, 1989), the patients had been treated with rHuEpo for an average of 28 weeks (range, 1 to 89 weeks).

Patients and Methods

One hundred patients from 20 pediatric nephrology centers had been included in the clinical trial and treated with rHuEpo by March 15, 1989. Table 19.1 lists the participating centers, with the respective number of patients and the responsible physicians. Of the 100 children,

51 were boys and 49 were girls, with an average age of 13 years (range, 2 to 20 years). The average previous duration of dialysis when entering the trial was 24 months (range, 1 to 144 months). Ninety patients were treated by hemodialysis (4 to 6 hours three times per week), and 10 were treated with continuous ambulatory peritoneal dialysis.

In 44 children, the primary diseases that had caused end-stage renal failure were hereditary nephropathies: cystinosis in 8, kidney hypoplasia or dysplasia in 17, nephronophthisis in 5, polycystic kidney disease in 4, Malta fever in 2, oligomeganephronia in 3, Goodpasture syndrome in 1, Bor syndrome in 1, Alport syndrome in 2, and oxalosis in 1. In 15 children, the primary diseases were congenital nephropathies: ureterovesical reflux in 6, megalocystic/megalourethral urethral valve in 5, chronic pyelonephritis in 4. In 41 children, the primary diseases were acquired nephropathies.

Before the start of rHuEpo therapy, the mean hemoglobin value was 6.3 g/dl (range, 5.7 to 7.0), the average hematocrit was 19.3 (range, 17.2 to 21.1), and the mean corpuscular hemoglobin concentration was 34.7 g/dl (range, 33.4 to 36.0). The average corrected reticulocyte value was 0.42 percent (range, 0.20 to 0.68). These data demonstrate that, despite the transfusions, the children suffered from severe normochromic hypoproliferative anemia before rHuEpo therapy.

Of the 100 children with renal failure who were treated with rHuEpo, 87 were transfusion-dependent when they entered the trial; 62 had received a minimum of 600 ml of blood during the 6 months preceding the trial. The average frequency of transfusion was 44 days (range, 11 to 120 days).

Children with end-stage renal failure who had renal anemia (hematocrit of less than 28), children who had been polytransfused (three transfusion units of ≥ 150 ml blood) during the preceding 6 months, and children with iron overload were included in the trial. Not included were children who had additionally been treated with cytostatic agents, hormone preparations, or immunosuppressants; children with systemic disease (e.g., tumor, epilepsy, diabetes mellitus); or children with folic acid, vitamin B_{12}, or iron deficiency. Another important criterion for nonparticipation was hard-to-control hypertension (changes in antihypertensive therapy during the preceding 4 months).

The Protocol of the Clinical Trials

After a 14-day run-in period during which the pretreatment values for the individual efficacy and safety parameters were repeatedly obtained, rHuEpo therapy was commenced. The patients included in the hemodialysis program were given rHuEpo three times per week intravenously, at the end of each hemodialysis. At the start of the trial, the initial dose was 100 units/kg body weight three times per week. As a result of experience in other clinical trials, because of the fact that there seemed to be a direct relationship between the development or aggravation of hypertension and the rate of increase in hematocrit, and also because there was no need for a fast correction of renal anemia, the initial dose was reduced to 80 units/kg and subsequently to 40 units/ kg (three times per week). This meant that 49 children received 100 units/kg three times per week, 24 children received 80 units/kg three times per week, and 17 children received 40 units/kg three times per week. The 10 CAPD patients on continuous ambulatory peritoneal dialysis were given 300 units of rHuEpo per kg intravenously once a week (2).

When the hematocrit was stable above 30 percent for a minimum of 2 weeks and when there was no further transfusion requirement (at the end of the correction period), the rHuEpo dosage was reduced to 30 units/kg three times per week. Further changes in the dosage were dependent upon the hematocrit and were made at the discretion of the participating physician.

Results

After rHuEpo therapy, a stimulation of erythropoiesis occurred. This was initially discerned through an increase in the reticulocyte count (Fig 19.1). With a 1-week delay, an increase in hematocrit was also observed, and the hematocrit was raised in all children included in the trial (Fig 19.2).

The weekly increase in hematocrit was dose-dependent. After the administration of 40 units/kg three times per week, the average increase was 0.64 percent; after the administration of 80 units/kg three times per week, the average increase was 0.72 percent; and after the administration of 100 units/kg three times per week, the average increase was 1.07 percent (Fig 19.3).

No significant difference in the hematocrit increase was observed between hemodialysis patients and patients on continuous ambulatory peritoneal dialysis. The response to rHuEpo showed very large individual differences, however. This may be accounted for by the multifactorial pathogenesis of renal anemia (12). The existence of different pathogenetic factors, such as absolute or functional iron deficiency, obscure

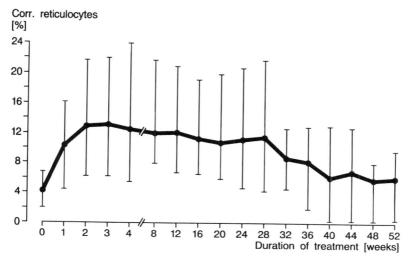

Figure 19.1. The course of corrected reticulocytes in children with end-stage renal failure during rHuEpo therapy (median and interquartile range).

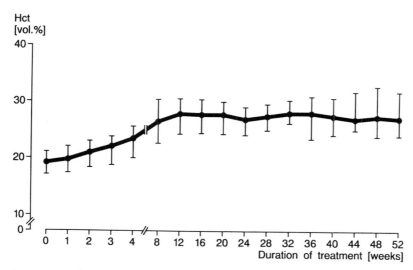

Figure 19.2. The course of the hematocrit (Hct) in children with end-stage renal failure during rHuEpo therapy (median and interquartile range).

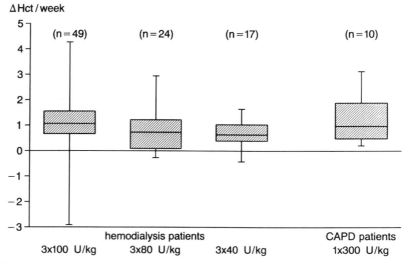

Figure 19.3. Increase in the hematocrit (ΔHct) per week in children with end-stage renal failure. CAPD, continuous ambulatory peritoneal dialysis.

blood loss, aluminum overload, secondary hyperparathyroidism, mye-lofibrosis, or the accumulation of possible erythropoiesis-inhibiting fac-tors, shows large individual differences (12).

During rHuEpo therapy, a reduction occurred in the transfusion-induced iron overload. This is demonstrated by the drop in serum ferritin levels. The iron stored in the reticuloendothelial system is mo-bilized and made available for erythropoiesis (2). The serum ferritin is a good measurement of the depot iron, and the transferrin saturation is an indication of the bioavailability of the iron (13). When the uptake of iron into the bone marrow is higher than the supply of iron (diet + iron mobilization from the depots + possible exogenous substitution), a functional iron deficiency may develop, even in polytransfused pa-tients (14–17). Figure 19.4 depicts the effect of transferrin saturation. At the 4th week, the 25th interquartile is at 15 percent and thus below the standard range. This means that more than 25 percent of the pa-tients developed a functional iron deficiency despite iron overload and exogenous iron substitution. This deficiency is in part responsible for the reduced response to rHuEpo (2) and accounts in part for the large fluctuations in the individual responses to rHuEpo (see also Fig 19.3).

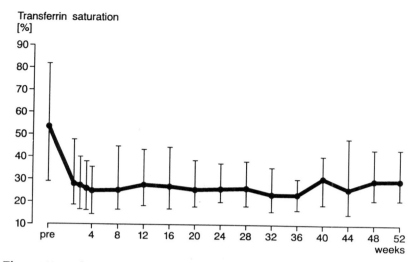

Figure 19.4. The course of transferrin saturation in children with end-stage renal failure before and during rHuEpo therapy. Pretreatment, $n = 84$; after 52 weeks, $n = 18$.

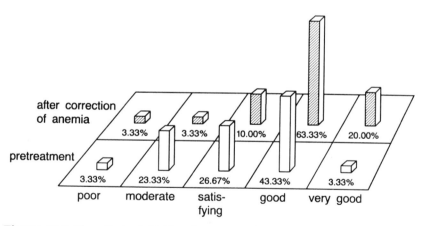

Figure 19.5. The effect of rHuEpo therapy on the appetite of children with end-stage renal failure ($n = 30$).

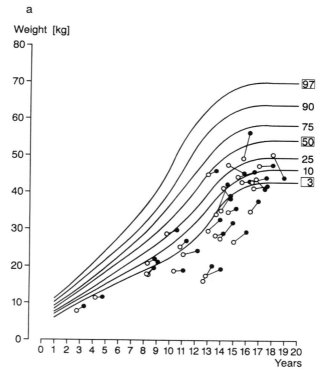

Figure 19.6. a, The effect of rHuEpo therapy on the body weight of girls with end-stage renal failure. (Duration of treatment: median, 277 days; range, 187 to 506 days; $n = 30$.) 0 = start of rHuEpo therapy.

The appetites of 30 of the 100 patients before and after the correction of renal anemia were evaluated by the same attending physician or nurse. A distinct improvement in appetite is evident under rHuEpo therapy (Fig 19.5). Almost all children gained weight during the trial (>180 days). The increase, however, is not disproportionate but runs mostly parallel to the age- and sex-specific percentile curves (Fig 19.6).

It is not known whether rHuEpo in itself has an effect on growth. Body measurements before and after therapy are available on 52 children (29 boys and 23 girls) who were treated with rHuEpo for an average of 238 or 243 days. The growth rates indicate that the children's growth accorded with the percentile curves, and there was no indication of an acceleration of growth (Fig 19.7). However, it is not yet possible to make a final evaluation of the effect on body growth of correcting

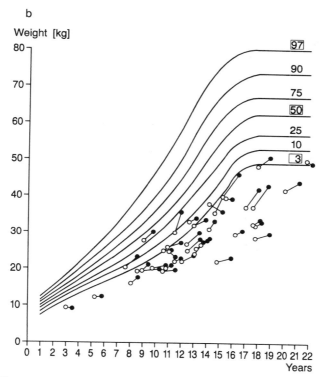

b, The effect of rHuEpo therapy on the body weight of boys with end-stage renal failure. (Duration of treatment: median, 287 days; range, 184 to 651 days; $n = 38$.) 0 = start of rHuEpo therapy.

renal anemia. When data from all of the children treated for 1 year or longer are available, an evaluation of the growth rate before as well as during rHuEpo therapy can be made.

Therapy with rHuEpo led to a distinct improvement in the general well-being of the children with end-stage renal failure. These data were obtained by questioning 30 of the 100 children before and after the correction of renal anemia by the same attending physician or nurse (Fig 19.8).

Ergometric investigations were performed on 10 children before and after the correction of renal anemia. The increase in hematocrit resulted in a significant increase in the maximal physical working capacity, to an average value of approximately 30 percent (Fig 19.9) (18).

The transfusion dependency of all children was eliminated with

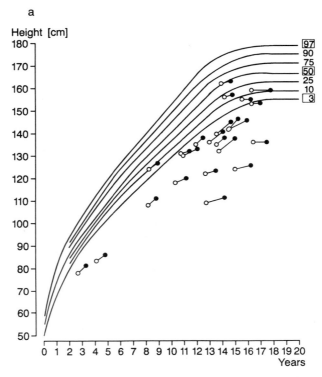

Figure 19.7. The effect of rHuEpo therapy on the growth of girls with end-stage renal failure. (Duration of treatment: median, 243 days; range, 195 to 520 days; $n = 23$.) 0 = start of rHuEpo therapy.

rHuEpo therapy. Figure 19.10 shows that, as of the 3rd month of therapy, no child with terminal renal insufficiency required further transfusions. The two transfusions in the 5th month were the results of acute events (shunt operation, intestinal surgery).

Information on cytotoxic antibodies before and after the correction of anemia in 34 children is available. Before the onset of rHuEpo therapy, cytotoxic antibodies were detectable in 21 children but not in 13 children. At the time of the interim evaluation (after an average of 28 weeks), cytotoxic antibodies were no longer detectable in 10 of the 21 primarily positive children; a significant reduction in titer was determined in 4 children. In another 4 of the 21 primarily positive children, the cytotoxic antibody titers remained unchanged, and an increase was

b

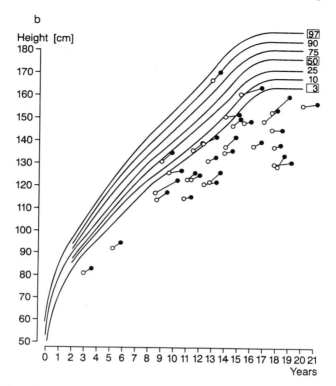

b, The effect of rHuEpo therapy on the growth of boys with end-stage renal failure. (Duration of treatment: median, 238 days; range, 182 to 607 days; $n = 29$.) 0 = start of rHuEpo therapy.

observed in 2 children. No further data are available on one primarily positive child.

Although rHuEpo therapy has highly beneficial effects (improvement in the physical working capacity, elimination of the requirement for transfusion, reduction in cytotoxic antibodies), it is accompanied by a number of side effects in children (Tables 19.2 and 19.3). The trial had to be discontinued for six children because of the adverse events. Two children died from the sequelae of pneumonia during the observation period; however, there is no indication of a causal relationship between rHuEpo therapy and the disease leading to death.

The most important adverse event observed during rHuEpo therapy is its effect on blood pressure. Although the blood pressure values re-

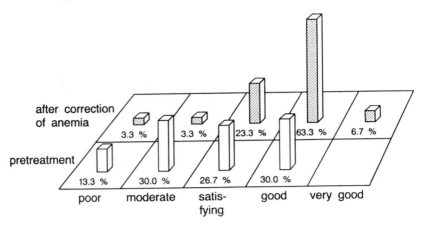

Figure 19.8. The effect of rHuEpo therapy on the well-being of children with end-stage renal failure ($n = 30$).

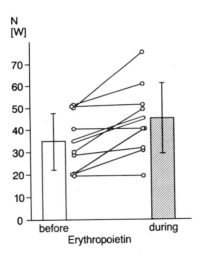

Figure 19.9. Physical working capacity (N [W]) in children with end-stage renal failure. □, before rHuEpo therapy; ▨, during rHuEpo therapy; $n = 9$.

mained virtually unchanged before and after the correction of renal anemia (before: systolic blood pressure, 127 ± 22 mm Hg; diastolic blood pressure, 77 ± 16 mm Hg; after: systolic blood pressure, 127 ± 26 mm Hg; diastolic blood pressure, 82 ± 20 mm Hg), some of the children showed a tendency toward an increase in blood pressure during rHuEpo therapy.

To be able to evaluate these results, investigators compared the chil-

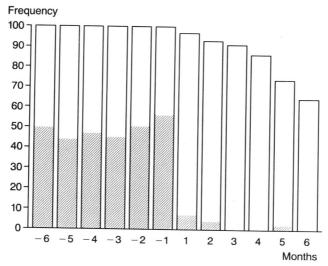

Figure 19.10. The frequency of monthly transfusions before and after rHuEpo therapy. ▨, transfusion; ☐, no transfusion.

Table 19.2. The Most Important Adverse Effects of rHuEpo Therapy Leading to Withdrawal from the Study

Adverse Effect	Number of Patients
Hypertension	2
Hypertensive crisis with seizure	1
Thrombosis of Hickman catheter	2
Death	2

dren's blood pressure values to age-appropriate blood pressures (19). The children were rated as hypotensive when their systolic blood pressure before the start of hemodialysis was below the fifth percentile; they were rated as hypertensive when their systolic or diastolic blood pressure was above the age-appropriate 90th percentile or when they underwent antihypertensive therapy. Children whose diastolic and systolic blood pressures were within the age-appropriate percentile curves and who did not receive antihypertensive therapy were rated as normoten-

Table 19.3. The Most Important Adverse Effects of rHuEpo Therapy Not Leading to Withdrawal from the Study

Adverse Effect	Number of Patients
Hypertension	19
Hypertensive crisis	2
Hypertensive crisis with seizure	4
Seizure	2
Shunt thrombosis	6
Thrombosis of Hickman catheter	1
Clotting in the extracorporeal system	7
Hyperkalemia	4

sive. In accordance with the above rating, 45 children were normotensive before the onset of rHuEpo therapy, 30 were hypertensive but did not receive antihypertensive therapy, and 25 were hypertensive with antihypertensive therapy (Fig 19.11).

During rHuEpo therapy, 14 of the 45 originally normotensive children became hypertensive; antihypertensive therapy was commenced in 7 of these children. In 31 of these 45 patients (69%), the blood pressure remained unchanged. In 6 of the 30 hypertensive patients who had not received antihypertensive therapy at the start of the trial, the blood pressure returned to normal, that is, they became normotensive. Blood pressure aggravation occurred in 5 patients, necessitating antihypertensive therapy.

In 2 of the 26 originally hypertensive patients who had undergone antihypertensive therapy before the start of rHuEpo therapy, antihypertensive therapy was discontinued during the course of the observation period. Antihypertensive therapy was reduced in 4 and remained unchanged in 8. The antihypertensive therapy had to be intensified, however, in 12 of these 26 children (46 percent) (Fig. 19.11).

In two originally hypertensive patients, the trial had to be discontinued because of uncontrollable hypertension (see Table 19.2). In one child, a 7-year-old boy, a generalized tonoclonic spasm was observed 34 days after the onset of rHuEpo therapy; the child's hematocrit had increased from 17 to 25 percent.

In another patient, a 17-year-old girl, aggravation of pre-existing (but well-controlled) hypertension occurred. Blood pressure surges during the first 5 weeks of rHuEpo therapy led to the discontinuation of rHuEpo therapy. The hematocrit changed only slightly throughout this period, however.

Temporarily severe blood pressure surges with corresponding clinical symptoms were observed in another 13 children. In these patients, rHuEpo therapy was usually discontinued; the blood pressure was then regulated through medication and the therapy was continued with a reduced dose of rHuEpo (an average of 30 units/kg three times per week).

These results indicate that the correction of renal anemia with rHuEpo should be commenced only in patients with stable blood pressure. Furthermore, the blood pressure should be carefully monitored in all children—and above all in children with pre-existing hypertension—during the 1st months of rHuEpo therapy.

In five children, generalized tonoclonic spasms were observed during the course of therapy. In three of these five, the spasms were part of a hypertensive crisis.

In a 10-year-old boy who had responded adequately to rHuEpo, petit mal seizures occurred briefly (for about 1 week) in the 5th month of therapy. This was confirmed by electroencephalography. The child's blood pressure was normal; the hematocrit fluctuated around 28 per-

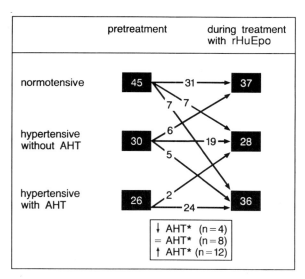

Figure 19.11. The blood pressure in children with end-stage renal failure during rHuEpo therapy. AHT, antihypertensive therapy.

cent at the time. The boy received antihypertensive therapy. Therapy with rHuEpo was continued; after 1½ years of therapy, the boy was doing well.

In six children, a thrombosis of the Cimino fistula or the arterio-venous shunt was observed. However, five of the Cimino fistulas were so-called fistulas-at-risk, that is, shunt occlusions had been observed before rHuEpo therapy, or there was poor blood flow or aneurysmatic vascular changes.

After 3 weeks of rHuEpo therapy, thrombosis of the Scribner shunt occurred in a 3-year-old boy whose response to rHuEpo was very good (change in hematocrit, approximately 2.5 percent per week). Because of the difficult vascular situation, a careful risk-benefit evaluation led to the discontinuation of rHuEpo therapy. In three other children, a Hickman catheter thrombosed; rHuEpo therapy was subsequently dis-continued in two of them. Thus, if a patient with a fistula-at-risk is to be treated with rHuEpo, a shunt revision should be performed in due course.

Clotting problems in the extracorporeal system were temporarily ob-served in seven children. These problems were solved by increasing the dosage of heparin. During rHuEpo therapy, the overall heparin dosage administered to the children was increased by an average of 20 percent compared to the run-in period.

The platelet count showed an approximately 20 percent increase at the start of the correction period (Fig 19.12). Although the platelet count dropped again during the course of the trial, it remained slightly elevated in comparison to the pretreatment values. In the two patients with platelet values greater than $500,000/mm^3$ during the run-in pe-riod, no further increase in platelet values occurred and no clinical com-plications ensued.

Overall, serum potassium levels remained unchanged during rHuEpo therapy. No increase in episodes of hyperkalemia was observed in the individual nephrology centers. In some patients with pre-existing prob-lems of hyperkalemia, however, these problems were aggravated as a result of improved appetite or a reduced compliance of the individual experiencing improved general well-being. In one center, the potassium value is therefore regularly checked in almost all children and the dialysate is adjusted to the potassium concentration. Hyperkalemia (serum potassium level of $\geqslant 8$ mmol/litre) was temporarily found in 4 children. Because of problems of hyperkalemia (serum potassium, 8.4 mmol/litre), 1 child had to undergo an additional dialysis. Fifty-nine children had received ion exchangers before the start of rHuEpo ther-

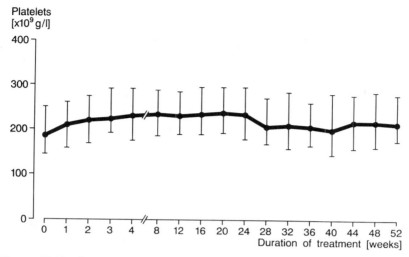

Figure 19.12. The course of the platelet count in children with end-stage renal failure during rHuEpo therapy (mean and interquartile range).

apy; in 12 of these, regular ion exchange therapy had to be commenced. Ion exchange therapy could, on the other hand, be reduced in 8 of the 59 children and discontinued in 5 children.

No significant increase in serum phosphate was observed. However, the dosage of phosphate binder had to be increased in 13 patients.

Conclusion

Therapy with rHuEpo resulted in a significant increase in the hematocrit in all children with end-stage renal failure. Transfusion dependency was eliminated in all children.

The iron overload was reduced by rHuEpo therapy in most of the previously polytransfused children. The results show that additional venesections are indicated only with extreme iron overload and evidence of iron-induced tissue damage.

Therapy with rHuEpo led to improved appetite in many of the children but not to a disproportionate increase in body weight. A final statement on the influence of the correction of renal anemia on body growth cannot yet be made, as the number of patients evaluated is still too small and the observation period too short. The results thus far indicate that the inhibition of renal growth is not influenced by the correction of renal anemia.

The most important complication observed was an increase in blood pressure, with blood pressure surges (with seizures in three cases) in a number of patients. Access thromboses may be expected in children with fistulas-at-risk. Before the start of rHuEpo therapy, the shunts or fistulas should be revised. A careful risk/benefit evaluation is necessary in these cases. Clotting in the extracorporeal circulation can easily be eliminated by an increase in the dosage of heparin.

Although no significant change in the serum potassium level was observed, the level should be checked regularly during the 1st months of rHuEpo therapy. A temporary increase in serum potassium levels in individual patients is likely to be the result of improved appetite or reduced compliance of the individual experiencing improved general well-being. The problem of possible hyperkalemia can easily be averted by increasing or initiating ion exchange therapy, by maintaining a careful diet, or by reducing the potassium concentration in the dialysate.

REFERENCES

1. Müller-Wiefel DE, Scigalla P. Specific problems of renal anemia in childhood. In: Koch KM, ed. Treatment of renal anemia with recombinant erythropoietin. Contrib Nephrol 1988;66:71–84.

2. Scigalla P, Bonzel KE, Bulla M, et al. Therapy of renal anemia with recombinant human erythropoietin in children with end-stage renal disease. Contrib Nephrol 1989;76:227–41.

3. Müller-Wiefel DE. Renale Anämie im Kindesalter: Untersuchungen zur Pathogenese und Kompensation. Stuttgart: Thieme, 1982.

4. Obrain RT. Iron overload: clinical and pathologic aspects in pediatrics. Semin Hematol 1977;14:115–25.

5. Holliday MA. Growth retardation in children with renal disease. In: Edelmann KL, ed. Pediatric kidney disease. Boston: Little, Brown, 1978: 331–41.

6. Mehls O, Ritz E, Gilli G, Kreusser W. Growth in renal failure. Nephron 1978;237–47.

7. Jacobs K, Shoemaker C, Rudersdorf RA, et al. Isolation and characterization of genomic and cona clones of human erythropoietin. Nature 1985; 313:806–10.

8. Lin FK, Suggs S, Lin CM, et al. Cloning and expression of the human erythropoietin gene. Proc Natl Acad Sci USA 1985;82:7580–4.

9. Goldwasser E, Jacobson LO, Fried W, Plzak LF. Studies on erythropoiesis, V: The effect of cobalt on the production of erythropoietin. Blood 1958;13:55–60.

10. Koch KM, Patyna D, Shaldon S, Werner E. Anemia of the regular hemodialysis patient and its treatment. Nephron 1974;12:405–19.

11. Williams JS, Stein JH, Ferris TF. Nandrolone decanoate therapy for patients receiving hemodialysis. Arch Intern Med 1974;134:289–92.

12. Eschbach JW, Adamson JW. Modern aspects of the pathophysiology of renal anemia. Contrib Nephrol 1988;66:63–70.

13. Finch CA. Erythropoiesis, erythropoietin, and iron. Blood 1982;60:1241–6.

14. Burghard R, Leititis J, Pallacks R, Scigalla P, Brandis M. Treatment of a seven-year-old child with end-stage renal disease and hemosiderosis by recombinant human erythropoietin. Contrib Nephrol 1988;66:139–48.

15. Bommer JW, Huber G, Tewes E, et al. Treatment of polytransfused hemodialysis patients with recombinant human erythropoietin. Contrib Nephrol 1988;66:131–8.

16. Winearls CG, Oliver DO, Pippard MJ, Reid C, Downing MR, Cotes PM. Effect of human erythropoietin derived from recombinant DNA on the anemia of patients maintained by chronic hemodialysis. Lancet 1986;2:1175–7.

17. Pippard MJ, Oliver D, Winearls C, Cotes PM. Iron metabolism during correction of anaemia in haemodialysis patients treated with erythropoietin [Abstract]. Br J Haematol 1988;69:105.

18. Zoellner K, Devaux S, Schmidt G, Roeseler E, Scigalla P, Wieczorek L. Korrektur der renalen Anämie mit rh-EPO bei terminal niereninsuffizienten Kindern. Presented at the 20th NephrologieKongreß, 1989, Bern.

19. André IL, Deschamps JP, Gueguen R. La tension artérielle chez l'enfant et l'adolescent. Arch Fr Pédiatr 1980;37:477–82.

Chapter 20

Recombinant Human Erythropoietin (Epoetin Alfa) in Patients with the Anemia of Prematurity

William C. Mentzer, Jr., Kevin M. Shannon, and Roderic H. Phibbs

The postnatal anemia that regularly appears in premature infants is one of the clinical settings in which recombinant human erythropoietin therapy is being evaluated. This anemia has two components. The first, "early" anemia, is a consequence of the fact that premature babies are often both very small and very sick, requiring assisted ventilation and other invasive supportive care. Because their blood volume is low (as little as 50 ml), consistent with their small size, anemia is a common result of the frequent blood sampling required to monitor their clinical status. A recent survey of 20 consecutive infants admitted to neonatal intensive care at the University of California at San Francisco disclosed that an average of 38.9 ml was removed for laboratory tests during the 1st week of life (1). The need to assure an adequate capacity for oxygen delivery despite blood loss from frequent blood sampling accounts for the majority of the red cell transfusions given in the nursery.

A second type of anemia develops in premature babies after the immediate perinatal period. This has been called the "anemia of prematurity" and is characterized by a progressive fall in the hemoglobin concentration, reticulocytopenia, and bone marrow erythroid hypoplasia (2–4). The central factor responsible for the anemia is an incompletely met requirement for the synthesis of new red cells to expand the red cell mass in the rapidly growing infant and to replace short-lived senescent fetal red cells and red cells lost when blood specimens are obtained for laboratory testing. The inadequate erythropoietic response in these infants is thought to be due in large part to inappropriately low levels of circulating erythropoietin.

The anemia of prematurity is responsible for 20 to 30 percent of the red cell transfusions given in most high-risk nurseries. Because affected infants have a well-defined condition, are clinically stable, would benefit from the avoidance of transfusions, and seem to lack an adequate capacity to synthesize erythropoietin, they represent an excellent group for clinical trials of recombinant human erythropoietin (rHuEpo) to correct anemia and prevent transfusions.

The Erythropoietic Requirements of the Growing Fetus and Preterm Infant

To keep pace with growth, erythropoiesis must be much more active in the developing fetus than in the normal child or adult. During the third trimester, fetal body mass triples, from about 1200 g to about 3600 g. Because the fetal circulation includes the fetal side of the placenta, which is highly vascular, the absolute requirement for an increase in red cell mass is even greater than that implied by the consideration of weight alone. Because of the contribution of the placenta, fetal blood volume is approximately 155 ml/kg body weight, compared to 83 ml/kg in the newborn and 75 ml/kg in the child or adult (5–7). Furthermore, the fetal hematocrit and hemoglobin level rise during the second and third trimesters to meet increasing demands for oxygen transport in a relatively hypoxic environment (8,9). Figures 20.1 to 20.3 depict the changes in hemoglobin concentrations and hematocrit, reticulocyte count, and erythroblast count, respectively, that occur during the latter half of gestation.

The partial pressure of oxygen (Po_2) of umbilical vein blood en route from the placenta to the fetus, the most highly oxygenated blood in the fetal circulation, is only 35 to 40 torr. Compensating for this state of relative hypoxemia are the high hemoglobin concentration characteristic of later fetal life and the predominance of hemoglobin F. The left-shifted oxygen dissociation curve of hemoglobin F allows a much higher oxygen saturation (about 85 percent) at a Po_2 of 35 torr than would occur with hemoglobin A. These two factors combine to increase the oxygen content of fetal blood to a satisfactory level. That the presence of hemoglobin F may be less crucial for fetal oxygen transport than previously thought is suggested by observations in severe alloimmune hemolytic disease. Affected fetuses receive intrauterine transfusions us-

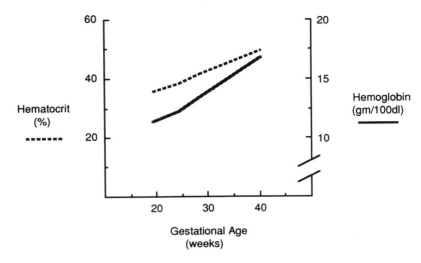

Figure 20.1 Change in the hematocrit and hemoglobin concentrations with gestational age in the human fetus. *Source: Data from Reference 9*

ing compatible adult donor red blood cells that contain hemoglobin A, not F. Often, when delivery is at or near term, virtually all circulating red cells are of donor origin, but adverse effects of hemoglobin A-containing red cells on oxygen transport in utero are not evident.

Except for the need to supply extra red cells for the placental circulatory system, the erythropoietic requirements of the prematurely born infant are quite similar to those of fetuses of equivalent gestational age who remain in utero. At birth, the hemoglobin concentration and hematocrit are lower than at term, in proportion to the degree of prematurity (Fig 20.1). Once the stresses of the immediate postnatal period are overcome and adequate nutritional intake is established, rapid growth ensues and infants gain weight at the rate of 1 to 2 percent per day. The red cell mass must increase concomitantly to maintain a stable hematocrit. Furthermore, in premature babies, the red cell life-span is only half that found in adults (11), so replacement of senescent red cells imposes a greater burden during early postnatal existence. Finally, the removal of blood for laboratory testing is a virtually universal feature of neonatal care but is a rarity before birth (although fetal blood sampling for diagnostic testing is gaining in popularity).

The Regulation of Fetal Erythropoiesis

As in other mammals, the earliest site of erythropoiesis in the developing human embryo is within the yolk sac. By 6 to 8 weeks of ges-

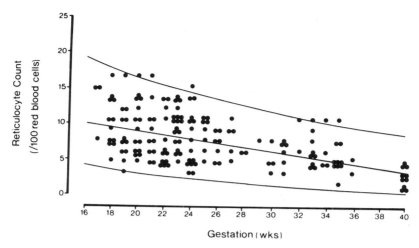

Figure 20.2. Change in the reticulocyte count in fetal umbilical cord blood with gestational age. *Source: Reference 10*

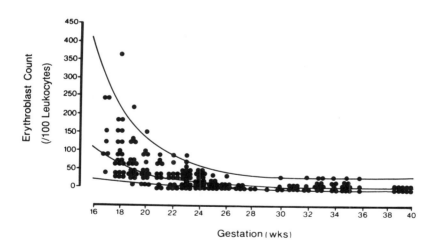

Figure 20.3. Change in the erythroblast count in fetal umbilical cord blood with gestational age. *Source: Reference 10*

tation, the main site of erythropoiesis has shifted to the fetal liver, which continues to be a source of new red cells until shortly after birth. Bone marrow erythropoiesis gradually replaces hepatic erythropoiesis after about 20 weeks gestation (12,13).

The regulation of fetal erythropoiesis is not completely understood during early embryonic life. Hamster yolk sac erythroid precursors bear erythropoietin receptors that increase to a maximal number at day 10 of gestation and then decline, and erythropoietin is required for in vitro erythroid colony formation by yolk sac cells (14). Fetal mouse liver cells also bear erythropoietin receptors (15), suggesting that hepatic erythropoiesis may be regulated by erythropoietin. Human liver erythroid progenitors obtained from 7 to 8-week embryos generate erythroid bursts when cultured in vitro in the presence of erythropoietin alone, and, in this regard, they differ from erythroid progenitors from adults, which require not only erythropoietin but also granulocyte-macrophage colony-stimulating factor (GM-CSF) and interleukin 3 in the culture medium (16). On the other hand, in third trimester fetal lambs, abolition of circulating erythropoietin activity by injection of anti-erythropoietin antibodies into the fetal circulation inhibits bone marrow and splenic erythropoiesis but has no effect on hepatic erythropoiesis (17). Other factors may govern hepatic erythropoiesis, at least in the lamb.

Physiologic studies clearly indicate that the fetus is capable of endogenous synthesis of erythropoietin in response to hypoxia. For example, phlebotomy of fetal goats is soon followed by a rise in fetal serum levels of erythropoietin. Maternal serum erythropoietin levels do not change, and prior bilateral nephrectomy of the mother has no effect on the magnitude of the fetal response, eliminating any contribution of maternal erythropoietin synthesis to the phenomenon (18). Similarly, human cord blood and amniotic fluid erythropoietin levels are elevated when the fetus has encountered hypoxic stress in utero, as in Rh disease, infants of diabetic mothers, or infants with placental insufficiency (19–21). When fetuses with severe Rh disease are treated successfully by intrauterine transfusions with adult red cells, fetal serum erythropoietin levels, which are initially high, fall to normal, whereas maternal serum erythropoietin levels are normal initially and remain so despite the fluctuations in the fetal values (22).

The magnitude of the erythropoietin response to hypoxia in the fetus may be blunted. Erythropoietin levels in blood obtained from anemic fetuses at about 28 weeks gestation by cordacentesis showed only a modest elevation above levels obtained from nonanemic fetuses. The rise was greater in anemic newborns and greater still in adults who were anemic (22).

The evidence is contradictory as to whether erythropoietin can cross the placenta. Injection of human urinary erythropoietin into fetal goats was not followed by measurable changes in maternal erythropoietin levels (23). In sheep, no maternal-to-fetal transfer of radiolabeled recombinant erythropoietin could be demonstrated (24). The placenta of goats and sheep differs from that of humans. In human Rh incompatibility, where fetal erythropoietin levels are higher than maternal levels, maternal reticulocyte counts were higher than in a group of pregnant women who did not exhibit blood group incompatibility, suggesting fetal-to-maternal transfer of erythropoietin (25). After the injection of radiolabeled recombinant erythropoietin into pregnant mice, 7 to 10 percent of the labeled material is found in the fetal circulation (26). Erythropoietin receptors were recently discovered in the mouse placenta. Their role is unknown but may relate to a transport system for erythropoietin from mother to fetus or vice versa (27).

Physiologic and biochemical studies in rats, mice, and sheep indicate that, during the latter part of gestation, the fetal liver is the main source of erythropoietin (26,28,29). The switch from hepatic to the primarily renal production of erythropoietin characteristic of adults begins late in the third trimester in the sheep and is complete shortly after birth (30). Timing of the switch can be accelerated by the administration of thyroid hormone and retarded by its absence (in thyroidectomized lambs) (30). Fetal lamb livers transplanted into their nephrectomized mothers retain the capability to make erythropoietin in response to hypoxic stress induced by bleeding the ewes (31). Zanjani and co-workers suggested that unique aspects of the fetal circulation might favor hepatic rather than renal production of erythropoietin (30). As oxygenated umbilical vein blood passes through the portal sinus, much of it is shunted directly to the heart through the ductus venosus, leaving portions of the liver supplied by more hypoxic portal vein blood. Relatively profound hepatic hypoxia may allow the hepatic oxygen sensor to initiate hepatic erythropoietin production (30). At birth, placental blood no longer flows through the umbilical vein and the ductus venosus soon closes, leaving the portal vein and hepatic artery as the sole blood supply to the liver. Furthermore, initiation of respiration markedly increases the oxygen content of both the hepatic and the renal blood supply, perhaps favoring renal rather than hepatic erythropoietin production. The oxygen sensor in the fetal liver seems to be as sensitive as that in the adult kidney in that equivalent degrees of hypoxia in the fetal lamb or adult sheep induce equivalent rises in erythropoietin (18,28). In contrast, the adult liver seems to require a greater degree of hypoxia than the kidney to trigger erythropoietin production (32).

The limited information available indicates that hepatic erythropoietin production also occurs in human fetuses, with a transition to the kidney as the major source at the time of birth. Large amounts of erythropoietin messenger ribonucleic acid (mRNA) were found in a liver obtained from a human fetus at 20 weeks of gestation (33). Infants born with renal agenesis are not anemic, suggesting exposure to an extrarenal source of erythropoietin in utero (34).

The Anemia of Prematurity

After normal term birth, the hemoglobin concentration falls from a mean of 17 g/dl to a nadir of approximately 11 g/dl at 2 to 3 months of age (4). This decline represents normal physiologic adaptation to extrauterine life. Inflation of the lungs, developmental changes in the cardiovascular system, and replacement of fetal hemoglobin (hemoglobin F) by adult hemoglobin (hemoglobin A) act together to increase peripheral oxygen delivery markedly. There is little or no stimulus for erythropoietin production, the reticulocyte count falls, and the observed fall in hemoglobin values ensues. Interestingly, patients with anemia due to hereditary hemolytic conditions maintain relatively high reticulocyte counts during this period, which emphasizes that term babies are capable of responding appropriately to hypoxia. The normal physiologic decline in hemoglobin concentration is exaggerated in babies who are born prematurely (4). The smallest and most immature infants show the greatest fall in hemoglobin values (4). In contrast to the situation in term babies, this fall in hemoglobin concentration is frequently associated with signs of impaired oxygen delivery, including slowing of the rate of growth, tachycardia, and worsening of the apnea and bradycardia of prematurity (35–37). Transfusions are frequently given to symptomatic infants.

A number of studies examined erythropoietin production in the anemia of prematurity. Using a mouse bioassay, Buchanan and Schwartz (38) reported undetectable levels of erythropoietin in the sera of anemic infants. Stockman at al. (39) subsequently used a more sensitive radioimmunoassay to demonstrate that serum erythropoietin levels in babies with the anemia of prematurity were within and below the normal range for nonanemic adults but well below levels seen in anemic adults. Their data also suggested that erythropoietin production was regulated by tissue hypoxia because infants with over 70 percent hemoglobin F showed higher erythropoietin levels at any given hemoglobin concentration than did patients with predominantly hemoglobin A (39). Subsequent work confirmed that serum erythropoietin levels in premature babies are low for the degree of anemia present. The most anemic infants had the highest erythropoietin levels (39–43), whereas the smallest and most immature premature infants produced the least erythropoietin (40,42). One study found that serum erythropoietin concentrations were lowest during the 1st month of life and that a subsequent rise in erythropoietin levels correlated with advancing postconceptional age as well as with worsening anemia (40). Similarly, the erythropoietin responses of babies with postconceptional ages of 27 to 31 weeks were blunted when compared with more mature infants (42). A recent study showed that erythropoietin deficiency in the sera of anemic premature infants was unaccompanied by equivalent deficiencies in other erythropoietic stimulatory factors as assessed in an in vitro colony-forming system (44). Thus, the available data regarding erythropoietin production by premature babies indicate that it is (a) low despite a measurable decrease in mixed venous oxygen tensions and peripheral oxygen availability, (b) regulated appropriately as erythropoietin levels are inversely correlated with hemoglobin concentrations and are influenced by the percentage of fetal hemoglobin, and (c) most impaired in the least mature infants.

Additional evidence that the anemia of prematurity is due to "erythropoietin insufficiency" is provided by the findings of low reticulocyte counts and of bone marrow erythroid hypoplasia in affected infants (45,46). In this regard, the anemia of prematurity resembles the anemia of chronic renal failure. The potential for an adequate erythropoietin response seems to be present in premature infants. Studies of in vitro erythroid progenitor colony growth revealed large numbers of bone marrow colony-forming units-erythroid (CFU-E) (45) and circulating burst-forming units-erythroid (BFU-E) (43), and both classes of progenitors showed a normal dose-response curve to erythropoietin in vitro (43,45).

Taken together, the results of studies performed over the past 15 years suggest that the erythropoietic response to anemia in infants with the anemia of prematurity is limited by inadequate erythropoietin production rather than by inadequate erythroid marrow potential. These observations provide a solid rationale for clinical trials using rHuEpo in an attempt to reduce transfusion requirements by preventing (or correcting) anemia in premature babies.

It is interesting to speculate as to why growing premature infants do not release adequate amounts of erythropoietin in response to tissue hypoxia. Intrauterine erythropoiesis at a similar stage of development is both active and effective. As reviewed above, the available evidence indicates that the liver is the major site of intrauterine erythropoietin production. The hepatic sensor may well be adapted to the intrauterine environment, which is characterized by a low Po_2 and by a fetal circulatory pattern. If this is true, the profound changes that accompany premature delivery might act to shut off hepatic erythropoietin release. Although renal erythropoietin production is developmentally adapted to maintain peripheral oxygen delivery in the well-oxygenated postnatal environment, this response would be deleterious in utero as it might result in polycythemia. It would be advantageous to restrict the full appearance of renal erythropoietin production until approximately 40 weeks of gestation. Babies born prematurely would cease hepatic erythropoietin synthesis but be unable to compensate by releasing sufficient erythropoietin from their kidneys. Observations that the most immature infants have the lowest erythropoietin levels and experience the greatest decline in hemoglobin concentration after birth are consistent with this hypothesis (4,40,42).

Transfusion Therapy in the Anemia of Prematurity

As transfusion therapy is the standard against which the potential benefits of recombinant erythropoietin treatment will be compared in future clinical trials, its risks and indications are briefly outlined.

Risks

The risks associated with transfusion into the anemic premature infant include serious infection, graft-versus-host disease, and suppression of erythropoietin production. Transfusion-acquired cytomegalovirus can cause a potentially fatal systemic disease with severe protracted pneumonitis that may require prolonged assisted ventilation (47,48). The majority of transfusion-borne cases of pediatric AIDS in non-hemophiliac patients were acquired in the nursery (49). Because the immune system of the premature infant is not fully developed, graft-versus-host disease may occur after transfusion unless the donor blood is irradiated. Transfusions given near the physiologic nadir in hemoglobin concentration that otherwise would reactivate erythropoiesis may suppress the release of erythropoietin and delay the natural recovery from the anemia of prematurity (50).

Indications for Transfusion

The stable, growing, asymptomatic preterm infant does not seem to need transfusions to correct mild to moderate anemia (51). However, an anemic infant whose weight declines despite adequate caloric intake will usually begin to gain weight again if transfused (35,52). Worsening of periodic breathing and apnea (a disorder of control of respiration common to preterm infants) is relieved by correction of anemia in some infants (35,37) but not in others (53). One recent study found that the presence of a low-grade lactic acidosis distinguished those anemic infants who were likely to respond to transfusion (54).

When infants have serious cardiopulmonary disease, the need for transfusion cannot be defined simply in terms of hemoglobin level or arterial oxygen content (which will depend on Po_2 and hemoglobin oxygen affinity as well as hemoglobin concentration) because these variables do not fully reflect oxygen requirements, which will vary with the state of the disease. Alverson and co-workers studied the effects of transfusion on oxygen transport and oxygen consumption in infants with cardiopulmonary disease. They found that the degree of improvement in these physiologic variables was directly related to the level of oxygen consumption before transfusion and not to the pretransfusion hemoglobin level (55).

Transfusion therapy may also be needed to maintain adequate circulating blood volume, particularly when infants are in acute hypovolemic shock immediately after birth because of blood loss to the placental circulation (56,57). Blood is also lost during the 1st weeks of life because of blood letting for laboratory studies. Some institutions replace blood removed for laboratory studies every time 10 percent of the total blood volume has been removed. Others wait for anemia to develop and then administer packed cell transfusions. There are no data to show that one approach is better than the other or that either one is beneficial.

The sick preterm infant is thought to do better if the circulating red cells contain adult rather than fetal hemoglobin. Two controlled trials in premature infants shortly after birth studied the effects of exchange transfusion which, without altering hematocrit, replaced fetal red cells (high hemoglobin F) with adult red cells (hemoglobin A) (58,59). The improved survival rate in treated infants compared to the controls was attributed to the lower oxygen affinity of hemoglobin A, which allows better oxygen off-loading in the capillaries (60). The presumed offsetting advantage of hemoglobin F in utero, that of enhancing oxygen uptake in the placenta, is no longer important after birth because capillary and venous Po_2 are much higher in the lungs than in the placental venous blood. Even in infants with serious pulmonary disease, oxygen and ventilator therapy can still raise the Po_2 to a level that will ensure more than 95 percent saturation of adult hemoglobin.

The above considerations indicate why red blood cell transfusions are an essential component of modern neonatal intensive care. At the University of California, San Francisco, the operating and recovery rooms combined are the only unit that administers more transfusions than the nursery. Recent improvements in supportive care increased the survival rate of tiny premature babies (those weighing less than 750 g at birth). Because these very low birthweight infants generally require the largest number of transfusions, blood use is likely to increase in the future. On the basis of recent California perinatal data, we estimate that nurseries administer 125,000 to 250,000 erythrocyte transfusions each year in North America. In addition to requiring a large number of transfusions, premature infants compete with other "high risk" populations for scarce resources such as cytomegalovirus-negative blood products (48). Clearly, alternatives to the use of blood products would be highly desirable.

The Potential Use of Recombinant Erythropoietin

The questions of who to treat and when hinge on the issue of which infants will require transfusions for the anemia of prematurity. In our experience, essentially all infants weighing less than 1000 g at birth and approximately 50% of those under 1500 g require one or more transfusions for anemia beyond the first 2 weeks of life. Effective treatment with rHuEpo offers the most potential benefit to these patients. Because small, premature babies are extremely likely to require transfusions, it is appealing to begin a rHuEpo study at birth. However, because these tiny babies have a large number of medical problems, are frequently unstable, and have large phlebotomy requirements, it would be difficult to assess beneficial or adverse effects of rHuEpo. For these reasons, we adopted relatively strict entry criteria in a recently completed pilot study (61). Infants had to be at least 10 days of age, clinically stable with minimal ventilatory requirements, tolerating enteral feedings, and have minimal ongoing phlebotomy requirements. With additional experience, we hope to begin treating patients at birth.

We believe that the duration of rHuEpo therapy should be determined by the developmental age of the infant. Because premature infants eventually "learn" to produce endogenous erythropoietin as they mature, it can be estimated that very immature infants may require 8 to 10 weeks of therapy, with larger prematures receiving rHuEpo for 4 to 6 weeks. The optimal duration of treatment can be defined only on the basis of clinical trials.

Although data derived from studies in adults and children with renal failure offer guidelines as to the appropriate dose of rHuEpo, premature infants are unique in a number of respects. As outlined earlier, it is necessary for a premature baby to approximately double the red cell mass to maintain a constant hemoglobin concentration during the first 2 months of life. Thus, the level of stimulation of erythropoiesis seen in adults with renal failure (a rise in hematocrit from 20 to 35 percent over 6 to 8 weeks) while receiving 150 units of rHuEpo per kg 3 times each week (62) would lead to a stable or falling hematocrit in a growing premature baby because of the rapid growth rate. Data from studies in newborn animals also support the use of relatively high doses of rHuEpo. Radiolabeled erythropoietin is cleared more rapidly from plasma after intravenous injection, has a greater distribution volume, and exhibits a more rapid terminal $T_{1/2}$ in newborn lambs than in adult sheep (63). The peak serum erythropoietin concentrations achieved in neonatal monkeys given 100 or 250 units of intravenous rHuEpo twice weekly were approximately 2½ times lower than levels in adult monkeys (64). Also, treated and untreated neonatal monkeys showed similar increases in total body hemoglobin concentrations during treatment. In contrast, treated adult animals achieved higher hemoglobin values than control animals. These findings verify a time-honored principle of clinical research in neonatology, that the responses of infants often cannot be inferred from results in adults and older children.

One aspect of neonatal erythropoiesis, defined in the monkey trial, which suggests that the results must be extrapolated with caution to human infants is the fact that erythropoiesis during the perinatal period is quite active in both control and treated animals, although it is relatively low in human premature and term babies. A final consideration in determining a starting dose of rHuEpo is the fact that blood sampling for laboratory tests imposes an additional challenge on the erythropoietic tissues of the growing premature baby. All of these factors argue that premature babies might require relatively large doses of rHuEpo, but safety is an overriding concern in this vulnerable patient population. For this reason, in our initial pilot study we administered only 100 units of rHuEpo per kg body weight twice each week (61). Higher doses of rHuEpo are clearly required for an optimal therapeutic effect.

There are three compelling reasons to use a double-blind, placebo-controlled design in all clinical trials of rHuEpo in premature babies. First, small premature babies have a high rate of medical complications, including acute and chronic pulmonary insufficiency, apnea and bradycardia, intraventricular hemorrhage, feeding intolerance and necrotizing enterocolitis, retrolental fibroplasia, a high risk of infection, and death. Without concurrent controls, it will be impossible to determine whether any of these problems is influenced by treatment with rHuEpo. Second, unlike patients with renal failure, premature babies eventually produce adequate amounts of erythropoietin. In the absence of a matched control group, it will be impossible to determine whether observed increases in hemoglobin concentrations or reticulocyte counts are a consequence of rHuEpo therapy or are due to the onset of endogenous erythropoietin production. Finally, the critical end point of therapeutic intervention with rHuEpo is whether or not treatment decreases the use of erythrocyte transfusions. Because there are no well-established clinical criteria for transfusions in the anemia of prematurity (65), it is likely that knowing whether or not a given infant is receiving rHuEpo might influence the decision to administer a transfusion. It therefore seems essential that the neonatologists caring for these patients be blinded.

Halperin and co-workers reported a group of seven premature infants who were treated with recombinant human erythropoietin for 4 weeks (66). Infants received 25, 50, or 100 units/kg three times each week. All babies were at least 3 weeks old, and six of seven weighed over 1250 g. The authors described a rapid rise in absolute reticulocyte counts and, importantly, a decrease in serum iron levels and transferrin saturations. Although the trial was conducted as an open label study and did not include controls, the authors noted that the onset of reticulocytosis was earlier and that hemoglobin concentrations were higher than those in a reference population of premature infants managed at the same hospital in recent years.

In our pilot study (61), 20 babies were randomly assigned to receive either rHuEpo (100 units/kg two times per week) or placebo for 6 weeks. These infants were much smaller than the group studied by Halperin and associates: all weighed less than 1250 g at birth and had a mean weight of 930 g at entry. There were no differences between treated and control infants with respect to hemoglobin concentrations, reticulocyte counts, transfusion requirements, or growth. There were also no rHuEpo-related changes in white blood cell or platelet counts. Most babies were followed for 6 months from completion of treatment, and we have seen no long-term adverse effects. Treated infants had a normal onset of endogenous erythropoietin production and showed normal erythropoiesis during the follow-up period. In our preliminary analysis, there is a trend toward higher reticulocyte counts on days 7 and 14 in treated infants. In addition, in a subgroup of 9 otherwise healthy babies who had <20 ml of blood removed for laboratory tests, none of 4 infants treated with erythropoietin received transfusions, whereas 3 of 5 infants in the placebo group received a transfusion. The observation of an initial rise in reticulocyte count in the treatment group suggests that iron, or some other factor, might have become limiting after an initial burst of erythropoiesis. Iron studies were not carried out in this trial because the amount of blood required was felt to be prohibitive. On the basis of these early results, we conclude that rHuEpo can be safely administered to premature infants at the dose studied. Pilot studies that incorporate substantially higher doses of rHuEpo and include prospective evaluations of iron status are in progress. Preliminary analysis of a study of this sort that we just completed (67) and of a similar study by Ohls and Christensen (68) indicates that higher doses of rHuEpo are effective.

ACKNOWLEDGMENTS

This work was supported in part by grants from the R. W. Johnson Pharmaceutical Research Corporation and the NIH (DK32094).

The opinions and assertions expressed herein are those of the authors and are not to be construed as official or as necessarily reflecting the views of the Department of the Navy or of the naval service at large.

REFERENCES

1. Shannon KM. Anemia of prematurity: progress and prospects. Am J Pediatr Hematol Oncol 1990;12:14–20.
2. Schulman I. The anemia of prematurity. J Pediatr 1959;54:663–7.
3. Stockman JA III. Anemia of prematurity. Clin Perinatol 1977;4:239–57.
4. Dallman PR. Anemia of prematurity. Ann Rev Med 1981;32:143–60.
5. Linderkamp O. Placental transfusion: determinants and effects. Clin Perinat 1982;9:559–92.
6. Usher R, Shephard M, Lind J. The blood volume of the newborn infants and placental transfusion. Acta Paediatr 1963;52:497–512.
7. Yao AC, Moinian M, Lind J. Distribution of blood between infant and placenta after birth. Lancet 1969;2:871–3.

8. Bratteby L. Studies on erythro-kinetics in infancy. IX. Prediction of red cell volume from venous haematocrit in early infancy. Acta Paediatr Scand 1968;57:125–31.

9. Forestier F, Daffos F, Galacteros F, et al. Hematological values of 163 normal fetuses between 18 and 30 weeks of gestation. Pediatr Res 1986;20:342–6.

10. Nicolaides KH, Thilaganathan B, Mibashan RS. Cordocentesis in the investigation of fetal erythropoiesis. Am J Obstet Gynecol 1989;161:1197–2000.

11. Pearson HA. Life-span of the fetal red blood cell. J Pediatr 1967; 70:166–71.

12. Oski FA, Naiman JL. Hematologic problems in the newborn. 3rd ed. Philadelphia: WB Saunders, 1982.

13. Brown MS. Fetal and neonatal erythropoiesis. In: Stockman JA III, Pochedly C (eds). Developmental and neonatal hematology. New York: Raven Press, 1988;39–56.

14. Boussios T, Bertles JF, Goldwasser E. Erythropoietin: receptor characteristics during the ontogeny of hamster yolk sac erythroid cells. J Biol Chem 1989;264:16017–21.

15. Tojo A, Fukamachi H, Kasuga M, Urabe A, Takaku F. Identification of erythropoietin receptors on fetal liver erythroid cells. Biochem Biophys Res Commun 1987;148:443–8.

16. Valtieri M, Gabbianelli M, Pelosi E, et al. Erythropoietin alone induces erythroid burst formation by human embryonic but not adult BFU-E in unicellular serum-free culture. Blood 1989;74:460–70.

17. Zanjani ED, Mann LI, Burlington H, Gordon AS, Wasserman LR. Evidence for a physiologic role of erythropoietin in fetal erythropoiesis. Blood 1974;44:285–90.

18. Zanjani ED, Peterson EN, Gordon AS, Wasserman LR. Erythropoietin production in the fetus: role of the kidney and maternal anemia. J Lab Clin Med 1974;83:281–7.

19. Finne PH. Erythropoietin levels in cord blood as an indicator of intrauterine hypoxia. Acta Paediatr Scand 1966;55:478–89.

20. Widness JA, Susa JB, Garcia JF, et al. Increased erythropoiesis and elevated erythropoietin in infants born to diabetic mothers and in hyperinsulinemic rhesus fetuses. J Clin Invest 1981;67:637–42.

21. Thomas RM, Canning CE, Cotes PM, et al. Erythropoietin and cord blood haemoglobin in the regulation of human fetal erythropoiesis. Br J Obstet Gynecol 1983;90:795–800.

22. Widness JA, Weiner CP, Giller RH, et al. Increasing plasma erythropoietin response to anemia during development [Abstract]. Pediatr Res 1990; 27:153A.

23. Zanjani ED, Gordon AS. Erythropoietin production and utilization in fetal goats and sheep. Isr J Med Sci 1971;7:850–6.

24. Widness JA, Schmidt RL, Chesnut DH. Lack of maternal to fetal transfer of ^{125}I-erythropoietin in sheep [Abstract]. Pediatr Res 1990;27:269A.

25. Finne PH. On placental transfer of erythropoietin. Acta Paediatr Scand 1967;56:233–42.

26. Koury MJ, Bondurant MC, Graber SE, Sawyer ST. Erythropoietin messenger RNA levels in developing mice and transfer of ^{125}I-erythropoietin by the placenta. J Clin Invest 1988;82:154–9.

27. Sawyer ST, Krantz SB, Sawada K. Receptors for erythropoietin in mouse and human erythroid cells and placenta. Blood 1989;74:103–9.

28. Zanjani ED, Poster J, Burlington H, Mann LI, Wasserman LR. Liver as the primary site of erythropoietin formation in the fetus. J Lab Clin Med 1977;89:640–4.

29. Clemons GK, Fitzsimmons SL, DeManincor D. Immunoreactive erythropoietin concentrations in fetal and neonatal rats and the effects of hypoxia. Blood 1986;68:892–9.

30. Zanjani ED, Ascensao JL, McGlave PB, Banisadre M, Ash RC. Studies on the liver to kidney switch of erythropoietin production. J Clin Invest 1981;67:1183–8.

31. Flake AW, Harrison MR, Adzick NS, Zanjani ED. Erythropoietin production by the fetal liver in an adult environment. Blood 1987;70:542–5.

32. Fried W. The liver as a source of extra renal erythropoietin production. Blood 1972;40:671–7.

33. Jacobs K, Shoemaker C, Rudersdorf R, et al. Isolation and characterization of genomic and cDNA clones of human erythropoietin. Nature 1985; 313:806–10.

34. Halvorsen K, Haga P, Halvorsen S. Regulation of erythropoiesis in the foetus and neonate. In: Nakao K, Fisher JW, Takaku F, eds. Erythropoiesis. Proceedings of the Fourth International Conference on Erythropoiesis. Baltimore: University Park Press, 1975:349–56.

35. Wardrop CAJ, Holland BM, Veale KEA, et al. Nonphysiological anemia of prematurity. Arch Dis Child 1978;53:855–60.

36. Usher R. The special problems of the premature infant. In: Avery GP, ed. Neonatology: pathophysiology and management of the newborn. Philadelphia: JB Lippincott, 1975:157–88.

37. Joshi A, Gerhardt T, Shandloff P, Bancalalri B. Blood transfusion effect on the respiratory pattern of premature infants. Pediatrics 1987;80:79–84.

38. Buchanan GR, Schwartz AD. Impaired erythropoietin response in anemic premature infants. Blood 1974;44:347–52.

39. Stockman JA III, Garcia JF, Oski FA. The anemia of prematurity: factors governing the erythropoietin response. N Engl J Med 1977;296:647–50.

40. Brown MS, Phibbs RH, Garcia JF, Dallman RP. Postnatal changes in erythropoietin levels in untransfused premature infants. J Pediatr 1983;103: 612–7.

41. Brown MS, Phibbs RH, Garcia JF, Dallman PR. Decreased response of plasma immunoreactive erythropoietin to "available oxygen" in anemia of prematurity. J Pediatr 1984;105:793–8.

42. Stockman JA III, Graeber JE, Clark DA, et al. Anemia of prematurity: determinants of erythropoietin response. J Pediatr 1984;105:786–92.

43. Shannon KM, Naylor GS, Torkildson JC, et al. Circulating erythroid progenitors in the anemia of prematurity. N Engl J Med 1987;317:728–33.

44. Ohis RK, Liechty KW, Turner MC, Christensen RD. Erythroid "burst promoting activity" in patients with the anemia of prematurity [Abstract]. Pediatr Res 1990;268A:1589.

45. Rhondeau SM, Christensen RD, Ross MP, et al. Responsiveness to recombinant erythropoietin of marrow erythroid progenitors in infants with anemia of prematurity. J Pediatr 1988;112:935–40.

46. Gairdner D, Marks J, Roscoe JD. Blood formation in infancy. Part IV. The early anemia of prematurity. Arch Dis Child 1955;30:203–11.

47. Spector SA. Transmission of cytomegalovirus among infants in hospital documented by restriction-endonuclease-digestion analysis. Lancet 1983;1: 378–81.

48. Yaeger AS, Grumment FC, Itafleigh EB, et al. Prevention of transfusion-acquired cytomegalovirus infections in newborn infants. J Pediatr 1981;98: 281–7.

49. Falloon J, Eddy J, Weiner L, Pizzo PA. Human immunodeficiency virus infection in children. J Pediatr 1989;114:1–30.

50. Brown MS, Phibbs RH, Dallman PR. Postnatal changes in fetal hemoglobin, oxygen affinity and 2,3-diphosphoglycerate in previously transfused preterm infants. Biol Neonate 1985;48:70–87.

51. Blank JP, Sheagreu TH, Vajaria J, et al. The role of RBC transfusions in the premature infant. Am J Dis Child 1984;138:831–3.

52. Stockman JA, Clark DA. Weight gain: a response to transfusion in selected preterm infants. Am J Dis Child 1984;138:828–30.

53. Keyes WG, Donohue PK, Spivak JL, et al. Assessing the need for transfusion of premature infants and the role of hematocrit, clinical signs, and erythropoietin level. Pediatrics 1989;84:412–7.

54. Ross MP, Christensen RD, Rothstein G, et al. A randomized trial to develop criteria for administering erythrocyte transfusions to anemic preterm infants 1 to 3 months of age. J Perinatol 1990;9:246–53.

55. Alverson DC, Isken VH, Cohen RS. Effect of booster blood transfusions on oxygen utilization in infants with bronchopulmonary dysplasia. J Pediatr 1988;113:722–6.

56. Fay RA. Feto-maternal haemorrhage as a cause of fetal morbidity and mortality. Br J Obstet Gynaecol 1983;90:443–6.

57. Phibbs RH. What is the evidence that blood pressure monitoring is useful? In: Lucey JF, ed. Problems of neonatal intensive care units (Report of the 59th Ross Conference on Pediatric Research). Columbus, Ohio: Ross Laboratories, 1969:71–89.

58. Delivoria-Papadopoulos M, Miller LD, Forster RE II, et al. The role of exchange transfusions in the management of low-birth-weight infants with and without severe respiratory distress syndrome. I. Initial observations. J Pediatr 1976;89:273–8.

59. Gottuso MA, Williams ML, Oski FA. The role of exchange transfusions in the management of low-birth weight infants with and without severe respiratory distress syndrome. II. Further observations and studies of mechanisms of action. J Pediatr 1976;89:279–85.

60. Rigel KP, Versmold H. Postnatal blood oxygen transport, with special respect to idiopathic respiratory distress syndrome. Bull Physio-Pathol Respir 1973;9:1533–48.

61. Shannon KM, Mentzer WC, Abels RI, et al. Recombinant human erythropoietin in anemia of prematurity: preliminary results of a double-blind placebo controlled pilot study. J Pediatr 1991 (in press).

62. Eschbach JW, Egrie JC, Downing RM, et al. Correction of the anemia of end-stage renal disease with recombinant erythropoietin: results of a combined Phase I and II clinical trial. N Engl J Med 1987;316:73–8.

63. Widness JA, Veng-Pederson P, Modi N, Schmidt RL, Chestnut RL. Increased elimination of erythropoietin in neonatal sheep [Abstract]. Pediatr Res 1990;27:56A.

64. George JW, Bracco CA, Shannon KM, et al. Age related differences in

erythropoietic response to recombinant human erythropoietin: comparison in adult and infant rhesus monkeys. Pediatr Res 1990;28:567–71.

65. Stockman JA III. Anemia of prematurity. Current concepts in the issue of when to transfuse. Pediatr Clin North Am 1986;33:111–28.

66. Halperin DS, Wacker P, Lacourt G, et al. Effects of recombinant human erythropoietin in infants with the anemia of prematurity: a pilot study. J Pediatr 1990;116:779–86.

67. Shannon KS, Mentzer WC, Abels RI, et al. Intensive treatment of the anemia of prematurity with recombinant human erythropoietin. Submitted for publication.

68. Ohls RK, Christensen RD. A randomized trial of erythropoietin administration versus erythrocyte transfusion in patients with the anemia of prematurity (Abstract). Clin Res 1991;39:12A.

Chapter 21

Recombinant Human Erythropoietin (Epoetin Alfa) in Autologous Blood Donors and Perisurgical Patients

Lawrence T. Goodnough

Blood Banking in a Changing Environment

Blood banking has undergone a period of significant change. This multidisciplinary field, now known as transfusion medicine, has had to respond to new demands and new expectations on the part of clinicians, regulatory and accreditation agencies, funding organizations, and patients. The developments of plastic blood containers and of aphoresis instruments, for example, have led to the transfusion of blood components rather than of whole blood, so one blood donor can potentially supply blood components for many blood transfusion recipients. The transfusion practices of physicians, however, have not kept pace with these technological advances. For example, the use of fresh-frozen plasma increased 10-fold nationally from 1970 to 1980 (1). Although some of the increased use of blood components can be attributed to the transfusion support of increasingly complex treatments in cancer medicine, trauma, transplantation, and the intensive care setting, one inescapable conclusion is that many patients are receiving modified whole blood equivalents but now at a cost of more blood donor exposures for each patient. This realization led the National Institutes of Health to sponsor consensus conferences on the use of fresh-frozen plasma (1), platelet transfusion therapy (2), and perioperative red cell transfusion (3) to address transfusion practice issues. Additionally, the Joint Committee on Accreditation of Health Care Organizations mandated the audit of every transfused patient against established guidelines during a defined period (4) to ensure that transfusion of blood and blood components meets transfusion practice guidelines.

Simultaneously, the acquired immunodeficiency syndrome (AIDS) has been recognized as a disease transmissible by the transfusion of blood and blood products. More than 2200 AIDS cases attributable to blood transfusion had been reported through January 1, 1989 (5). Although AIDS has brought blood safety into focus for the public, blood transfusion has always been known to carry risks from other potential complications, including hepatitis C, hepatitis B, alloimmunization, transfusion reaction, immunologic suppression, and iron overload. The need for a dialogue concerning these risks between the transfusing physician and the potential transfusion recipient led to a recommendation by the American Association of Blood Banks that informed consent be obtained and documented before an elective or anticipated blood transfusion (6).

If the process is to be effective, early involvement of the patient in such a dialogue is necessary. In addition to an explanation of the relative risks and benefits of blood transfusion, alternatives should be presented (7). One alternative is to perform no transfusion, as with a patient who refuses blood because of religious beliefs (8); another possibility is the re-evaluation of the postoperative "transfusion-trigger hematocrit" in elective surgical patients (9), also addressed in the National Institutes of Health Perioperative Red Cell Transfusion Consensus Conference (3). A third example is the use of pharmacologic agents to reduce or avoid homologous blood transfusion. The use of recombinant human erythropoietin (rHuEpo) therapy in the surgical patient is the focus of this review, with particular emphasis on the use of rHuEpo in autologous blood donation before elective surgery.

Erythropoietin Therapy in Autologous Blood Donation

Preoperative autologous blood donation is a transfusion practice that has been widely endorsed (10–12) for two reasons: the patient's own blood is the safest blood (13), and blood procured in anticipation of an elective operation will add to the national blood inventory (14,15). A third benefit of autologous blood donation is that this practice has a positive effect on physician transfusion behavior. Physicians accept lower nadir and discharge hematocrits in surgical patients who have predonated autologous blood, suggesting a lowering of the transfusion-trigger hematocrit (16).

Patients scheduled for elective orthopedic surgery are particularly well suited for enrollment in an autologous blood donation program because the need for perioperative blood transfusion is significant and can be anticipated. Autologous blood predeposit programs at hospitals with active orthopedic surgical services, as at our hospital, have seen a more than 10-fold increase in activity over the last 3 years (17). The percentage of participation of elective patients scheduled for hip and knee procedures for which blood is typed and crossmatched increased from 5 percent to more than 60 percent during the last 3 years in our program. The percentage of such patients who receive transfusions of homologous blood has been reduced to 14 percent, compared to 41 percent of patients who undergo elective orthopedic surgery without autologous blood donation. The safety, utilization, and efficacy of this practice as an alternative to homologous blood transfusion has now made autologous blood donation a standard of practice in elective orthopedic surgery (17).

One unit of autologous blood can be procured from a patient every 72 hours until 72 hours before operation, as long as the hematocrit stays at least 33 percent (American Association of Blood Bank Standards [18]); iron supplementation is routinely given (19). Many units of autologous blood can potentially be procured over periods of up to 42 days (the maximal storage interval for liquid blood). Limitations in predonating the amount of autologous blood necessary to avoid subsequent need for homologous blood transfusion include physician (surgeon) underordering (16), the effective autologous blood storage period (i.e., the date of surgery scheduling until the date of surgery) (20), iron-restricted erythropoiesis (19), and the endogenous erythropoietin response to serial phlebotomy (21).

The early experience in our program suggested that, because physicians were underordering autologous blood (16), subsequent homologous blood exposure was not minimized (22). The problem of physician underordering was corrected by a continuing medical education program that consisted of a series of grand rounds lectures to departments of surgery, medicine, and anesthesia (23). Our recommendation to referring surgeons was that the number of autologous units requested should approximate the number of blood units normally requested for type and crossmatch for the surgical procedure; this approach was also suggested by others (24). Analysis of patients treated after the education program showed that patients who successfully predonated the requested amount of autologous blood had a likelihood of receiving homologous blood that declined from 12 of 42 (29 percent) to 6 of 52 (12 percent) to 1 of 51 (2.1 percent) over a 2-year period (20). However, the education program had no influence on the effective autologous blood storage interval, which remained a mean of approximately 21 days at our institution.

Another potential limitation to the procurement of adequate autologous blood is iron-restricted erythropoiesis (25). It has long been apparent that supplemental iron therapy must be given to ensure rapid regeneration of blood after phlebotomy (26). Although studies have shown the efficacy of this approach with long-term supplementation (27), the effectiveness of short-term oral iron therapy and the compliance of patients prescribed iron salt therapy with known side effects (28) are unresolved issues for autologous blood donor programs. A prospective audit of 72 consecutive iron-treated adults enrolled in our autologous blood donor program showed that, although all 27 male patients successfully predonated the requested amount of autologous blood, 15 (33 percent) of 45 female patients were deferred and unable to predonate the requested amount of autologous blood (29). Iron studies in the 15 deferred patients compared to the 57 nondeferred patients revealed significantly lower storage, circulating, and total body iron estimates, as well as higher free erythrocyte protoporphyrin levels in the deferred group. Additionally, the initial mobilizable red blood cell (and iron) mass for autologous blood donors was found to be predictive of the success of procuring the requested amount of autologous blood. A significant percentage of donors who are unable to donate the requested amount of autologous blood potentially have iron-restricted erythropoiesis if oral iron absorption is not adequate (29). Subsequent studies have indicated that premenopausal women, in particular, need alternatives for iron supplementation in autologous blood donation (30).

A further potential limitation to the procurement of adequate autologous blood is the endogenous erythropoietin response to serial phlebotomy. Until the recent development of a radioimmunoassay for serum erythropoietin (31), valid quantitative measurements of erythropoietin were limited to the research laboratory and were virtually unavailable to the clinician. Serial measurements of serum immunoreactive erythropoietin levels in autologous blood donors showed that, although a rise in serum immunoreactive levels can be demonstrated, the increase is not significantly above the upper limit of normal (26 units/litre) for the assay (29,32). It has long been known that the relationship between an increasing degree of anemia and the endogenous erythropoietin response is linear (33); with the development of radioimmunoassay for erythropoietin, however, it has been more recently appreciated that this linear relationship holds true only for significantly anemic patients; for mild anemias (hemoglobin of more than 10.5 g/dl), endogenous eryth-

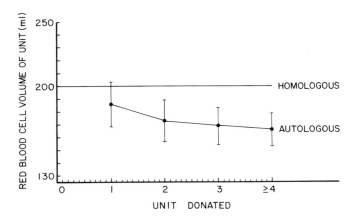

Figure 21.1. The relationship between the number of autologous blood units donated and the mean red cell volume. The mean red cell volume of homologous blood units donated by men and women is also indicated.

ropoietin levels do not correlate with the degree of anemia and rarely rise above the normal range (34). The slow compensatory response in autologous blood donors can be demonstrated clinically by the fall in hematocrits of autologous blood donors; as seen in Figure 21.1, the calculated red cell mass of autologous units by autologous donors reveals a significant fall over the 3-week course of phlebotomy. Because of this anemia, 20 percent of autologous blood units have a red cell mass less than the 95 percent confidence interval for the red cell mass of homologous blood units (35).

Because understorage of autologous blood increases the likelihood of subsequent homologous donor exposure (20), a prospective, randomized, double-blind trial of rHuEpo therapy was undertaken in adult autologous blood donors scheduled for elective orthopedic surgery for which ≥3 units of blood was requested (36). Patients received either rHuEpo (600 units/kg of body weight) or placebo intravenously twice a week for 21 days, during which time collection of 6 units of blood between 25 and 35 days before surgery was attempted according to standards of the American Association of Blood Banks (18). All patients received iron sulfate (325 mg orally three times daily). Forty-seven patients completed the study. The 24 patients in the placebo group and the 23 patients in the rHuEpo group were no different in age, sex, types of surgical procedures, or duration of hospitalization. The 23 rHuEpo-treated patients donated 125 units (5.4 ± 0.2 units, mean ± SE) compared to 99 units donated by 24 placebo patients (4.1 ± 0.1 units). As shown in Figure 21.2a, male patients treated with rHuEpo donated 42 percent more red blood cell mass per patient over the study duration than did male patients treated with placebo (1097 vs. 776 ml, respectively). Similarly, female patients treated with rHuEpo donated 29 percent more red blood cell mass per patient (809 ml) than did female patients treated with placebo (627 ml) (Fig 21.2b). Mean red cell volume per autologous blood unit collected at the third and fourth donations was significantly higher in the rHuEpo-treated group (174 ml) compared to the placebo group (156 ml); analysis of red blood cell volume showed that 23 (24 percent) of 99 units from placebo-treated donors had <154 ml of red blood cells (American Association of Blood Banks minimal standards for homologous blood units [18]), compared to 15 (12 percent) of 125 units from rHuEpo-treated donors. When donation was analyzed according to sex, the men (5.9 ± 01.2 vs. 4.6 ± 0.6 units) and women (4.9 ± 0.6 vs. 3.9 ± 0.5 units) in the rHuEpo group donated significantly more units than did the men and women in the placebo group. In men, the effect of rHuEpo was seen in an increased hematocrit (Fig 21.3a) and in the number of units successfully donated (71 of 72 [99 percent] possible units compared to 41 of 54 [76 percent] possible units in the placebo group). Similarly, in women, the effect of rHuEpo was seen in the successful donation of 54 of 66 units (82 percent) compared to 58 of 90 (64 percent) possible units in the placebo group, as well as an increased hematocrit (Fig 21.3b). Significant differences between placebo- and rHuEpo-treated patients were noted for hematocrit levels by the third study visit (7.2 ± 0.8 days) and for reticulocyte responses by the second study visit (3.5 ± 0.6 days). Platelet counts in the rHuEpo and placebo groups were not different: 296 ± 17 and 321 ± 14 × $10^3/mm^3$ initially and 367 ± 23 and 360 ± 22 × $10^3/mm^3$ after the study.

The relationship between amount of iron available for erythropoiesis and the number of autologous blood units donated in this study showed a better correlation with the initial level of mobilizable circulating iron (calculated from initial body weight and hematocrit, $r^2 = 0.70$) than with the initial level of mobilizable stored iron (calculated from initial serum ferritin, $r^2 = 0.50$). The correlation between mobilizable circulating iron levels and successful donation was strongest among rHuEpo-treated women ($r^2 = 0.90$) and placebo-treated women ($r^2 = 0.73$). The five premenopausal women in the rHuEpo group successfully donated 21 (70 percent) of 30 possible units compared to 18 (60 percent) of 30 possible units in the five premenopausal placebo patients

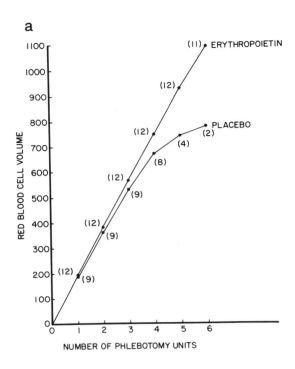

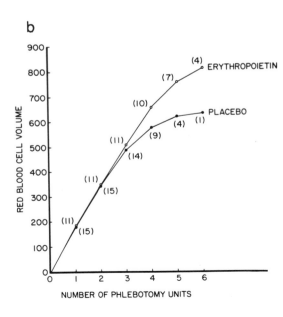

Figure 21.2. The cumulative red cell volumes procured per male patient (a) and per female patient (b). The number of patients at each donation is indicated in parentheses. Mean cumulative time in days for each visit: 3.5 for visit 1, 7.2 for visit 2, 10.6 for visit 3, 14.2 for visit 4, 17.6 for visit 5, 20.9 for visit 6.

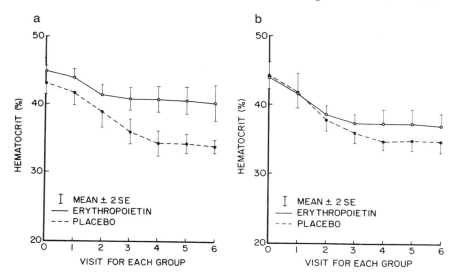

Figure 21.3. The mean hematocrit values for male patients (a) and for female patients (b) in each treatment group before the study and at visits 1 to 6. *Source: Reference 37*

($P > 0.05$). Mobilizable circulating iron levels were not correlated with successful donation in men. These results indicate that iron-restricted erythropoiesis depends on both mobilizable iron compartments (stored and circulating); in women, the ability to compensate for lower stored iron is hindered by a generally smaller circulating iron compartment; in men, however, circulating iron is generally not a limitation because stored iron is adequate. As the efficacy of erythropoietin therapy is to increase the production of circulating iron, either from storage iron or from orally absorbed iron, this analysis suggests that, as long as sufficient iron is absorbed orally, the subgroup for whom erythropoietin would be particularly effective are individuals with small circulating iron (red blood cell) volumes, such as small or anemic individuals, particularly women and pediatric patients.

The efficacy of rHuEpo therapy in the autologous blood donor setting can be seen not only in enhanced autologous blood procurement, but also in hematocrit during the subsequent surgical admission. Mean admission (38.6 ± 1.2 vs. 35.2 ± 0.9 percent) and discharge (33.5 ± 0.7 vs. 30.5 ± 0.7 percent) hematocrits were significantly higher in the rHuEpo-treated than in the placebo-treated patients, respectively. These differences were also significant when analyzed for men and women.

In addition, only 1 (4 percent) of the 23 rHuEpo-treated patients was unable to donate at least 4 units, compared to 7 (29 percent) of the 24 placebo-treated patients. The small number of study patients precluded showing a difference in subsequent homologous blood transfusion exposure; one rHuEpo-treated patient received transfusion of 2 homologous units, whereas two placebo-treated patients received 5 homologous units. A subsequent clinical trial is evaluating the efficacy of rHuEpo therapy in autologous donor patients with pre-existing anemia (hematocrit < 39 percent) to address this issue.

Erythropoietin Therapy in the Perisurgical Setting

In addition to a role in autologous blood donation before elective surgery, rHuEpo therapy also has potential applications in "nonelective" surgical settings in which preoperative autologous blood donation is not practical. Examples of these surgical settings include nonelective orthopedic surgery, vascular procedures, and coronary artery bypass graft procedures, where blood loss is significant and blood transfusions are commonly required. The potential effect of rHuEpo therapy on transfusion medicine in these settings is significant; for example, the majority of the 250,000 patients who undergo coronary artery bypass grafting receive transfusion, and these represent nearly 10 percent of the estimated 3.2 million recipients of red cell transfusions annually (38,39). Animal studies showed that rHuEpo therapy in baboons stimulates significant erythropoiesis pre- and postoperatively compared to placebo-treated controls (40). Based on the study results of rHuEpo therapy in autologous blood donors, reticulocytosis would be expected after 3.5 days of rHuEpo therapy and a change in hematocrit would be expected by 7.2 days of rHuEpo therapy (36). An analysis of the kinetics of the hematocrit change in autologous blood donors receiving rHuEpo at each visit allows the differences between the placebo and rHuEpo groups to be examined with respect to time. Table 21.1 contains estimates of the depletion and repletion rates of erythropoiesis depending on whether an autologous blood unit was or was not donated on the previous visit. The model on which these estimates are based studies hematocrit on visit 1 as a function of the hematocrit on visit $(i - 1)$ and whether or not blood was donated on visit $(i - 1)$. The model has two branches depending on the action taken on the previous visit. That is, if no blood was donated on visit $(i - 1)$, then the hematocrit increased r_i percent by visit i. If blood was donated on visit $(i - 1)$, then the hematocrit decreased d_i percent by visit i. The cumulative hematocrit percentage

Table 21.1. The Effect of Erythropoietin Therapy and Erythropoiesis

Days of rHuEpo Treatment	Depletion Rate*			Replacement Rate†		
	Placebo, %	rHuEpo, %	Σ (Δ)	Placebo, %	rHuEpo, %	Σ (Δ)
3.5	−3.468	−2.800	0.668	3.100	2.633	−0.467
7.2	−2.838	−0.970	2.536	1.850	3.250	0.933
10.6	−1.821	−0.774	3.583	0.000	0.950	1.883
14.2	−1.150	−0.406	4.327	1.254	3.000	3.629
17.6	−2.230	−0.701	5.856	1.794	4.100	5.935
20.9	−0.300	−0.123	6.033	1.582	2.683	7.036
			Δ = 6.033			Δ = 7.036
		Total Difference = 13.069%				

Source: Reference 37
*If blood was donated during the prior visit.
†If blood was not donated during the prior visit.

differences between placebo- and rHuEpo-treated patients is 6.03 percent (depletion rate) plus 7.04 percent (replacement rate), or 13.07 percent over a 21-day treatment course. Similar estimates for the erythropoietic effect of rHuEpo therapy can be calculated from Table 22.1 for shorter periods of administration. For example, 14 days of rHuEpo therapy can be estimated to result in 4.3 percent + 3.6 percent = 7.9 percent hematocrit (over 2 blood units) of erythropoietic effect. Thus, perisurgical treatment with rHuEpo can be anticipated to result in the erythropoietic equivalence of several units of homologous blood transfusion. Clinical trials of perisurgical rHuEpo therapy are currently under way to address this issue.

Conclusion

Erythropoietin shows considerable promise as a pharmacologic alternative to homologous blood transfusion in the surgical patient. Animal and human studies to date indicate that erythropoietin facilitates autologous blood procurement before elective surgery and increases surgical admission hematocrits in rHuEpo-treated patients and that erythropoietin therapy can stimulate erythropoiesis postoperatively as well as preoperatively. It is anticipated that ongoing clinical trials will further define clinical applications of erythropoietin designed to minimize or eliminate the need for homologous blood transfusions in the perisurgical period.

ACKNOWLEDGMENT

The author gratefully acknowledges Mark Von Tress, Ph.D., for providing helpful data analysis.

REFERENCES

1. National Institutes of Health Consensus Conference. Fresh frozen plasma: indications and risks. JAMA 1985;253:551–3.
2. National Institutes of Health Consensus Conference. Platelet transfusion therapy. JAMA 1987;257:1777–80.
3. National Institutes of Health Consensus Conference. Perioperative red cell transfusion. JAMA 1988;260:2700–3.
4. Blood usage review (Ms.6.1.5). In: Accreditation manual for hospitals (AMH). Chicago: Joint Commission on Accreditation of Health Care Organizations, 1988:120.
5. Goodman R, ed. Morbidity and mortality weekly report. Atlanta: Centers for Disease Control, 1989;38:229–36.
6. Campbell S, ed. AABB issues recommendations on informed consent for transfusion. AABB Newsbriefs, Jul 1986:1–3.
7. Goodnough LT, Shuck JM. Review of risks, options and informed consent for blood transfusion in elective surgery. Am J Surg 1990;159:602–9.
8. Gould SA, Rosen AL, Sehgal LR, et al. Fluosol-DA as a red cell substitute in acute anemia. N Engl J Med 1986;314:1653–6.
9. Friedman BA, Burns TL, Schork MA. An analysis of blood transfusion of surgical patients by sex: a quest for the transfusion trigger. Transfusion 1980;20:179–88.
10. Council on Scientific Affairs. Autologous blood transfusions. JAMA 1986;256:2378–80.
11. Campbell S, ed. AABB establishes national autologous resource center. AABB Newsbriefs, May 1987:1–3.
12. Mintz P. Autologous transfusion endorsed. JAMA 1985;254:507.
13. Surgenor DM. The patient's blood is the safest blood. N Engl J Med 1987;316:542–4.
14. Haugen K, Hill E. Large scale autologous blood program in a community hospital. JAMA 1987;257:1211–4.
15. Toy PTCY, Strauss R, Stehling L, et al. Predeposit autologous blood for elective surgery: a multi-center study. N Engl J Med 1987;316:517–20.
16. Wasman J, Goodnough LT. Effect of autologous blood donation for elective surgery on physician transfusion behavior. JAMA 1987;258:3135–7.
17. Goodnough LT, Schafron D, Marcus RE. The impact of autologous blood donation in orthopaedic surgical practice. Vox Sang 1990;59:65–9.
18. Holland P, ed. Standards for blood banks and transfusion services. 13th ed. Arlington, Virginia: American Association of Blood Banks, 1989:40.
19. Finch S, Haskins O, Finch CA. Iron metabolism. Hematopoiesis following phlebotomy. Iron as a limiting factor. J Clin Invest 1950;29:1078–86.
20. Goodnough LT, Wasman J, Corlucci K, Chernosky A. Limitations to do-

nating adequate autologous blood prior to elective orthopaedic surgery. Arch Surg 1989;124:494–6.

21. Finch CA. Erythropoiesis, erythropoietin and iron. Blood 1982;60:1241–6.

22. Goodnough LT. Autologous blood donation. JAMA 1988;259:2405.

23. Hull A, Wasman J, Goodnough LT. Effects of a CME program on physicians' transfusion practices. Acad Med 1989;64:681–5.

24. Axelrod FB, Pepkowitz SH, Goldfinger D. Establishment of a schedule of optimal preoperative collection of autologous blood. Transfusion 1989;29:677–80.

25. Jacobs P, Finch CA. Iron for erythropoiesis. Blood 1971;37:220–30.

26. Coleman DH, Stevens AR, Dodge HT, Finch CA. Rate of blood regeneration after blood loss. Arch Intern Med 1953;92:341–8.

27. Simon TL, Hunt WC, Garry PJ. Iron supplementation for menstruating female blood donors. Transfusion 1984;24:469–72.

28. Skikne B, Lynch S, Borek D, Cook J. Iron and blood donation. Clin Haematol 1984;13:271–387.

29. Goodnough LT, Brittenham GM. Limitations of the erythropoietic response to serial phlebotomy: implications for autologous blood donor programs. J Lab Clin Med 1990;115:28–35.

30. Goodnough LT, Price TH, Rudnick S. Iron-restricted erythropoiesis as a limitation to autologous blood donation in the erythropoietin-stimulated bone marrow. J Lab Clin Med (in press).

31. Egrie JC, Cotes PM, Lane J, et al. Development of radioimmunoassays for human erythropoietin using recombinant erythropoietin as tracer and immunogen. J Immunol Methods 1987;99:235–41.

32. Kickler TS, Spivak JL. Effect of repeated whole blood donations on serum immunoreactive erythropoietin levels in autologous donors. JAMA 1988;260:65–7.

33. Adamson JW. The erythropoietin/hematocrit relationship in normal and polycythemic man: implications of marrow regulation. Blood 1968;32:597–609.

34. Erslev AJ, Caro J. Physiologic and molecular biology of erythropoietin. Med Oncol Tumor Pharmacother 1986;3:159–64.

35. Goodnough LT, Bravo J, Hsueh Y, Keating L, Brittenham G. Red blood cell volume in autologous and homologous blood units: implications for risk/benefit assessment for autologous blood "crossover" and directed blood transfusion. Transfusion 1989;29:821–2.

36. Goodnough LT, Rudnick S, Price TH, et al. Increased preoperative collection of autologous blood with recombinant human erythropoietin therapy. N Engl J Med 1989;321:1163–8.

37. Goodnough LT. Erythropoietin as a pharmacologic alternative to blood transfusion in the surgical patient. Transfusion Med Rev 1990;4:288–96.

38. Goodnough LT, Johnston MFM, Toy PTYC, et al. The variability of transfusion practise in coronary artery bypass surgery. JAMA 1991;265:86–90.

39. Killip T. Twenty years of coronary bypass surgery. N Engl J Med 1988;319:366–8.

40. Levine EA, Gould SA, Rosen AL, et al: Perioperative recombinant human erythropoietin. Surgery 1989;106:432–8.

Chapter 22

Recombinant Human Erythropoietin (Epoetin Alfa) in Patients with the Anemia of Chronic Disease

Sanford B. Krantz, Frederick Wolfe,
I. Jon Russell, Robert T. Means, Jr.,
and Joseph A. Boccagno

The anemia of chronic disease accompanies infectious, inflammatory, or neoplastic diseases and is second only to iron deficiency as the most common anemia (1). It is characterized by a shortened red cell survival, an impaired release of iron from the reticuloendothelial system, and a greatly reduced response of the marrow to anemia (2). The hemolytic component, however, is minimal, and the major factor in the anemia is a lack of adequate marrow response.

Erslev et al. (3) reported subnormal erythropoietin levels, measured by bioassay, in the anemia of chronic inflammation, but subsequently reported that erythropoietin levels measured by radioimmunoassay were appropriate for the degree of anemia (4). Erythropoietin levels were considered appropriate for the anemia of rheumatoid arthritis by one group (5), but three other groups demonstrated lower than expected levels (6–8). In addition, this laboratory reported a blunted erythropoietin response in patients with rheumatoid arthritis compared to patients with other anemias (9). These observations suggest that the anemia of rheumatoid arthritis and perhaps the anemias of other chronic inflammatory or neoplastic disorders might respond to the administration of exogenous erythropoietin. However, a primary defect in the anemia of chronic disease must still reside in an abnormal response of the bone marrow to erythropoietin because erythropoietin levels are generally above normal in these conditions. Whether the abnormal marrow would respond to higher erythropoietin levels was untested and unknown in human beings, so we initiated a study of the effect of recombinant human erythropoietin (rHuEpo) on the anemia of patients with rheumatoid arthritis. The investigation has shown that rHuEpo can completely correct this anemia.

Methods

The Selection of Patients

A full description of this study has been submitted for publication (10), but the present chapter is written to provide additional detail and commentary. Seventeen patients, aged 25 to 73 years, all female except one, were studied at five institutions. All had hematocrits of 34 percent or less, and all met the American Rheumatism Association criteria for rheumatoid arthritis (11). Patients with severe allergic disorders, seizures, asthma, renal disease, hepatitis, other inflammatory conditions, malignancy, uncontrolled hypertension, ischemic heart disease, peptic ulcer disease, neutropenia, hemolytic anemia, or thrombocytopenia were excluded. The protocol was approved by the institutional review boards of the participating centers, and patients gave fully informed consent before entry.

Patients were screened at baseline with a complete medical history and physical examination, ophthalmologic and audiometric evaluations, chest roentgenography, electrocardiography, routine hematology, serum chemistries (including a hepatitis battery, a reticulocyte count, serum ferritin, serum iron and iron-binding capacity, serum folate, and serum B_{12}), occult blood in the stool, routine urinalysis, and coagulation tests. A small fraction of the patients at one institution had chromium 51-labeled red cell mass studies and bone marrow aspirates for morphology, cytogenetics, and progenitor cell culture (12).

Study Design

The study consisted of a double-blind, randomized, placebo-controlled phase and an open maintenance phase. During the acute phase, patients were observed for a baseline period of 2 weeks, during which they received ferrous sulfate, 300 mg three times daily, which was continued throughout the study. The patients were then randomized to receive placebo or one of three doses of rHuEpo (50, 100, or 150 units/kg) three times per week intravenously over 5 minutes. The chosen therapy was continued for 8 weeks or until the hematocrit exceeded 40 percent for men or 35 percent for women. Patients were then offered the option of participating in a 24-week open label study during which all patients received rHuEpo that could be increased or decreased to maintain a hematocrit of 40 percent in men or 35 percent in women. A response to rHuEpo was arbitrarily defined as an increase of 6 hematocrit units, whereas correction of anemia was defined as reaching a hematocrit of 40 percent in men or 35 percent in women. Hematocrit, hemoglobin, and reticulocyte counts were obtained biweekly during the acute phase and weekly thereafter. Serum chemistries, iron, iron-binding capacity, and ferritin values were measured every 2 weeks. Baseline screening, ^{51}Cr-labeled red cell volumes, and bone marrow testing were repeated at the end of the acute phase just before maintenance treatment began. Eleven patients completed the open label, maintenance study.

In Vitro Studies

Erythroid colony- and burst-forming units-erythroid (CFU-E, BFU-E), granulocyte-monocyte colony-forming units (CFU-GM), and megakaryocyte colony-forming units (CFU-Mk) were assayed by the plasma clot method (13–15) using the marrow cells of two patients before and at the end of the acute phase of treatment with rHuEpo. Assays were performed on light-density, nonadherent, and T-cell-depleted marrow fractions (15). This method of preparation was chosen to minimize variations caused by different amounts of blood drawn during marrow aspiration. The plating cell concentrations were 0.2, 0.4, 0.2, and 2.0 × 10^5 per millilitre of medium for CFU-E, BFU-E, CFU-GM, and CFU-Mk, respectively. Enumeration of hematopoietic colonies was performed using standard criteria. All cultures were performed with six replicates, and the results were reported as means ± SEM. Progenitor cell and ^{51}Cr-labeled red cell mass studies were evaluated using Student's t-test. A coefficient of variation for the red cell mass determination was estimated to be 8 percent.

Results

Hematologic Responses

The responses of 17 rheumatoid arthritis patients entered into the double-blind, randomized, placebo-controlled 8-week trial of rHuEpo, followed by the 24-week open maintenance phase, are shown in Table 22.1. During the initial 8-week study, 13 patients received rHuEpo and 4 received placebo. Four patients responded to rHuEpo with a 6-unit

Table 22.1. The Response of Rheumatoid Arthritis Patients to Recombinant Human Erythropoietin

	Total	rHuEpo 150 units/kg	100 units/kg	50 units/kg	Placebo
Number of patients	17	1	6	6	4
Number responding (8-wk randomized phase)	4	1	2	1	0
Percentage responding (8-wk randomized phase)	31	100	33	17	0
Additional responses/ patients entered (open maintenance phase)	8/8	0/0	4/4	1/1	3/3
Nonresponders	5	0	0	4	1

Note: Response to therapy: An increase from the mean baseline hematocrit of at least 6 percentage points or correction of anemia (hematocrit $\geq$ 40 percent in males or 35 percent in females).

or more increase in the hematocrit: 1 of 1 who received 150 units/kg, 2 of 6 who received 100 units/kg, and 1 of 6 who received 50 units/kg. None of the 4 patients who received placebo had such a response.

When the patients were entered into the open maintenance phase, which permitted increased time of treatment and increased dosage of rHuEpo, 8 of 8 additional responses to rHuEpo were evident in patients who had previously not responded. Of the 4 patients who had previously not responded to placebo, only 3 entered the maintenance phase, but all 3 responded, showing that they were capable of responding when they received the hormone. Altogether, 4 patients did not respond to rHuEpo, but they received only the smallest dose (50 units/kg) for the shortest period (8 weeks). One patient, who received placebo for 8 weeks, elected not to enter the maintenance phase, so she never received rHuEpo. Thus, 12 of 16 rheumatoid arthritis patients who received rHuEpo had a response and 11 of 12 attained a normal hematocrit.

Two patients, who were previously reported (12), had ^{51}Cr-labeled red cell volumes performed initially and 8 weeks after receiving rHuEpo at 100 units/kg three times per week intravenously (Table 22.2). Both had significant increases in their red cell volumes. This test was performed to determine whether a true increase in the number of red cells had occurred rather than a decrease in the plasma volume. In addition, marrow progenitor cell assays for CFU-E, BFU-E, and CFU-Mk showed statistically significant increases over the pretreatment values, and one

Table 22.2. Values for Selected Variables before and after the Administration of rHuEpo to Two Women with Rheumatoid Arthritis and Anemia

	Patient 1		Patient 2	
	Pre-rHuEpo	Post-rHuEpo	Pre-rHuEpo	Post-rHuEpo
Red cell mass (ml)	1076	1379*	1317	1870[†]
Plasma volume (ml)	2532	2540[‡]	2905	2713[‡]
MCV (fl)	79	77	71	69
Serum iron (μg/dl)	7	7	5	55
TIBC (μg/dl)	285	324	498	300
Serum ferritin (μg/litre)	55	32	23	5
Marrow iron	Present	Absent	Absent	Absent
Assay findings (10^5 marrow cells)[§]				
CFU-E	304 ± 21	848 ± 17[‡]	185 ± 28	313 ± 28[‡]
BFU-E	38 ± 4	93 ± 11[‡]	36 ± 3	65 ± 4[‡]
CFU-GM	89 ± 7	151 ± 9[‡]	133 ± 13	128 ± 8[§]
CFU-Mk	40 ± 5	96 ± 12[‡]	69 ± 4	93 ± 9[‡]

Source: Reference 12
Note: rHuEpo, recombinant human erythropoietin (100 units/kg intravenously, three times per week for 8 weeks); MCV, mean corpuscular volume; TIBC, total iron-binding capacity; CFU-E, colony-forming units—erythroid; BFU-E, burst-forming units—erythroid; CFU-GM, colony-forming units—granulocyte/macrophage; CFU-Mk, colony-forming units—megakaryocyte.
*$P < 0.05$, by Student's t-test.
[†]$P < 0.01$, by Student's t-test.
[‡]Not significant.
[§]Assays were performed as described under "Methods." Values are means ± SEM.

patient also responded with a significant increase in CFU-GM as well (Table 22.2). No significant change was noted in either patient's white blood cell or platelet counts.

In almost all cases, the serum iron/total iron-binding capacity ratio was low, as expected with the anemia of inflammatory disease. A serum ferritin of less than 60 μg/litre, which suggests iron deficiency in the anemia of chronic disorders (16,17), was present in eight patients who responded to rHuEpo. However, these patients were treated with ferrous sulfate, 300 mg three times per day, beginning 2 weeks before rHuEpo administration, and the mean hematocrits and reticulocyte counts (31 percent, 1.2 percent) for the eight patients did not change significantly (29.9 percent, 1.9 percent; $P > 0.05$) with iron therapy alone. In addition, one patient's serum ferritin value was corrected without the hematocrit being increased during the placebo period before rHuEpo administration (10); in two female patients, the hematocrits increased to 49 to 50 percent, which is above normal and is unlikely to be due to iron treatment. In three patients, the hematocrits declined to pre-rHuEpo levels after cessation of rHuEpo treatment. These observations indicate that the patients responded to rHuEpo rather than to the iron.

Representative Cases

Three representative cases illustrate patient responses to rHuEpo. The first was a 73-year-old man who had had rheumatoid arthritis for 7 years with an initially low rheumatoid factor titer of 1:20 (18). The arthritis became more severe in 1984 with a weight loss of 7 kg, lethargy, and a substantial rise in the rheumatoid factor titer of 1:2560. At that time, the hematocrit was 35 percent. The patient was treated with hydroxychloroquine, 400 mg, and ibuprofen, 2400 mg, each day, which was continued throughout the rHuEpo treatment period. The arthritis continued to be active, and his hematocrit stabilized at 32.5 percent. The patient was begun on rHuEpo at 100 units/kg, three times per week intravenously, and his hematocrit gradually increased over 8 weeks to 44 percent (Fig 22.1). Throughout this time his serum ferritin was within the normal range, indicating that iron deficiency was not present. When the rHuEpo was discontinued, the hematocrit declined to 33 percent in 11 weeks and was essentially the same 8 months later.

The second patient was a 31-year-old woman who presented with a 1-year history of prolonged morning stiffness and polyarticular pain. Her joint symptoms involved her wrists, metacarpophalangeal joints, knees, and ankles. She had been treated with ibuprofen, 2400 mg, and prednisone, 5 mg, each day. Examination showed that many of her metacarpophalangeal joints and both wrists, knees, and ankles were warm and swollen but exhibited no deformity. There were no palpable nodules. Her rheumatoid factor titer was positive at 1:640, and the Westergren sedimentation rate was 49 mm/hour. Her antinuclear antibodies were weakly positive at 1:80 with a homogeneous pattern, but fractionation serologic tests (anti-SSA, anti-SSB, anti-Smith, anti-RNP, anti-DNA) were all negative. In addition, the plasma complement C3 and C4 levels were not depressed. Her white blood count was 6800/μl, with a hematocrit of 30.4 percent. Ibuprofen and prednisone were discontinued and replaced with naproxen, 500 mg, orally two times per day.

Three months later this patient entered the rHuEpo study with a stable hematocrit of 31.5 percent (Fig 22.2). She was randomized to the placebo group, and her hematocrit at the end of 8 weeks was 33 percent. She then began to receive open label rHuEpo at 50 units/kg, three times per week intravenously, and by 5 weeks her hematocrit was 37 percent.

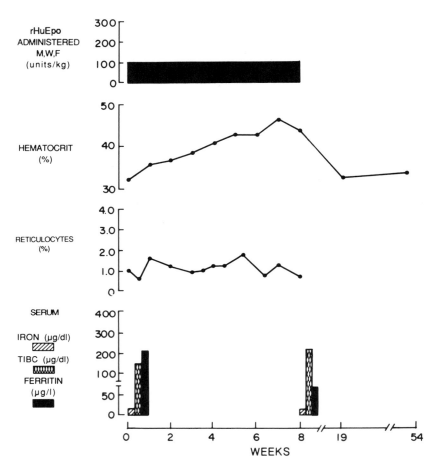

Figure 22.1. The response of a 73-year-old man with active rheumatoid arthritis to rHuEpo, 100 units/kg, three times per week intravenously. Although the iron/total iron-binding capacity ratio was low, as commonly seen in the anemia of chronic disorders, the serum ferritin was normal. In 8 weeks, the patient's hematocrit rose from 32.5 percent to 44 percent. After rHuEpo was discontinued, the hematocrit declined to 33 percent. TIBC, total iron-binding capacity. *Source: Reference 18. Reprinted with permission of the publisher, AlphaMed Press, Dayton, Ohio.*

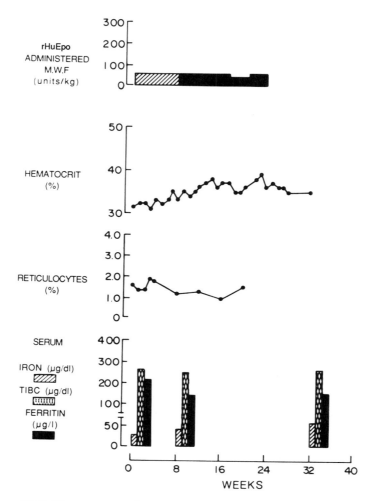

Figure 22.2. The response of a 31-year-old woman with active rheumatoid arthritis to rHuEpo, 50 units/kg, three times per week intravenously. Serum ferritins were normal, although the iron total/iron-binding capacity ratios were low. The patient started the rHuEpo randomized study with a hematocrit of 31.5 percent and received placebo (▨) for the first 8 weeks. At the end of that period, the hematocrit was 33 percent. Open label rHuEpo therapy was begun and led to an increase in the hematocrit to 37 percent by 5 weeks and to 39 percent by 16 weeks of treatment. TIBC, total iron-binding capacity.

Her rHuEpo dosage was briefly reduced to 25 units/kg, three times per week intravenously, because her hematocrit had risen above the arbitrary limit of 35 percent. Later the dose was increased to 50 units/kg, three times per week intravenously for several weeks, and then was discontinued. The peak hematocrit was 39 percent. In both of these patients, the increase in hematocrit clearly seemed to result from rHuEpo therapy.

The third patient was a 41-year-old woman who first developed symptoms of rheumatoid arthritis at the age of 37 years. Her symptoms began in the metatarsophalangeal joints. The swelling and tenderness later spread to the hands, where there was significant involvement of the proximal interphalangeal joints and the metacarpophalangeal joints. Ankle involvement and discomfort in both knees, shoulders, wrists, and the jaw soon followed. The patient was first seen in the arthritis clinic 1.5 years after the onset of rheumatoid arthritis. At the time of the initial visit, the patient complained of fatigue, headache, sore throat, loss of appetite, and anorexia. Four hours of morning stiffness was noted. Swelling and tenderness were found scattered across the proximal interphalangeal, the metacarpophalangeal, and the metatarsophalangeal joints. Both wrists were tender, motion of the right shoulder was restricted, and swelling was present at the left ankle. The sedimentation rate was 45 mm/hour, and the rheumatoid factor was positive at a dilution of 1:2560. The hematocrit was 35 percent.

The patient was started on naproxen and auranofin. The hematocrit fell to 31 percent during the subsequent 3 months, but 6 months later she was improved clinically and psychologically. She had no morning stiffness, and only two joints with active disease were noted. The sedimentation rate had fallen to 25 mm/hour, and the hematocrit had risen to 38 percent. Aspirin at 3900 mg/24 hours was substituted for naproxen. At that time, the onset of 2+ proteinuria prompted discontinuation of the oral gold.

The subsequent worsening of her condition led to the initiation of hydroxychloroquine therapy 1 year before rHuEpo treatment. However, her disease continued to be active throughout the year and her hematocrit dropped to 30 percent with a sedimentation rate of 53 mm/hour. Two weeks before rHuEpo therapy, the hematocrit was 36 percent. Ferrous sulfate, 300 mg three times daily, was begun. Two weeks later, at the initiation of rHuEpo treatment, 100 units/kg, three times per week intravenously, the hematocrit was only 34 percent (Fig 22.3). rHuEpo was continued for 32 weeks during which the arthritis remained active, but the hematocrit reached 48 to 49 percent on three consecutive tests.

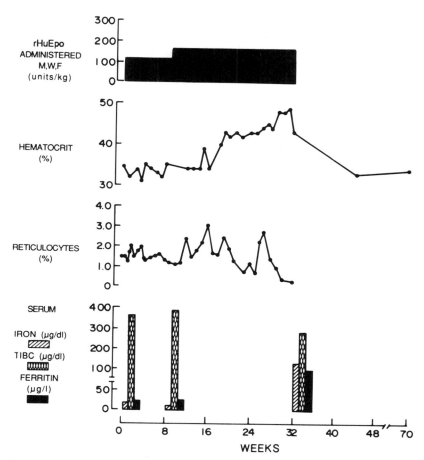

Figure 22.3. The response of a 41-year-old woman with active rheumatoid arthritis to rHuEpo. The patient had a low iron/total iron-binding capacity ratio and a low serum ferritin. She was begun on ferrous sulfate (300 mg, three times per day), and her hematocrit, which was initially 36 percent, was even lower (34 percent) 2 weeks later. Ferrous sulfate was continued and rHuEpo was begun (100 units/kg, three times per week intravenously for 8 weeks, and 150 units/kg thereafter). The hematocrit eventually rose to above-normal levels (48 to 49 percent), and the rHuEpo was discontinued. At that time the serum ferritin was 97 μg/litre, but the hematocrit soon declined to 33 percent. The above-normal hematocrit while receiving rHuEpo and its subsequent decline after the cessation of rHuEpo treatment indicate that the patient's increased erythropoiesis resulted from the administration of recombinant hormone. TIBC, total iron-binding capacity.

During this time, there were no significant changes in the overall clinical status of the patient except for the hematologic status. Three months after the termination of rHuEpo treatment, the hematocrit had fallen again to 33 percent and the clinical data continued to reflect active rheumatoid arthritis. The patient's serum ferritin also increased to a normal level during this period, but the abnormal elevation of the hematocrit to 48 to 49 percent in a woman with rheumatoid arthritis and the decline of the hematocrit after discontinuation of the rHuEpo cannot be explained by the enhanced iron stores. No effect on the white cell or platelet counts was observed in any of the patients.

No serious or unusual adverse experiences, increases in blood pressure, seizures, or discontinuations due to adverse effects occurred with rHuEpo therapy of these rheumatoid arthritis patients. Serial evaluation of the patient's activities of daily living was obtained by using a modified version of a standardized, self-report health assessment questionnaire (19,20), and the patients' overall sense of musculoskeletal pain was assessed by a visual analog pain scale (21). No significant changes in these measures were found despite correction of the anemia.

Discussion

These studies demonstrate that rHuEpo can completely correct the anemia of chronic disease that occurs in patients with rheumatoid arthritis. Not only were the hematocrits increased, but the ^{51}Cr-labeled red cell masses of two patients and the numbers of CFU-E and BFU-E in the bone marrow were also increased. No important adverse events were encountered, and the drug appeared entirely safe. However, no improvement in the quality of life was observed in these particular patients. This could be due to the amount of physical activity required by the study because the patients had to return for evaluation and intravenous therapy three times per week. Alternatively, only a minor fraction of the rheumatoid arthritis patients' fatigue might be due to their anemia. It is also possible that the period of maintained normal hemoglobin was too short because it has been shown that 24 additional weeks of hemoglobin maintenance at 10.7 g/dl led to an increase in aerobic exercise capacity and anaerobic threshold (22). Nevertheless, the study clearly demonstrates the effectiveness of rHuEpo in correcting the anemia of inflammation, and this may be of particular benefit to selected patients with rheumatoid arthritis. Increasing numbers of these patients are having prosthetic joint surgery. Those who wish to predonate blood before surgery could do so with the use of rHuEpo (23). Because the preoperative hematocrit seems to determine the risk at surgery (24) and blood transfusions still carry finite risks, rHuEpo could be used pre- and perioperatively to provide a normal hematocrit. It could also prepare the bone marrow to compensate better for hemorrhage to reduce the risk of surgery and of homologous blood transfusions.

These results also suggest that rHuEpo may be useful in treating severe anemia in other patients with a wide variety of inflammatory diseases such as AIDS, chronic tuberculosis, fungal infections, bacterial endocarditis, abscesses, regional enteritis, and ulcerative colitis. The anemia of chronic disease present in patients with cancer seems to have a similar pathogenesis related to tumor necrosis factor (25,26), and current studies indicate that rHuEpo may be able to correct this anemia as well (27).

In contrast to patients on hemodialysis who respond to rHuEpo with a high, prompt, sustained increase in corrected reticulocyte count within 1 or 2 weeks (28), our patients had very small increases in the number of reticulocytes. The increase in reticulocyte count may be due to the correction of erythropoietin deficiency in the renal patients, leading to the rescue of large numbers of CFU-E that otherwise would die without the hormone (29). In rheumatoid arthritis, there is no deficiency of the hormone, but some component of the disease process can apparently be overcome by an excess of rHuEpo. Schooley et al. (30) showed that interleukin 1 suppresses CFU-E growth in vitro and that this can be overridden by large concentrations of rHuEpo. Interleukin 1 is elevated in the sera and joint fluids of rheumatoid arthritis patients, and the amount of elevation is inversely proportional to the anemia (31). Thus, rHuEpo is most likely overcoming an inhibition of erythropoiesis by interleukin 1, and perhaps other accessory cytokines, in this disease. Because erythropoietin levels are elevated in rheumatoid arthritis, fewer additional CFU-E would be available for rescue.

The reason for the increase in CFU-GM and CFU-Mk during rHuEpo therapy is unknown, but the same phenomenon has been observed in patients with end-stage renal disease (32). This is, therefore, not likely to be a specific consequence of the anemia of chronic inflammation but rather a general response to rHuEpo. Such responses could be due to the activation of accessory cells or erythroid cells by rHuEpo in a manner that enhances growth factor production (33). Alternatively, rHuEpo administration might lead to a feedback activation of the pluripotential stem cell. As late erythroid progenitors are stimulated to differentiate, earlier progenitors might be recruited to take their place. This might ultimately activate the pluripotential stem cell, leading to increased hematopoietic progenitor cells of all lineages. However, the CFU-GM and CFU-Mk might not undergo terminal differentiation because of a lack of additional factors required for further differentiation.

The dosages of rHuEpo and the duration of therapy required to achieve meaningful increases in the hematocrits of rheumatoid arthritis patients varied considerably. An extensive study of several hundred hemodialysis patients with end-stage renal disease showed that two thirds of the patients responded in 4 weeks and that 5 percent showed a response only after 10 to 19 weeks of treatment (34,35). Whereas three-fourths of the hemodialysis patients required no more than 125 units of rHuEpo per kg, three times per week intravenously, to maintain their hematocrits at 33 to 35 percent, 17 percent required 150 to 500 units/kg three times per week intravenously. This large spread of response makes it impossible to be certain of any difference in response of the smaller number of rheumatoid arthritis patients that were studied. A much larger study is needed to identify any significant differences in the response time or required dose of the hormone for this group or any other group of patients compared to the renal patients.

In summary, this study provides clinical evidence of a role for rHuEpo in overcoming the pathogenetic factors that produce the anemia of rheumatoid arthritis.

ACKNOWLEDGMENTS

This study was supported by the Ortho Pharmaceutical Corporation; by grants DK-15555, RR-95, and T32-07186 from the National Institutes of Health; by research funds from the Department of Veterans Affairs; and by the Joe C. Davis Hematology Research Fund. Dr. Means is an Associate Investigator of the VA Career Development Program.

REFERENCES

1. Lee GR. The anemia of chronic disease. Semin Hematol 1983;20:61–80.

2. Cartwright GE. The anemia of chronic disorders. Semin Hematol 1966;3:351–75.

3. Erslev AJ, Carol J, Miller O, Silver R. Plasma erythropoietin in health and disease. Ann Lab Clin Sci 1980;10:250–7.

4. Erslev AJ, Wilson J, Caro J. Erythropoietin tiers in anemic nonuremic patients. J Lab Clin Med 1987;109:429–33.

5. Biregaard G, Hallgren R, Caro J. Serum erythropoietin in rheumatoid

arthritis and other inflammatory arthritides: relationship to anemia and the effect of anti-inflammatory treatment. Br J Haematol 1987;65:479–83.

6. Ward HP, Gordon R, Pickett JC. Serum levels of erythropoietin in rheumatoid arthritis. J Lab Clin Med 1969;74:93–7.

7. Pavlovic-Kentera V, Ravidic R, Milenkovic P, Marinkovic D. Erythropoietin in patients with anemia in rheumatoid arthritis. Scand J Haematol 1979;23:141–5.

8. Hochberg MC, Arnold CM, Hogans BB, Spivak JL. Serum immunoreactive erythropoietin in rheumatoid arthritis: impaired response to anemia. Arthritis Rheum 1988;31:1318–21.

9. Baer AN, Dessypris EN, Goldwasser E, Krantz SB. Blunted erythropoietin response to anemia in rheumatoid arthritis. Br J Haematol 1987;66: 559–64.

10. Pincus T, Olsen NJ, Russell IJ, et al. A multicenter study of correction of anemia in rheumatoid arthritis using recombinant human erythropoietin. Am J Med 1990;89:161–8.

11. Arnett FC, Edworthy SM, Block DA, et al. The American Rheumatism Association 1987 revised criteria for the classification of rheumatoid arthritis. Arthritis Rheum 1988;31:315–24.

12. Means RT, Olsen NJ, Krantz SB, et al. Treatment of the anemia of rheumatoid arthritis with recombinant human erythropoietin: clinical and in vitro studies. Arthritis Rheum 1989;32:638–42.

13. Dessypris EN, Krantz SB, Roloff JS, Lukens JN. Mode of action of the IgG inhibitor of erythropoiesis in transient erythroblastopenia of childhood. Blood 1982;59:114–23.

14. Dessypris EN, Clark DA, McKee LC, Krantz SB. Increased sensitivity to complement of erythroid and myeloid progenitors in paroxysmal nocturnal hemoglobinuria. N Engl J Med 1983;309:690–3.

15. Dessypris EN, Gleaton JH, Sawyer ST, Armstrong OL. Suppression of maturation of megakaryocyte colony forming units in vitro by a platelet-released glycoprotein. J Cell Physiol 1987;130:361–8.

16. Hansen TM, Hansen NE, Birgens HS, Holund B, Lorenzen I. Serum ferritin and the assessment of iron deficiency in rheumatoid arthritis. Scand J Rheumatol 1983;12:353–9.

17. Hansen TM, Hansen NE. Serum ferritin as indicator of iron responsive anemia in patients with rheumatoid arthritis. Ann Rheum Dis 1986;45:596–602.

18. Krantz SB, Sawyer ST, Sawada K-I, Wolfe F, Boccagno J. Erythropoietin: receptors and clinical use in rheumatoid arthritis. Int J Cell Cloning 1990; 8(Suppl 1):181–98.

19. Fries JF, Spitz PW, Kraines RG, Holman HR. Measurement of patient outcome in arthritis. Arthritis Rheum 1980;23:137–45.

20. Pincus T, Sammey JA, Soraci SA, Wallston KA, Hammon NP. Assessment of patient satisfaction in activities of daily living using a modified Stanford Health Assessment Questionnaire. Arthritis Rheum 1983;26:1346–53.

21. Huskisson EC. Measurement of pain. J Rheumatol 1982;9:768–9.

22. Mayer G, Thum J, Cada EM, Stummvoll HK, Graf H. Verhalten der aeroben und anaeroben Leistungsfähigkeit chronischer Hämodialysepatienten unter einer Dauertherapie mit rekombinantem humanem Erythropoietin. Nephron 1989;51(Suppl 1):34–8.

23. Goodnough LT, Rudnick S, Price TH, et al. Increased preoperative col-

lection of autologous blood with recombinant human erythropoietin therapy. N Engl J Med 1989;321:1163–8.

24. Carson JL, Poses RM, Spence RK, Bonavita G. Severity of anaemia with operative mortality and morbidity. Lancet 1988;1:727–9.

25. Balkwill F, Osborne R, Burke F, et al. Evidence for tumor necrosis factor/cachetin production in cancer. Lancet 1987;2:1229–32.

26. Johnson RA, Waddelow TA, Caro J, Oliff A, Roodman GD. Chronic exposure to tumor necrosis factor in vivo preferentially inhibits erythropoiesis in nude mice. Blood 1989;74:130–8.

27. Henry DH, Rudnick SA, Bryant E, et al. Preliminary report of two double blind, placebo controlled studies using recombinant erythropoietin (rHuEpo) in the anemia associated with cancer [Abstract]. Blood 1989;74(Suppl 1):6A.

28. Eschbach JW, Egrie JC, Downing MR, Browne JK, Adamson JW. Correction of the anemia of end-stage renal disease with recombinant human erythropoietin. N Engl J Med 1987;316:73–8.

29. Koury MJ, Bondurant MC. Erythropoietin retards DNA breakdown and prevents programmed death in erythroid progenitor cells. Science 1990;248:378–81.

30. Schooley JC, Kullgren B, Allison AC. Inhibition by interleukin-1 of the action of erythropoietin on erythroid precursors and its possible role in the pathogenesis of hypoplastic anemias. Br J Haematol 1987;67:11–7.

31. Eastgate JA, Symons JA, Wood NC, Grinlinton FM, de Giovine FS, Duff GW. Correlation of plasma interleukin 1 levels with disease activity in rheumatoid arthritis. Lancet 1988;2:706–9.

32. Dessypris EN, Graber SE, Krantz SB, Stone WJ. Effects of recombinant erythropoietin on the concentration and cycling status of human marrow hematopoietic progenitor cells in vivo. Blood 1988;72:2060–2.

33. Sytkowski AJ, O'Hara C, Vanasse G, et al. Characterization of biologically active, platelet-derived growth factor-like molecules produced by murine erythroid cells in vitro and in vivo. J Clin Invest 1990;85:40–6.

34. Eschbach JW, Abdulhadi MH, Browne JK, et al. Recombinant human erythropoietin in anemic patients with end-stage renal disease. Results of a Phase III multicenter clinical trial. Ann Intern Med 1989;111:992–1000.

35. Adamson JW. The promise of recombinant human erythropoietin. Semin Hematol 1989;26(Suppl 2):5–8.

Chapter 23

Recombinant Human Erythropoietin (Epoietin Alfa) in Patients with AIDS and AZT-induced Anemia

David H. Henry and Robert I. Abels

Anemia is a common problem associated with human immuno-deficiency virus (HIV) infection. Approximately 10 percent of asymptomatic HIV-infected persons are anemic. With progression of the infection, anemia is increasingly common, rising to 20 percent in untreated patients with AIDS-related complex and 75 percent in those with full-blown AIDS (1). It is estimated that 1 to 2 million Americans are currently infected with HIV. More than 100,000 cases of AIDS have been diagnosed to date; 300,000 cases are projected by the end of 1992 (2). The anemia may be severe enough to require transfusion for the palliation of symptoms, especially if the patient is taking azidothymidine (AZT).

This chapter discusses the anemia of AIDS, with particular attention to its etiology, its exacerbation with AZT, and its potential treatment with recombinant human erythropoietin (rHuEpo) in place of transfusion.

The Etiology of AIDS-related Anemia

All three classic mechanisms of anemia may play a role in the anemia of AIDS: decreased production, increased destruction, and blood loss. Decreased bone marrow production is by far the most important mechanism and may occur for several reasons in the same patient.

The first and fundamental cause of the underproductive anemia is the HIV infection itself. Although the virus has not yet been convincingly isolated from red cell progenitors or precursors, the CD34 pluripotent stem cell can be directly infected with the HIV in vitro (3). Furthermore, Donohue et al. demonstrated that the growth of erythroid progenitor cells from HIV-infected patients is markedly retarded in HIV antibody-positive serum but is normal in HIV-negative serum. This suggests that the HIV infection has caused some change in the red cell membrane antigen that is recognized by the HIV antibody, leading to the suppression of red cell growth (4).

HIV infection also causes a wholesale change in the growth factor and cytokine environment necessary for proper erythropoiesis in the bone marrow (5,6). Erythropoietin is the most important growth factor for erythropoiesis and is usually inadequate for the degree of anemia in the HIV-infected patient. Spivak et al. assayed erythropoietin levels in 55 anemic AIDS patients not receiving AZT. They found that erythropoietin levels were either not elevated at all or not elevated to the extent that would ordinarily be expected (7). This finding was confirmed in a multicenter study of anemic AIDS patients not receiving AZT (8). The reason for inadequate levels of erythropoietin may be somehow related to the HIV itself but is more likely just another example of the inadequate erythropoietin response often seen in the anemia of chronic disease. The anemia of chronic disease is characterized by a modest shortening of red cell survival, poor iron reutilization by the bone marrow, and usually an inadequate erythropoietin response (9). Figure 23.1 illustrates the relationship between the hematocrit and erythropoietin titers in "normal" patients with iron deficiency and the titers in patients with the anemia of chronic disease. In the anemia of chronic disease, the erythropoietin response to anemia seems to be blunted (see Chapter 11).

As the immunosuppression secondary to HIV infection progresses, opportunistic infections become increasingly common and can affect the bone marrow directly or indirectly. Both tuberculosis and *Mycobacterium avium-intracellulare* have been observed or cultured from bone marrow aspirates. Anemia and leukopenia are especially common when patients are taking AZT and develop *Mycobacterium avium-intracellulare* infection (10). Several fungal infections can involve the marrow, including histoplasmosis, coccidioidomycosis, and cryptococcus. Systemic viral infections suppress erythropoiesis indirectly, but direct suppression of the bone marrow has been documented only by cytomegalovirus and herpes simplex virus. Toxoplasmosis, commonly associated with infection in the central nervous system, can also infect the bone marrow.

A wide range of drugs is used to treat or palliate the patient with HIV.

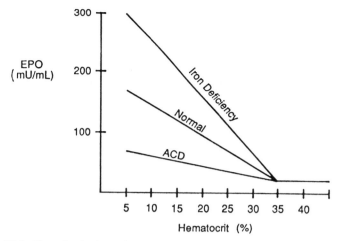

Figure 23.1. Hypothetical erythropoietin response to anemia. ACD, anemia of chronic disease; EPO, erythropoietin. *Source: Data from References 7–9*

When anemia develops, it can be difficult to be certain which medication is responsible, but those most likely to be involved include antibiotics (especially those containing sulfur moieties) and AZT.

AZT is currently the only medication approved by the Food and Drug Administration to treat patients with AIDS. Unfortunately, it has a significant number of side effects, the most important of which is anemia. In the original placebo-controlled trial, the development or exacerbation of anemia was significantly more common with AZT than with placebo (38 percent vs. 13 percent), and the frequency of anemia requiring transfusion was much higher in the AZT-treated cohort (31 percent vs. 11 percent) (11). AZT retards the replication of HIV by inhibiting HIV's essential enzyme for replication, reverse transcriptase. A complementary DNA copy of the HIV RNA cannot be made properly because of AZT's inhibition of this enzyme, but AZT can also inhibit normal host cell DNA polymerase function. AZT's bone marrow toxicity may come from the particular sensitivity of bone marrow DNA polymerases to its action. Generally, a macrocytosis is seen as the anemia develops, but in a small percentage of patients the mean cell volume does not increase. These patients usually develop a more severe anemia, suggesting that there may be two mechanisms of AZT-induced anemia.

Finally, in as many as 30 percent of AIDS patients, the B_{12} level is low (12). In some AIDS patients, a gastropathy with poor basal acid secre-

tion may partly explain this observation (13). Even so, overt megalo-
blastic anemia does not occur, and the anemia does not tend to correct
with parenteral supplementation of B_{12}. In vitro data suggest that AZT's
toxic effect on the marrow may be exacerbated by B_{12} deficiency, but
clinical studies with AZT and B_{12} to examine this issue have not yet been
performed (14).

Two other possible mechanisms of anemia in AIDS patients are peripheral destruction of red cells or blood loss. Overt hemolytic anemia
is rare, although positivity to Coombs' test is not. Several authors have
reported positive direct antiglobulin tests in as many as 45 percent of
patients (15,16). In general, however, only about 10 percent of unselected patients will be Coombs-positive, and this is probably secondary
to the nonspecific hypergammaglobulinemia associated with AIDS and/
or antibody formation from multiple previous blood transfusions. Although blood loss can occur, it is usually not the main mechanism of
anemia. In some patients, it can be significant if thrombocytopenia or
bleeding from a gastrointestinal lesion is present.

The Treatment of Anemia

Transfusion

Until now, the treatment of anemia in AIDS patients has been by
blood transfusion, but this is not without its problems. At the very least,
it is inconvenient for the patient, whether the transfusion is performed
in the hospital or at home. Blood transfusion also poses several risks to
the patient. First, there is the potential for a transfusion reaction; some
20 percent of patients receiving transfusions experience chills, fever,
itching, rash, or hives, often requiring medication. Also, despite the
careful screening of donors and testing of blood units, there is still an
almost 2 percent chance of transmitting any type of hepatitis with a
single blood transfusion (17).

Perhaps the most troubling issue surrounding blood transfusion in
AIDS patients is the possibility that transfused blood causes immunosuppression. Since Opelz and Terasaki first reported longer renal transplant survival in patients who received transfusions before surgery,
there has been intense interest in the area of homologous blood transfusion and its effect on the recipient's immune function (18). After the
renal transplant observation, a major controversy developed in the on-
cology literature regarding whether perioperative blood transfusion adversely affected the cancer patient's time to recurrence and overall
survival. In two reviews on the subject, there was still a lack of agree-

ment, as none of the studies was prospective or controlled (19,20). However, a number of immunologic changes can be demonstrated after repeated blood transfusion, including decreased CD4 helper lymphocyte count, decreased CD4/CD8 helper suppressor lymphocyte ratio, decreased natural killer cell count, and decreased macrophage/monocyte function (20). These changes do not occur with autologous blood transfusion.

Two studies raised the possibility of further immunosuppression in HIV-infected patients as a consequence of blood transfusion. Blumberg and Heal reviewed published reports of subsequent blood transfusion histories in patients who were HIV infected from a blood transfusion. They found a twofold greater rate of progression to full-blown AIDS in those patients who subsequently received *uninfected* plasma or whole blood vs. just packed red cells (21). Ward et al. reported a somewhat similar experience in patients who acquired HIV infection from a single contaminated blood transfusion. They found that the time to progression to AIDS was much shorter in those patients who subsequently received more *uninfected* units of blood at the time of HIV infection than in those who received less (22). Further studies are necessary to confirm these findings, but these immunologic and clinical observations strongly suggest a potential role for transfusion to further harm the immune system of the patient who is already infected with the HIV.

Clinical Trials with Recombinant Human Erythropoietin

Given the drawbacks associated with transfusion, an alternative form of therapy for the anemia of AIDS would be preferable. As discussed above, the erythropoietin levels are usually inadequate for the degree of anemia in the HIV-infected patient. With the advent of rHuEpo and its success as replacement therapy in the anemia of chronic renal failure, clinical trials were initiated to test the efficacy and safety of rHuEpo as replacement therapy in anemic AIDS patients.

Four prospective, double-blind, placebo-controlled, multicenter studies were initiated in anemic AIDS patients taking AZT. Table 23.1 outlines the study designs. In each trial, the hematocrit, transfusion requirement, and quality of life were measured. The results from the first study have been analyzed, and the details are given below (23). The results from the other three studies are still not final, but some preliminary data are available.

Sixty-three patients were entered into the first study. Table 23.2 shows the patients' demographics. Baseline patient parameters of hematocrit, erythropoietin level, transfusion requirement, and AZT dos-

Table 23.1. Clinical Trials of rHuEpo in AZT/AIDS-related Anemia

Study	Dose, units/kg (rHuEpo vs. Placebo, 3 Times per Week)	Route*	Duration, wk
1	100	IV	12
2	100	SC	12
3	150	SC	12
4	200	SC	12

*IV, intravenously; SC, subcutaneously.

Table 23.2. Demographics of Patients in Study 1

	rHuEpo ($n = 29$)	Placebo ($n = 34$)
Sex		
Male	29	33
Female	0	1
Race		
Caucasian	27	31
Black	1	2
Other	1	1
Median age (yr)	37.6	39.8

age were not significantly different at entry into the study; these are outlined in Table 23.3. A surprise finding was the distribution of baseline erythropoietin values as a function of the hematocrit (Fig 23.2). Some erythropoietin values were much higher than would be expected in anemic AIDS patients according to the model of the anemia of chronic disease. Apparently, AZT can cause some patients to develop a striking elevation in erythropoietin. A regression line of the erythropoietin response to anemia is drawn through the data in Study 1 (Fig 23.2) and shows a steep erythropoietin response to anemia. For comparison, a regression line for anemic AIDS patients *not* taking AZT is superimposed on the data points in Figure 23.2 and shows the typical blunted erythropoietin response seen in the anemia of chronic disease. Others observed the same exaggerated increase in erythropoietin in some anemic

Table 23.3. Baseline Parameters of Patients in Study 1

Parameter	rHuEpo (n = 29)	Placebo (n = 34)
Mean hematocrit	28.0	28.7
Mean level of erythropoietin, mU/ml	397.2	448.9
Number of patients requiring transfusion before therapy	23 (79%)	27 (79%)
Mean number of units transfused per patient per month before therapy	1.7	1.9
Mean daily AZT dose, mg	726	753

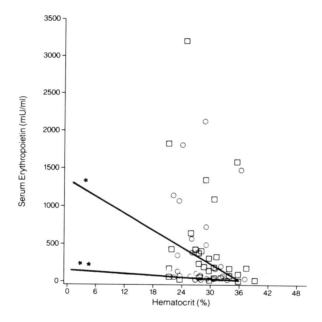

Figure 23.2. Prestudy serum erythropoietin and hematocrit values in AIDS patients taking AZT (Study 1). *, regression line for Study 1 patients; **, regression line for non-AZT patients with AIDS, for comparison (7, 8). Circles indicate rHuEpo treatment; squares, placebo. *Source: Some data from References 7 and 8*

Table 23.4. Baseline Characteristics of Patients in Study 1 by Level of
Erythropoietin

Characteristic	Level of Erythropoietin	
	Low (≤500 mU/ml) (*n* = 48)	High (>500 mU/ml) (*n* = 13)
Mean hematocrit	28.9	27.1
Mean cell volume*	98.4	88.5
During 3 mo before study		
Number of patients receiving transfusions	37 (77%)	13 (100%)
Mean number of units per patient per month	1.5	3.2
Mean daily AZT dose, mg	749	670

*Significantly different at $P < 0.05$.

patients taking AZT (7). A level of 500 mU/ml was chosen from the data
in Study 1 as a cutoff, separating "high" from "low" levels of erythropoietin, because it gave the best statistical fit to discriminate between
those patients who were or were not likely to respond to rHuEpo. Thir-
teen (21 percent) patients had erythropoietin levels of more than 500
mU/ml, and 48 (79 percent) had erythropoietin levels less than or equal
to 500 mU/ml. As one might expect, the patients with the lower erythropoietin levels were more likely to respond to rHuEpo therapy because
they had a greater erythropoietin "deficiency" than those with higher
levels of erythropoietin.

The reason for the spectacular increase in erythropoietin in some
patients taking AZT is not clear, but it may have to do with the activity
of AZT at the DNA level. Some chemotherapy can also act directly on
DNA, and a brief burst in erythropoietin has been reported in some
leukemic patients receiving pulse chemotherapy (24). Whether AZT
and chemotherapy alter the production or catabolism of erythropoietin
or act via entirely different mechanisms remains to be determined.

When several patients' parameters were analyzed separately according to high or low baseline erythropoietin, some important differences
were noted (Table 23.4). The red cell size as measured by the mean cell
volume was very different between the two groups. A macrocytosis was
noted in the low-erythropoietin group, as is common in most patients
taking AZT, but did not occur in the high-erythropoietin group. There
was no difference in the reticulocyte count to explain this difference in

mean cell volume between groups. In addition, there was a difference in the transfusion requirement between the two groups as measured by the numbers of units transfused per patient per month. The low-erythropoietin group had a much lower transfusion requirement than the high-erythropoietin group. Again, these observations suggest a fundamental difference in the mechanism of AZT-induced anemia depending on whether it is associated with a high or low level of erythropoietin.

The analysis of the final results from Study 1 are shown in Tables 23.5 and 23.6. Table 23.5 depicts the number of units of blood being transfused on a daily basis at the beginning and at the end of the study. There was a significant decrease in the transfusion requirement of the rHuEpo-treated patients whose baseline level of erythropoietin was less than or equal to 500 mU/ml. Specifically, there was a 36 percent decline in the transfusion requirement of the rHuEpo-treated patients vs. a 63 percent increase in the placebo-treated patients. In the patients whose baseline levels of erythropoietin were greater than 500 mU/ml, there was no significant change in the transfusion requirement between the rHuEpo- and the placebo-treated groups.

In Table 23.6 the data from Study 1 are displayed according to the number of patients who received transfusions each month. Again, in

Table 23.5. The Number of Units Transfused in Study 1

Group	n	At Entry into Study*	At Conclusion of Study†
All patients			
rHuEpo	29	1.74	1.48
Placebo	34	1.87	2.58
Low level of erythropoietin (≤500 mU/ml)			
rHuEpo	22	1.31	0.84‡
Placebo	26§	1.68	2.74
High level of erythropoietin (>500 mU/ml)			
rHuEpo	7	3.10	3.50
Placebo	6§	3.32	2.78

*Mean number of transfused units per patient per month during the 3 months before entry into the study (baseline).

†Mean number of transfused units per patient at the completion of the 3rd month or when the patient left the study.

‡Significantly fewer ($P < 0.05$) than the placebo group.

§Values of endogenous erythropoietin are not available for two patients in the placebo-treated group. Therefore, these patients are not accounted for in either the low- or the high-erythropoietin group but are included with all patients.

Table 23.6. The Number of Patients Who Received Transfusions in Study 1

Group	n	At Entry into Study*	At Conclusion of Study†
All patients			
rHuEpo	29	23	11
Placebo	34	27	21
Low level of erythropoietin (≤500 mU/ml)			
rHuEpo	22	16	5‡
Placebo	26§	21	17
High level of erythropoietin (>500 mU/ml)			
rHuEpo	7	7	6
Placebo	6§	6	4

*Number of patients who received transfusions during the 3 months before entry into the study (baseline).

†Number of patients who received transfusions during the last month of participation in the study.

‡Significantly fewer ($P < 0.05$) than the placebo group.

§Values of endogenous erythropoietin are not available for two patients in the placebo-treated group. Therefore, these patients are not accounted for in either the low- or the high-erythropoietin group but are included with all patients.

the low-erythropoietin group (≤500 mU/ml), there was a significant decrease in the number of patients requiring transfusion in the rHuEpo-treated group. No improvement in the transfusion requirement was seen in the treatment group with high erythropoietin levels (>500 mU/ml) at entry into the study.

Inasmuch as AZT has such a profound tendency to cause or exacerbate AIDS-related anemia, an analysis of the comparability of AZT dosage in different groups was critical for the investigators to be certain that the outcome of the study was due to rHuEpo and not to AZT. The AZT dosage over time is shown in Table 23.7. Not surprisingly, there was a trend from the beginning to the end of the study to decrease the AZT dosage in all patients, but there was no statistical difference in the AZT dosage of any group at any time during the course of the study.

The issues of quality of life and safety were evaluated during the study. A questionnaire assessing the quality of life was administered to all patients at the beginning and end of Study 1. The three parameters of energy level, work capacity, and overall quality of life were assessed. In the low-erythropoietin group only, there was a trend toward improvement in energy level and overall quality of life which approached but did not quite reach statistical significance. The rHuEpo treatment was also extremely well tolerated. As shown in Table 23.8, there was no difference in side effects between rHuEpo and placebo, demonstrating that the side effects observed were due to the patients' underlying disease and not to rHuEpo.

After the 12-week double-blind phase of Study 1, all patients were allowed to enter an open label phase with an escalation of the rHuEpo dosage each month to a maximum of 500 units/kg intravenously (or subcutaneously) three times per week. During this phase, the decrease in transfusion requirement continued in all patients with low levels of

Table 23.7. The Average Daily Dosage of AZT in Study 1

Group	n	AZT Dose at Entry into Study*	AZT Dose at Conclusion of Study†
All patients			
rHuEpo	29	726	580
Placebo	34	753	652
Low level of erythropoietin ($\leq$500 mU/ml)			
rHuEpo	22	784	619
Placebo	26‡	720	672
High level of erythropoietin (>500 mU/ml)			
rHuEpo	7	543	457
Placebo	6‡	819	528

Note: There were no significant between-group differences.
*Baseline.
†Average daily dosage of AZT, either during the last month (obtained upon completion of the study) or earlier if the patient left the study before the 3rd month.
‡Values of endogenous erythropoietin are not available for two patients in the placebo-treated group. Therefore, these patients are not accounted for in either the low- or the high-erythropoietin group but are included with all patients.

Table 23.8. The Number of Patients with Adverse Effects in Study 1

Effect	rHuEpo	Placebo
Pyrexia	11 (38%)	11 (32%)
Fatigue	5 (17%)	7 (21%)
Asthenia	5 (17%)	7 (21%)
Rash	7 (24%)	5 (15%)
Headache	7 (24%)	4 (12%)
Diarrhea	5 (17%)	6 (18%)

Note: No significant difference.

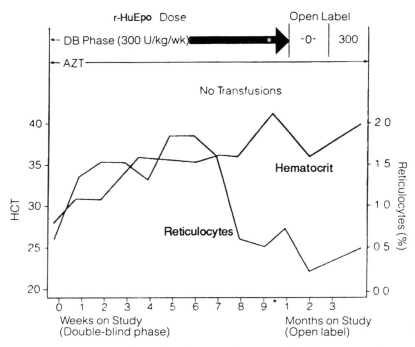

Figure 23.3. Patient with low baseline erythropoietin level (83 mU/ml). *, early entry into open label phase after reaching target hematocrit. DB, double-blind; U, units.

erythropoietin (≤500 mU/ml), but the high-erythropoietin (>500 mU/ml) group continued to be refractory to rHuEpo and required transfusions at the same frequency.

Figure 23.3 graphically displays data from Study 1 on a patient in the low-erythropoietin group who responded to rHuEpo during the double-blind phase. Figure 23.4 displays data on a patient in the high-erythropoietin group who did not respond to rHuEpo during either the double-blind phase or the open label dose-escalation phase. When the patient stopped AZT secondary to side effects, its discontinuation had a profound effect on the reticulocyte count and the hematocrit.

Three other prospective, double-blind, placebo-controlled multicenter studies of anemic AIDS patients taking AZT have been completed, and detailed analyses of each study are pending. A preliminary summary of all four studies, representing a total of 255 patients, is available.

A meta-analysis of the pooled results was performed and again revealed that a baseline erythropoietin value of 500 mU/ml was the best predictor of hematologic response. In the low-erythropoietin group (≤500 mU/ml), there was a 40 percent decrease in the transfusion requirement and a 4-point increase in the hematocrit in the rHuEpo-treated patients. This result was highly statistically significant. In the high-erythropoietin group (>500 mU/ml), there was no improvement in the transfusion requirement or the hematocrit in the rHuEpo-treated patients. Thus, it seems that an anemic AIDS patient taking AZT who has an erythropoietin level of more than 500 mU/ml already has an adequate erythropoietin response. The administration of additional rHuEpo up to the maximum used in these studies (500 units/kg intravenously or subcutaneously three times per week) to stimulate the bone marrow further is unlikely to achieve a hematologic response.

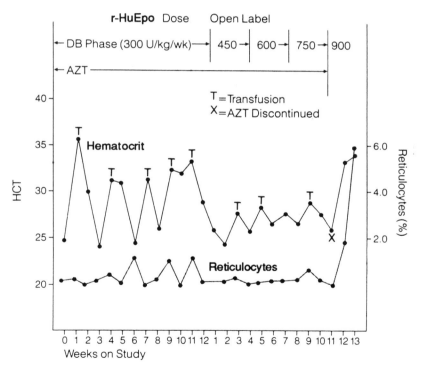

Figure 23.4. Patient with high baseline erythropoietin (1860 mU/ml). DB, double-blind.

Conclusion

Recombinant human erythropoietin can be safely used in AIDS patients. It can increase the hematocrit and decrease the requirement for transfusion in anemic AIDS patients taking AZT whose baseline levels of erythropoietin are less than or equal to 500 mU/ml. The appropriate starting dosage is between 100 and 200 units/kg intravenously or subcutaneously three times per week. Escalation of the dosage in the low-erythropoietin group may achieve additional hematologic improvement. At the dosage used in these studies (up to a maximum of 500 units/kg intravenously or subcutaneously three times per week), no hematologic benefit was achieved in patients with high baseline levels of erythropoietin (>500 mU/ml).

REFERENCES

1. Zon LI, Groopman JE. Hematologic manifestations of the human immune deficiency virus (HIV). Semin Hematol 1988;25:208–18.
2. AIDS Weekly Surveillance Report. U.S. AIDS Program, Center for Infectious Diseases, Centers for Disease Control. January 8, 1990.
3. Folks TM, Kessler SW, Orenstein JW, et al. Infection and replication of HIV-1 in purified progenitor cells of normal human bone marrow. Science 1988;242:919–22.
4. Donahue RE, Johnson MM, Zon LI, et al. Suppression of in vitro hematopoiesis following human immunodeficiency virus infection. Nature 1987;326:200–3.
5. Laurence J, Gottlieb AB, Kunkel HG. Soluble suppressor factors in patients with acquired immune deficiency syndrome and its prodrome: elaboration in vitro by T lymphocyte-adherent cell interactions. J Clin Invest 1983;72:2072–81.
6. Murray HW, Rubin BY, Nasur H, et al. Impaired production of lymphokines and immune (gamma) interferon in the acquired immunodeficiency syndrome. N Engl J Med 1984;310:883–9.
7. Spivak JL, Barnes DC, Fuchs E, Quinn TC. Serum immunoreactive erythropoietin in HIV-infected patients. JAMA 1989;261:3104–7.
8. Data on file, Ortho Biotech Corp., Raritan, New Jersey.
9. Lee GR. The anemia of chronic disease. Semin Hematol 1983;20:61–80.
10. Diagnosis and Management of HIV Disease: A Reference Manual. Burroughs Wellcome, 1988.
11. Richman DD, Fischl MA, Grieco MH, et al. The toxicity of azidothymidine (AZT) in the treatment of patients with AIDS and AIDS-related complex. N Engl J Med 1987;317:192–7.
12. Herbert V. B_{12} deficiency in AIDS [Letter]. JAMA 1988;260:2837.
13. Kotler DP, Gaetz HP, Lange M, Klein EB, Holt PR. Enteropathy associated

with the acquired immunodeficiency syndrome. Ann Intern Med 1987;101: 421–8.

14. Herzlich BC, Mohammad R, Nawabi I, Herbert V. Synergy of inhibition of DNA synthesis in human bone marrow by azidothymidine plus deficiency of folate and/or B_{12}? Am J Hematol 1990;33:177–83.

15. Toy PTC, Reid ME, Burns M. Positive direct antiglobulin test associated with hyperglobulinemia in acquired immunodeficiency syndrome. Am J Hematol 1985;19:145–50.

16. McGinniss MH, Macher AM, Rook AH, et al. Red cell autoantibodies in patients with acquired immune deficiency syndrome. Transfusion 1986;26: 405–9.

17. Bove JR. Transfusion-associated hepatitis and AIDS: what is the risk? N Engl J Med 1987;317:242–5.

18. Opelz TG, Terasaki PI. Poor kidney-transplant survival in recipients with frozen blood transfusions or no transfusions. Lancet 1974;2:696–8.

19. Wu HS, Little AG. Perioperative blood transfusions and cancer recurrence. J Clin Oncol 1988;6:1348–54.

20. Perkins HA. Transfusion-induced immunologic unresponsiveness. Transfusion 1988;2:196–203.

21. Blumberg N, Heal JM. Transfusion and recipient immune function. Arch Pathol Lab Med 1989;113:246–53.

22. Ward JW, Bush BS, Perkins HA, et al. The natural history of transfusion-associated infection with human immunodeficiency virus. N Engl J Med 1989; 321:947–52.

23. Fischl M, Galpin JE, Levine JD, et al. Recombinant human erythropoietin for patients with AIDS treated with zidorudine. N Engl J Med 1990; 322:1488–93.

24. Piroso E, Erslev AJ, Caro J. Inappropriate increase in erythropoietin titers during chemotherapy. Am J Hematol 1989;32:248–54.

Chapter 24

Summary and Conclusions

Allan J. Erslev, John W. Adamson,
Joseph W. Eschbach, and Christopher G. Winearls

The aim of this monograph on erythropoietin is to provide an account of the events that led to the transformation of a concept of red cell regulation into an effective treatment of many anemias. Each chapter is authored by investigators who were involved in this transformation and who are still at work on elucidating the origin, kinetics, action, and regulation of this growth hormone. In this concluding chapter, the editors briefly review the preceding chapters and add some personal comments on the challenges and problems of the future therapeutic use of recombinant erythropoietin.

Summary of Preceding Chapters

In the first chapter, Allan Erslev traces the history of erythropoietin from astute observations in the mountains of Mexico during the 19th century via physiologic identification, chemical purification, genetic cloning, and mass production to its clinical application.

Following this introduction, Joan Egrie and Jeffrey Browne describe the molecular biology of erythropoietin and outline the methods used to identify its gene and harness it for mass production of recombinant erythropoietin. These methods were used almost simultaneously by two biotechnology laboratories, Genetics Institute in Massachusetts and Amgen in California. They both identified short strings of amino acid and constructed a large number of matching oligonucleotide sequences which in turn were used as probes to identify the gene in a human genomic library. This gene was cloned in mammalian cells and shown to direct the synthesis of a glycoprotein with the structural, immunologic, and biologic properties of human DNA. The probes were also used to identify human erythropoietin mRNA in fetal liver tissue and monkey and mouse mRNA in hypoxic kidney preparations. The mRNA was made to produce its corresponding complementary DNA (cDNA) by incubation with reverse transcriptase.

These studies led to the exact determination of the five exons and four introns in the erythropoietin gene and elucidation of its transcription and translation. There is extensive homology among human, monkey, and mouse genes and their erythropoietins. Interestingly, the rate of evolution as estimated by the number of substitutions is approximately equal to that of α and β globins. The practical consequence of this work was the transfection of the gene into Chinese hamster ovary cells, with the subsequent production of an almost unlimited amount of recombinant human erythropoietin.

In Chapter 3, Eugene Goldwasser describes the primary and secondary structure of erythropoietin isolated from humans, monkeys, and mice. The primary amino acid sequence in humans consist of 193 amino acids including a 27-residue leader sequence and a terminal arginine that is split off after translation. As expected because of overlapping in vivo activities, there is a striking homology among the three erythropoietin species, especially in the 5' upstream sequence, in the first exon and in the first intron. The secondary structure is affected by disulfide bonds and by one O-linked and three N-linked oligosaccharide branches. Removal of the terminal sialic acid affects in vivo life-span but not in vitro activity, whereas complete carbohydrate removal causes a loss of about one half of biologic activity. Attempts, however, to identify the biologically active site have not been successful.

The regulation of the gene expression and the genetic and cellular localization of erythropoietin biosynthesis are dealt with in the next chapters. Studies described by Jaime Caro, Stephen Schuster, and Sylvia Ramirez (Chapter 4) on the messenger RNA of erythropoietin established the liver as the primary site of erythropoietin production in fetal life and, as first suggested by Jacobson and co-workers, established the kidney as the primary site in the adult. Based on ''run-on'' experiments on nuclei derived from normal and hypoxic kidneys, these authors suggested that the increase in erythropoietin synthesis after hypoxia is due to an increased rate of transcription rather than translation. This augmentation of transcription may be caused by a DNA-binding protein released by hypoxia and capable of activating a regulatory promoter. The striking homology among species upstream and downstream of exon 1 suggested that this may be the site for a regulatory promoter or enhancer, but recent studies of hepatoma cells have identified hypoxia-responsive enhancers in the 3' area.

In Chapter 5, studies aimed at identifying the cellular site for the activation of the erythropoietin gene are discussed by Stephen Koury, Mark Koury, and Maurice Bondurant. With the use of in situ hybridization of a genetic probe for erythropoietin, mRNA was identified in interstitial cells located in the inner renal cortex. These cells are situated close to but clearly separated from the proximal tubules, and preliminary studies suggested that they are endothelial in origin. Because the number of active cells rather than their degree of activation is proportional to the severity of anemic hypoxia, it is suggested that the cells are involved in an all-or-none mode of erythropoietin production.

In the next chapter, Armin Kurtz and Kai-Uwe Eckardt discuss the concepts of an oxygen sensor and the mechanism by which such a sensor could transmit information to the erythropoietin-producing interstitial cells. Although extrarenal hypoxia appears to influence renal erythropoietin production, the primary oxygen sensor must reside in the kidney inasmuch as isolated perfused kidneys synthesize erythropoietin in response to hypoxia. Because of the complex functional and structural anatomy, local oxygen tension varies widely within the kidney; however, the proximal tubules, with their large oxygen consumption, are the cells most likely to sense and respond to hypoxia. This possibility is strengthened by their close proximity to the interstitial cells assumed to be the erythropoietin-producing cells. Furthermore, the proximal tubular cells contain large amounts of heme proteins, which are suspected to play a role in oxygen sensing owing to their reversible allosteric change in response to hypoxia and their possible role in regulating hepatic production of erythropoietin. Kurtz and Eckardt review and discuss a number of metabolic indicators of hypoxia and their possible role in transforming low oxygen tension into signals activating erythropoietin synthesis.

In Chapter 7, John Adamson reviews the cellular kinetics of normal red cell production and discusses the effect of erythropoietin on these kinetics. It seems that erythropoietin acts as a general growth factor on erythroid progenitors and precursors in consort with other growth factors, such as interleukin 3 and granulocyte-macrophage colony-stimulating factor (GM-CSF). However, its main action is as a differentiating factor in the transformation of late erythroid progenitors (CFU-E) to early erythroid precursors (proerythroblasts). In the absence of erythropoietin, the DNA of the CFU-E degenerates and the cells die; in its presence, they proceed with their normal, possibly predestined, maturation. The specific signal transduced by the erythropoietin receptor complex is not known. Erythropoietin also has an effect on the synthesis of fetal hemoglobin, possibly by accelerating the transit from the stage of burst-forming units (BFU-E) to erythroblasts.

The action on erythroid progenitor cells demands the presence of specific erythropoietin receptors. In the next two chapters, Stephen Sawyer and Gordon Wong, Simon S. Jones, and Alan D. D'Andrea describe the physiology and molecular biology of such receptors. In Chapter 8, Sawyer outlines the identification of receptors both on the erythroleukemic cells induced in mice by the Friend leukemia virus and on normal human erythroid progenitors. After many trials and errors, mild iodinization of recombinant erythropoietin was found to lead to a biologically active and easily identified erythropoietin. Using this as a probe, one could show that responsive erythroid cells had about 1000 receptors, one half high activity and one half low activity receptors. As both types appear to be derived from the same gene, the difference is probably post-translational and possibly not of physiologic significance. The density of receptors on the surface of erythroid progenitor cells seems to increase gradually during the maturation of BFU-E to CFU-E, with a subsequent decrease during the maturation of precursor cells. Erythropoietin-receptor complex could be shown to be internalized by endocytosis, but the subsequent fate of either or both components is still unknown. Neither is it known exactly what the erythropoietin receptor complex triggers in the CFU-E to promote its differentiation to a pro-erythroblast. However, recent studies suggest that the complex prevents DNA disintegration and ensures cellular survival.

The structure of these receptors is described in great molecular detail by Wong and co-workers in Chapter 9. Using an erythropoietin-responsive mouse erythroleukemia cell line, these authors isolated the mRNA for an erythropoietin receptor, converted it into cDNA, and cloned it in a mammalian expression vector. The resulting recombinant plasmids were introduced into a mammalian host cell that in turn was examined for its ability to produce a surface protein capable of binding erythropoietin. The finally isolated murine receptor protein had a molecular mass of 55 kd and was composed of 507 amino acids. Although this molecular mass is quite different from that of the receptors described in the previous chapter, the difference may have been due to glycosylation. The mouse erythropoietin receptor gene was eventually used as a probe to isolate the human receptor gene, which was found to code for a protein with 508 amino acids and with an 82 percent homology with its murine counterpart.

The murine and human receptors consist of a transmembrane domain and of equal-sized extracellular and cytoplasmic domains. The extracellular domain appears to be capable not only of binding erythropoietin but also of binding an envelope glycoprotein on the Friend virus, which possibly explains the capacity of the virus to transform erythroleukemia cells to erythroblasts in the absence of erythropoietin.

Of additional interest is the fact that there is a considerable homology between these receptors and the extracellular domains of a number of growth factor receptors, including GM-CSF, G-CSF, and interleukins 2, 3, 4, 6, and 7. This has led to the concept of the existence of a closely related hemopoietin-receptor super family.

The pharmacokinetics and metabolism of erythropoietin in health and disease are described by Jerry Spivak and P. Mary Cotes in the next two chapters. Despite different cellular source, recombinant and native human erythropoietin are very similar if not identical in their amino acid sequence and in their glycosylation composition. The physiologic significance of the components of the carbohydrate chains is not known except for the fact that the ultimate sialic acid covers galactose radicals and prevents galactose receptors in the liver from causing hepatic endocytosis and catabolism of circulating erythropoietin. The pharmacokinetics of erythropoietin shows that the immediate volume of distribution approximates that of the plasma volume. This is followed by a dilution phase with erythropoietin entering extracellular spaces. The dilution phase has a half-life of a few minutes in rodents and 1 to 2 hours in humans. The subsequent elimination phase is slower, with a half-life in rodents of about 90 minutes and in humans of 6 to 9 hours. These half-lives are not related to biologic activity; they are the same for active and inactive erythropoietin, for homologous and heterologous erythropoietin, and for various levels of erythropoietin. The half-life, however, is longer after subcutaneous or intraperitoneal administration. This seems to be related to a slower but more sustained release from subcutaneous and intraperitoneal depots. Such a sustained release appears to be of advantage because a certain level of red cell production can be maintained by smaller amounts given subcutaneously than given intravenously.

The catabolic fate of erythropoietin is still unknown. The liver does not seem to clear erythropoietin, and renal clearance or degradation is quite low. Elimination by utilization in erythroid tissue has been a popular concept for many years, but it is a most unlikely mechanism as shown by a half-life that is not affected by the level of circulating erythropoietin or by the activity of erythroid tissue.

In Chapter 11, Cotes and Spivak review the relationship between erythropoietin titers and erythroid activity in both health and disease. They discuss the various in vivo and in vitro assays and conclude that immunologic assays are here to stay, either radioimmune or ELISA, as convenient and reliable methods. In the normal individual, there is a diurnal variation with a peak around midnight 40 percent above the morning trough. This oscillating pattern is not dependent on age or sex and is subject to considerable individual variations. Because of these variations, it has been impossible to show significant differences between the titers of normal adult men and those of women, newborns, or premature infants. In fetal life, increased titers have been related to fetal stress, but here again the "normal" levels vary greatly. Currently, determination of erythropoietin titers of amniotic fluid has not facilitated the management of precarious pregnancies.

In anemias, the erythropoietin titers increase exponentially as the hemoglobin concentration decreases, but again the individual variations are so large that it is impossible to predict the level of erythropoietin from measured hemoglobin or hematocrit. After acute blood loss, there is a brief increase in titers followed by a return almost to baseline values. The titers in patients with renal disease are lower than those expected for equally anemic patients with normal kidney function. Some of this erythropoietin (and all in anephric patients) is derived from extrarenal sources, primarily the liver. Patients with chronic inflammatory disorders, infections, and malignancies have erythropoietin titers that seem inappropriately low. This is also true for patients with malnutrition, which may explain some but not all of the decrease observed in patients with chronic, debilitating diseases.

In erythrocytosis the titer of erythropoietin is, as might be expected, increased in patients with hypoxic disorders and decreased in patients with endogenous overproduction of red cells, as in the clonal disorder polycythemia vera. Erythrocytosis may also be due to inappropriate overproduction of erythropoietin by renal cysts or tumors or by neoplasms in the liver or cerebellum. Idiopathic, often familial overproduction may also occur from unknown sources.

The next 10 chapters are devoted to the clinical use of recombinant erythropoietin as a replacement agent in patients with anemia due to renal disease and as a pharmacologic agent in patients with anemia due to various chronic illnesses. In the first of these chapters, Joseph Eschbach reports on the treatment of almost 450 hemodialysis patients with recombinant human erythropoietin produced by Amgen, Inc., and carrying the genetic designation of epoetin alfa and the trade name of Epogen. The patients were treated in 13 dialysis centers in the United States over a 3-year period from 1985 to 1988. Of the 449 patients who completed 12 weeks of therapy, 96 percent responded with an increase in the mean hematocrit from 22 percent to 35 percent. The treatment protocols were adjusted to the rise in hematocrit; after a hematocrit of 35 percent was reached, the maintenance dosage was about 75 units/kg three times a week intravenously. The need for transfusions ceased completely except for those required for emergency surgery. Tissue iron stores were decreased or, rather, shifted from the tissues into the red cell mass, and the overall quality of life improved significantly. Questionnaires were used to assess energy and activity levels, functional ability, sleep and eating behavior, satisfaction with health, sex life, and happiness. There was a marked improvement in all of these parameters; in the face of a continued need for dialysis, however, the quality of life was not restored to normal.

There were three major problems. The first was an absolute or relative iron deficiency necessitating oral iron replacement therapy in patients with ferritin values of less than 100 ng/ml. The second was hypertension with a blood pressure increase, which was experienced by about one third of the patients. The increase in blood pressure appeared to be unrelated to the speed at which the hematocrit rose or the dose of recombinant erythropoietin. The third problem was seizures, which were experienced by 4 percent of the patients and were usually associated with a sudden rise in blood pressure.

A potential concern had been that improved platelet function, as reflected by a shortening of the bleeding time after normalization of the hematocrit, would cause problems with clotting of the shunts. In this study, however, there were no major problems with vascular access, and the increase in platelet count was not significant. A second concern had been whether the rise in hematocrit would result in a decrease in dialyzer clearance because of the contraction in plasma volume. There was indeed a small rise in creatinine, phosphate, and potassium concentrations but not to the extent that the dialysis time had to be increased. Nevertheless, hyperkalemia did occur in some patients and resulted in the death of three noncompliant individuals. Eschbach concluded that recombinant human erythropoietin is effective, well tolerated, and safe as long as blood pressure and serum potassium are carefully monitored and managed. He felt that it should be part of the standard treatment in dialysis patients with hematocrits of less than 30 percent.

In a similar study in Japan, Tadao Akizawa and associates described the effect of recombinant human erythropoietin administered to 830 anemic patients with chronic renal failure, both on dialysis and predialysis. The optimal initial dosage was determined to be about 60 units/kg given intravenously three times a week. Recombinant erythropoietin was effective in 95 percent of cases, whereas androgen was effective in only 56 percent of patients. Furthermore, the erythropoietin group had none of the side effects such as hirsutism, vocal changes, and dermatitis that plagued the androgen recipients. When erythropoietin was given intraperitoneally in patients on continuous ambulatory peritoneal dialysis, the effect was more sustained and could be attained with lower doses. In no patient on dialysis or predialysis was there any evidence of aggravation of renal dysfunction despite the decrease in the circulating plasma volume.

About 6 percent of patients were poorly responsive to erythropoietin. In most of these, the cause was iron deficiency, chronic infection, or aluminum overload; in only seven cases was the cause not identified.

Outcome was assessed by a number of studies relating to quality of life, coagulation parameters, endocrinologic status, and electrolyte balance, but no significant changes were observed except for an improvement in bleeding time and a tendency to hyperkalemia. Side effects were less obvious in this series, with only 7 percent of patients experiencing an increase in blood pressure. No patient experienced seizures, and clotting of fistulas was no problem.

In Chapter 14, the Canadian experience with recombinant human erythropoietin (epoetin alfa) is summarized by Norman Muirhead, who directed a randomized, double-blind, placebo-controlled, multi-institutional trial. In this trial, the initial dosages of 100 units/kg three times per week intravenously had almost the same effect as 200 units/kg three times per week but were superior to the use of 50 units/kg three times per week. When changing the sequence of injections, the thrice weekly schedule was superior and more economical than a schedule based on larger doses given at less frequent intervals. In these studies, 90 percent of the treated patients reached a target hemoglobin and could be maintained at a reduced dose. The half-life of the recombinant erythropoietin ranged from 5.9 to 12 hours, with a mean of 6.6 hours. An elaborate study of the quality of life and exercise capacity showed the expected improvement as the hemoglobin concentration rose. Individual variations were great, however; although the improvement in general was clinically significant, there were exceptions, especially in the category of frustrations and sexual functions.

Hypertension was a problem even in the placebo group where 9 percent of patients required an increase or change in hypertensive medication. However, almost 27 percent of erythropoietin-treated patients experienced an increase in blood pressure. An attempt was made to correlate this increase with the presence or absence of native kidneys and the rate of rise in hematocrit, but no firm associations could be identified. Echocardiography studies suggested that, despite the increase in diastolic blood pressure, there was a beneficial effect of the normalized hematocrit on left ventricular function. Although most of the observations were similar to those experienced by United States and Japanese investigators, the Canadian team had problems with access failure far in excess of those observed in the two other countries.

The next chapter, authored by Joseph Sobota and Yoshihei Hirasawa, reports the experience with epoetin beta in the United States and Japan. Epoetin beta is (like epoetin alfa) a recombinant erythropoietin derived from the human gene and expressed in Chinese hamster ovary cells. The final isolation and purification from the supernatant fluid of these cells is patented and to a certain extent defines the difference claimed to exist between epoetin alfa (distributed by Amgen, Inc.) and epoetin beta (distributed by Genetics Institutes and its affiliates).

Although the results with epoetin beta reported by Sobota and Hirasawa are similar to those reported for epoetin alfa, there may be subtle differences of potential significance when both preparations are released for general use. Thus far, epoetin beta has been approved by the Food and Drug Administration in Japan and Europe but not in the United States.

The pharmacokinetics of epoetin beta, similar to those reported for epoetin alfa, seem to be the same in normal individuals and in individuals with the anemia of chronic renal disease. The half-life ranges from 4.4 to 11 hours and appears to be dose-dependent because the clearance time tends to decrease at higher titers. The distribution volume equals that of plasma.

The recombinant erythropoietin is usually administered intravenously. Studies of the effect of subcutaneous dosing, however, suggest that a delayed release from subcutaneous depots provides a more sustained plasma concentration. In one study, the total weekly maintenance dose of erythropoietin could be reduced by 37 percent when patients were converted from intravenous to subcutaneous administration.

Phase I studies in the United States and Japan established the safety of recombinant erythropoietin and showed the complete absence of antibody formation. They also showed a dose-dependent rise in the hemoglobin concentration of the recipients and elimination of the need for transfusions. In subsequent Phase II and III trials, the clinical effectiveness was confirmed in regard both to the rise in hemoglobin concentrations and to the associated improvement in the quality of life and exercise tolerance. There were numerous minor, insignificant adverse effects; when every ache and pain was included, it was found that two thirds of the patients (whether receiving 25 or 200 units/kg) had some problems. In most instances, however, these problems did not affect the participation of the patients and, furthermore, patients receiving placebo had almost the same number of mild adverse effects. The incidence of clotting of the shunts also happened to be no higher in the treated group than in the placebo group. Hypertension, which was observed with the same incidence as in previous studies of patients treated with epoetin alfa, was felt to be related to the rate of increase in hematocrit and was primarily a problem during the dose adjustment period.

In 80 percent of patients treated in the United States, the dose required for maintenance was 75 units/kg or less three times per week intravenously, with only 20 percent requiring higher doses. In Japan, 50 percent of patients could be maintained on 30 units/kg three times per week, 30 percent on 60 units/kg, and 20 percent on higher doses. As was the case for patients treated with epoetin alfa, iron deficiency occurred frequently. In more recent studies, iron was given routinely to patients with ferritin values of less than 100 ng/ml.

In Chapter 16, Christopher Winearls and co-workers report on the use of both epoetin alfa and epoetin beta in several multicenter trials in Europe. The first observations were made in a pilot study in London and Oxford and provided data for the 1986 paper in *Lancet* which, for the first time, described the clinical efficacy of recombinant human erythropoietin in dialysis patients.

The initial dosage was a cautious 3 units/kg three times per week, but lack of response led to more realistic dosing. Pharmacokinetic determinations in this groundbreaking study showed that the red cell mass increased in parallel with the increase in hematocrit and that red cell survival was not altered. Studies of the erythroid progenitor pools showed a decrease in BFU-E and somewhat surprisingly no change in the number of CFU-E.

Except for the first patient, who experienced a frightening hypertensive encephalopathy, there was no significant side effect in this early study of 15 patients. In the following Cilag multicenter study of epoetin alfa, 169 patients were entered and 126 were followed for at least 1 year. All patients responded with an increase in the hemoglobin concentration to 10 to 12 g, but some did not respond until after they had become iron repleted. The optimal starting dose was about 50 units/kg three times per week intravenously, producing a hemoglobin increase of about 1 g/dl/month.

Hypertension was a problem in 34 percent of the cases. In seven patients, seizures occurred, but these were not all hypertensive individuals. There was also an increased risk of clotting of the vascular access but, without placebo controls, the significance of these events could not be evaluated. A moderate increase of platelet counts was observed, and the authors suggested that this could have been caused by an associated decrease in tissue iron rather than by an active stimulation of megakaryocytes.

The studies described in the previous chapters were almost all conducted on dialysis patients. In Chapter 17, Brendan Teehan and coworkers review the results of erythropoietin treatment in predialysis patients. The overall results were most encouraging and, as could be expected, benefits and side effects were similar to those observed in patients on dialysis. The pharmacokinetic studies of half-life and distribution volume indicated that these parameters are the same for dialysis and predialysis patients and are actually no different from those observed in normal controls.

Because there is no easy intravenous access in predialysis patients, it was thought important to evaluate the effect of subcutaneous dosing. As expected, the peak level was lower after subcutaneous than intravenous administration but was more sustained and produced dose for dose at least the same and often an increased erythropoietic response.

Teehan et al. detail the results of a double-blind placebo-controlled multicenter study of 117 predialysis patients. Despite the previous data on subcutaneous dosing, the patients in this study all received their recombinant erythropoietin intravenously. The overall response in these patients in regard to both increases in hematocrit and performance and the occurrence of side effects were the same as in dialysis patients. Actually, the incidence of hypertension in the placebo group was almost as high (31 percent) as in the treated group (42 percent).

One major concern in this study was the possibility that residual renal function would be impaired by the concomitant decrease in plasma volume and glomerular filtration. However, this concern was not supported by studies of renal function, and there was no evidence of a detrimental effect on residual renal capacity.

The use of recombinant erythropoietin in 31 patients maintained by continuous ambulatory peritoneal dialysis is summarized by Iain Macdougall and associates. One half of the patients were treated with epoetin alfa in Oxford and London, and the other half were treated with epoetin beta in Cardiff. Erythropoietin was administered subcutaneously rather than intraperitoneally and was given in dosages ranging from 60 to 100 units/kg two times per week. Most patients reached the target hemoglobin value within 2 to 4 months. Of the few nonresponders, almost all had infectious peritoneal complications. Blood pressure elevations were noticed in almost half of the patients but were easily managed. There seemed to be no effect on peritoneal exchange function despite the increase in hematocrit.

The results from the use of recombinant human erythropoietin (epoetin beta) in 100 children followed in 20 pediatric nephrology centers in Europe are reported by Paul Scigalla (Chapter 19). These children were all dialysis-dependent, and 87 of them were also transfusion-dependent. As for adults, the therapy resulted in a significant increase in hematocrit in all children and complete elimination of transfusion dependency. Iron overload, when existing, was reduced, the appetite was increased, but growth retardation was not significantly affected. Blood pressure elevations were a problem in children as in adults and in three cases were associated with seizures. Clotting of vascular access occurred, but it was felt that it could be eliminated by an increase in the heparin dose. Hyperpotassemia was not observed in these carefully monitored children. Dr. Scigalla emphasized, however, that this is a potential problem that must be looked for carefully, especially in children who, because of an increase in appetite, may have a reduced compliance with diet.

The anemia of prematurity is the second category of anemias in which the administration of recombinant erythropoietin can be considered a replacement therapy. In Chapter 20, the pathogenesis of this anemia is discussed by William Mentzer, Kevin Shannon, and Roderic Phibbs. The erythropoietic demands during the last trimester are intense because of rapid expansion of the circulatory bed not only in the fetus but also in the highly vascular fetal side of the placenta. The fetal blood volume is actually 115 ml/kg as compared to 87 ml/kg in the newborn and 70 ml/kg in the adult. This erythropoietic demand is pres-

ent when erythropoietin synthesis switches from the liver to the kidney; even in normal infants there is a slight delay in this switch. In premature infants this delay is even more pronounced, and erythropoietin levels are low despite progressive anemia. This lack of a compensatory increase in red cell production is further aggravated by the frequent blood sampling required to monitor the clinical status in neonatal intensive care units. Consequently, transfusions are required in almost all of these babies, and there has been an interest in using recombinant erythropoietin to reduce the need for such blood supplements.

Mentzer et al. describe pilot studies in progress in which exogenous recombinant erythropoietin has resulted in a significant increase in reticulocytes but no measurable change in transfusion requirements. The demand for red cells in the rapidly growing and repeatedly venesectioned infant may be more than can be met by exogenous erythropoietin, but even a slight reduction in transfusion requirements is a worthy goal.

With recombinant human erythropoietin established as an effective replacement agent in patients with renal failure, it has become important to determine whether it is also effective as a pharmacologic agent in normal and anemic individuals. The use of recombinant human erythropoietin to increase the rate of red cell production in normal or near normal individuals is described by Lawrence Goodnough in Chapter 21. Increased red cell production would make it possible for persons to be bled repeatedly and to have their own blood set aside for use during a subsequent elective operation. Current blood donor regulations permit the procurement of 1 unit every 3 days as long as the hematocrit is greater than 33 percent. The effect of recombinant human erythropoietin on the efficiency of autodonation of blood was examined in a randomized and double-blind trial in adult autologous blood donors scheduled for elective orthopedic surgery. The patients received either erythropoietin, 600 units/kg of body weight, or placebo intravenously two times per week for 21 days. All patients received iron sulfate by mouth, and donations were permitted only if the hematocrit was more than 33 percent. The 24 placebo patients donated an average of 4.1 units, while the 23 patients receiving recombinant erythropoietin donated an average of 5.4 units. Because the hematocrit was higher in the erythropoietin-treated patients, the average red cell mass in each donated unit was 174 ml as compared to 156 ml in the placebo group. Women donated fewer units with lower hematocrits per unit; however, the relative difference between erythropoietin-treated and placebo patients was the same as for the male subjects. At surgical admission, the hematocrits were significantly higher in the erythropoietin-treated group than in the placebo group.

The effectiveness of erythropoietin in accelerating red cell production in normal or near normal subjects indicates that it can also be used to augment the red cell mass in patients undergoing nonelective surgery. Clinical trials of perisurgical therapy with recombinant erythropoietin are in progress in several surgical centers.

The use of recombinant human erythropoietin to treat the anemia in patients with intact kidneys and intact endogenous erythropoietin production is explored by Sanford Krantz and associates in Chapter 22. In theory, exogenous erythropoietin should eliminate the anemic hypoxia necessary as a driving force for increased erythropoietin production and also supplement an inadequate production of erythropoietin. In preliminary studies, these authors, as well as other investigators, have shown that erythropoietin production in patients with various chronic disease, although increased, is less than expected for patients without chronic disorders and with normally functioning kidneys. The reason for this blunted erythropoietin response is not known. It probably plays at least in part a pathogenetic role in the anemia of chronic diseases and especially in the anemias associated with rheumatoid arthritis. Because of this observation, a placebo-controlled study of 17 patients with rheumatoid arthritis and moderately severe anemia was undertaken. The doses administered ranged from 50 mU/kg to 150 mU/kg three times per week intravenously in the treated group of patients. Neither the patients in the placebo group nor the patients receiving 50 mU/kg responded. After the doses were adjusted adequately, 11 of 12 treated patients achieved normal hematocrits. Unfortunately but not unexpectedly, there was no significant improvement in the quality of life, a parameter probably determined by factors other than the level of hemoglobin concentration. Nevertheless, the normalization of hemoglobin concentration was of great value in patients who, because of elective orthopedic surgery, desired to predonate blood. Krantz et al. also mention the increasing number of studies in which the use of recombinant erythropoietin had been of value in anemic patients suffering from other chronic diseases, such as ulcerative colitis and solid tumors.

The final chapter, by David Henry and Robert Abels, outlines a multiinstitutional study of the effect of recombinant human erythropoietin in anemic AIDS patients treated with azidothymidine (AZT). In preceding studies, it had been shown that endogenous erythropoietin production in many such patients is blunted, similar to the situation in patients with rheumatoid arthritis. The anemia of AIDS patients, however, is also caused by a direct effect of the human immunodeficiency virus on bone marrow cells and by direct AZT-induced suppression of red cell production. Dr. Henry describes the results of one study of 63 patients and alludes to results from three trials in progress. Endogenous erythropoietin values in these anemic patients showed a great variation, ranging from less than expected to more than expected values. All patients received 100 units/kg three times per week intravenously. The responders could be clearly separated from the nonresponders according to the level of endogenous erythropoietin production. Patients with an initial erythropoietin level of less than 500 mU/ml had a definite increase in the hematocrit and decrease in transfusion requirements, in contrast to the lack of response in the group with endogenous erythropoietin levels of more than 500 mU/ml. One goal in this study had been to increase or maintain AZT treatment by eliminating or ameliorating the anemia. At the end of the study, however, there was no significant difference in AZT dosage in the two groups. The quality of life was not significantly improved in the responding group, which is not surprising in view of the many problems experienced by these chronically ill patients. Blood pressure alterations and clotting abnormalities were not observed in any patient.

The Future of Erythropoietin Therapy

At present a large number of clinical trials of recombinant human erythropoietin are in progress in patients with anemias due to renal failure or other diseases. New questions as to indications and limitations are briefly summarized and commented upon here.

Anemia due to Renal Failure

In patients with chronic renal disease, there is no dispute as to the efficacy of erythropoietin in reversing the anemia, but there are still a number of unresolved issues. First, what is the most effective route and frequency of erythropoietin administration? Intravenous injections three times per week are convenient for the hemodialysis patient, but subcutaneous administration three times per week may in many patients provide the same results and at lower doses (1,2). Weekly injections may require larger doses (3), but daily subcutaneous injections may be not only the most physiologic but also the most effective method of administration (4). If this is confirmed in subsequent studies, the treatment of this hormone deficiency should be the patient's responsibility, just as is the case with insulin injections for diabetic patients. Unfortunately, in the United States, Medicare does not reimburse for self-administered drugs unless done by home dialysis patients; thus, 80 percent of dialysis patients are presently denied reimbursement for a cheaper and probably more effective means of erythropoietin treatment.

Second, what should be the initial dose of erythropoietin? Early clinical trials used relatively large doses (100–300 units/kg intravenously three times per week), which were associated with increasing diastolic blood pressure in 31 percent, seizures in 4 percent, and iron deficiency in 50 percent of patients. Present cost constraints imposed by Medicare in the United States have limited the initial doses to 50 units/kg or less three times per week. Studies of the incidence of complications in patients treated at lower doses are inconclusive, but only 70 percent of patients receiving the lower dose will achieve a satisfactory hematocrit of more than 33 percent. If the initial dose is ≥100 units/kg intravenously three times per week, however (5), the response rate is more than 90 percent. Although the response to erythropoietin is dose dependent, there is a wide individual response, even in the absence of iron deficiency or inflammatory illnesses. Thus far, there is no way to predict which patient will respond to low doses and which will require larger doses.

Third, what is the optimal hematocrit/hemoglobin target? The data are insufficient to answer this precisely, but energy and a sense of well being appear to improve and anginal pain often clears as soon as the hematocrit increases above 30 percent. Many patients claim that they continue to improve as the hematocrit increases toward 38 percent or the hemoglobin increases toward 12.5 g/dl. Why should the target not be the normal levels? Because of concerns that, at a normal hematocrit level, hypertension will be harder to control, the incidence of shunt closure will increase, and dialysis efficacy will decrease, a hematocrit of 30 to 33 percent has been chosen as the target.

Fourth, how can the development of hypertension and seizures be reduced or eliminated? Hypertension is most likely caused by an increase in red cell mass and not by the hormone per se (6), but its precise pathophysiologic mechanism has not been determined (7–9). Since the pressor response often resolves with time even though the hematocrit remains at its target level and since most patients do not develop this complication, some form of delayed autoregulation to the increasing red cell mass must occur. Lower doses of erythropoietin may produce a slower rise in hematocrit and allow more time for autoregulation to be initiated. Seizures are rare and are rarely associated with serious consequences, but they are terrifying. Although some are related to a sudden rise in blood pressure, others cannot be explained as hypertensive encephalopathy (10–12). It is possible that an excessive reduction in cerebral blood flow from elevated levels toward normal in patients responding to erythropoietin may result in a critical reduction in cerebral perfusion as the red cell mass increases (13). Seizures may therefore be ischemic as well as hypertensive.

Finally, should select red cell transfusions continue to be given for immunosuppression before renal transplantation? Although transplant survival may improve slightly by such "immunosuppression," there is a 15 percent incidence of sensitization due to a pretransplant transfusion. Elimination of transfusions by erythropoietin therapy has resulted in the gradual reduction of HLA antibody titers so that renal transplantation can be safely undertaken (14), but a controlled study in Finland failed to confirm this beneficial effect (15). A prospective study in which transfusions are prevented by erythropoietin therapy and therefore the incidence of HLA sensitization is reduced for first-time transplant recipients is necessary to resolve this issue.

Anemias due to Extrarenal Disorders

The clinical experience with erythropoietin in these anemias is not yet as extensive as that in the anemia of chronic renal failure, but much has been learned from clinical trials in progress. What has become apparent is that patients with chronic disorders associated with mild anemia and modestly elevated serum erythropoietin levels (less than 500 mU/ml) will respond to erythropoietin administered in doses only somewhat higher than those needed for the anemia of chronic renal failure. This has been observed in patients with rheumatoid arthritis, as outlined by Krantz and colleagues in their chapter, and also in patients with multiple myeloma or solid tumors or receiving chemotherapy (16–19). Because the anemia in many of these patients is quite asymptomatic, an improved concentration of hemoglobin not only is costly but also may merely be cosmetic. If such patients, however, have cardiovascular problems or are in need of surgery, erythropoietin therapy could be of great help.

In more severe anemias associated with higher endogenous serum erythropoietin levels, as in patients with myelodysplastic disorders, exogenous erythropoietin in conventional doses has been quite ineffective (20). Would such patients benefit from much larger doses? This is possible (21), but since there is a limit to the extent of red cell production, larger doses may not increase the rate of production further. However, they may reduce the degree of anemic hypoxia needed to generate erythropoietin from endogenous sources.

The recent application of growth factors to overcome bone marrow suppression has raised new issues about the use of erythropoietin in conjunction with these factors. Whether such combined therapy will lead to synergism or antagonism remains to be determined (22–24).

For the last 40 years the authors and editors of this monograph have been privileged to play a role in the elucidation of the physiology, biology, and clinical application of erythropoietin. It has been a challenging journey, and we hope that we have been able to transmit some of the excitement of this long voyage to our readers.

REFERENCES

1. Bommer J, Samtleben W, Koch KM, et al. Variations of recombinant human erythropoietin application in hemodialysis patients. Contrib Nephrol 1989;76:149–58.

2. McMahon FG, Vargas R, Ryan M, et al. Pharmacokinetics and effects of recombinant human erythropoietin after intravenous and subcutaneous injections in healthy volunteers. Blood 1990;76:1718–22.

3. Besarab A, Vlasses P, Caro J, et al. Subcutaneous (SC) administration of recombinant human erythropoietin (H-rEPO) for treatment of ESRD anemia [Abstract]. Kidney Int 1990;37:236.

4. Granolleras C, Branger B, Beau MC, Deschodt G, Alsabadani B, Shaldon S. Experience with daily self-administered subcutaneous erythropoietin. Contrib Nephrol 1989;76:143–8.

5. Eschbach JW, Adamson JW. The pathophysiology and treatment of the anemia of chronic renal failure. Curr Nephrol (in press).

6. Eschbach JW. Erythropoietin-associated hypertension [Reply]. N Engl J Med 1990;323:999–1000.

7. Nonnast-Daniel B, Deschodt G, Brunkhorst R, et al. Long-term effects of treatment with recombinant human erythropoietin on haemodynamics and tissue oxygenation on patients with renal anaemia. Nephrol Dial Transplant 1990;5:444–8.

8. Satoh K, Masuda T, Ikeda Y, et al. Hemodynamic changes by recombinant erythropoietin therapy in hemodialyzed patients. Hypertension 1990;15:262–6.

9. Macdougall IC, Lewis NP, Saunders MJ, et al. Long-term cardiorespiratory effects of amelioration of renal anaemia by erythropoietin. Lancet 1990;335:489–93.

10. Brown AL, Tucker B, Baker LRI, Raine AEG. Seizures related to blood transfusion and erythropoietin treatment in patients undergoing dialysis. Br Med J 1989;299:1258–9.

11. Temple RM, Eadington DW, Swainson CP, Winney R. Seizure related to erythropoietin treatment in patients undergoing dialysis. Br Med J 1990;300:46.

12. Edmunds ME, Walls J, Tucker B, et al. Seizures in haemodialysis patients treated with recombinant human erythropoietin. Nephrol Dial Transplant 1989;4:1065–9.

13. Johnson WJ, McCarthy JT, Yanagihara T, et al. Effects of recombinant human erythropoietin on cerebral and cutaneous blood flow and on blood coagulability. Kidney Int 1990;38:919–24.

14. Grimm PC, Sinai-Trieman L, Sekiya NM, et al. Effects of recombinant human erythropoietin on HLA sensitization and cell mediated immunity. Kidney Int 1990;38:12–8.

15. Koskimies S, Lautenschlager I, Grönhagen-Riska C, Häyry P. Erythropoietin therapy and the antibody levels of highly sensitized patients awaiting kidney transplantation. Transplantation 1990;50:707–9.

16. Ludwig H, Fritz E, Kotzmann H, Höcker P, Gisslinger H, Barnas U. Erythropoietin treatment of anemia associated with multiple myeloma. N Engl J Med 1990;322:1693–9.

17. Bunn HF. Recombinant erythropoietin therapy in cancer patients. J Clin Oncol 1990;8:949–51.

18. Oster W, Herrmann F, Gamm H, et al. Erythropoietin for the treatment of anemia of malignancy associated with neoplastic bone marrow infiltration. J Clin Oncol 1990;8:956–62.

19. Matsumoto T, Endoh K, Kamisango K, et al. Effect of recombinant human erythropoietin on anti-cancer drug-induced anaemia. Br J Haematol 1990;75:463–8.

20. Jacobs A, Bowen DT, Calligan D. The treatment of anaemia in the myelodysplastic syndrome with human recombinant erythropoietin. Br J Haematol (in press).

21. Stebler C, Tichelli A, Dazzi H, et al. High-dose recombinant erythropoietin for treatment of anemia in myeloblastic syndromes and paroxysmal nocturnal hemoglobinuria: a pilot study. Exp Hematol 1990;18:1204–8.

22. Schooley JC, Kullgren B, Allison AC. Inhibition by interleukin-1 of the action of erythropoietin on erythroid precursors and its possible role in the pathogenesis of hypoplastic anaemias. Br J Haematol 1987;67:11–7.

23. Johnson CS, Cook CA, Furmanski P. In vivo suppression of erythropoiesis by tumor necrosis factor-α (TNF-α): reversal with exogenous erythropoietin (EPO). Exp Hematol 1990;18:109–13.

24. Clibon U, Bonewald L, Caro J, Roodman GD. Erythropoietin fails to reverse the anemia in mice continuously exposed to tumor necrosis factor-alpha in vivo. Exp Hematol 1990;18:438–41.

Index

Abels, R., 448
Abscesses, erythropoietin therapy for, 415
Access failure. *See* Vascular access failure
Acetazolamide, 191
Acquired immunodeficiency syndrome (AIDS):
  anemia associated with. *See* Anemia, AIDS-related
  antibiotic therapy for, 421
  azidothymidine (AZT) therapy for, 420–422. *See also* Azidothymidine (AZT)
  Coombs-positive patients with, 422
  erythropoietin therapy for, 423–432
  pediatric, 382
  transfusion-transmitted, 382, 393
Actinomycin D, 60
Acute blood loss, 187. *See also* Blood loss
Acute fetal hypoxia, 191
Acute pulmonary insufficiency, in premature infants, 386
Adamson, J. W., 102, 437
Adenosine:
  messenger role of, in oxygen sensing, 92–95
  triphosphatase (ATPase), 91
  triphosphate (ATP), 91–92, 191
Administration of erythropoietin. *See* Human recombinant erythropoietin (rHuEpo), methods of administering
Adults, plasma erythropoietin concentration in, 189–190
African green monkey kidney cells, erythropoietin gene expression in, 134
Age:
  diurnal variation not related to, 440
  plasma erythropoietin concentration related to, 189
Aglyco erythropoietin, 35, 37, 47–48, 119. *See also* Deglycosylation of erythropoietin
AIDS. *See* Acquired immunodeficiency syndrome (AIDS)
Akizawa, T., 442
Alkaline phosphatase, 219
Allergic reactions, 308

Alloimmunization, transfusion-induced, 393
Alpha-amanitin, 59
Alport syndrome, 357
Aluminum bone disease, 234
Aluminum overload, 339, 360, 442
Alverson, D. C., 383
Ambulatory peritoneal dialysis:
  continuous. *See* Continuous ambulatory peritoneal dialysis (CAPD)
  erythropoietin therapy for. *See* Erythropoietin therapy, in patients on ambulatory peritoneal dialysis
American Association of Blood Banks, 393, 394, 396, 397
American Rheumatism Association, 405
Amgen, Inc., 117, 212, 216, 220, 291, 435, 441, 443. *See also* Epogen (epoetin alfa)
Amino acid sequences. *See also* Erythropoietin gene; Protein sequences
  of erythropoietin, 147, 148
  by Hopp and Woods method, 48–49
  conservation in, across species, 42–43
  homology of, 31
  hydrophilicity value for, 48
  identification and isolation of, 21–32, 115
  probable antigenic site in, 48
  of human erythropoietin, 25–28, 33, 41–43, 46–48
  hydrophilicity value for, 48
  intron/exon junction sites in, 25
  lysine in, 42
  of human recombinant erythropoietin, 269
  of human urinary erythropoietin, 269
  of human versus murine erythropoietin receptors, 147, 148
  leader, 42
  of monkey erythropoietin, 33, 41–43
  of mouse erythropoietin, 33, 41–43
Amniotic fluid, plasma erythropoietin in, 190–191
Anabolic steroids, mepitiostane, 229
Anaerobic muscle metabolism, effect of erythropoietin therapy on, 236. *See also* Exercise tolerance